Maternal-Child Nursing Test Success

D1214652

Ruth A. Wittmann-Price, PhD, RN, CNS, CNE is chairperson and professor at Francis Marion University (SC) Department of Nursing. Dr. Wittmann-Price has been an obstetrical/women's health nurse for 32 years. She earned her MS as a Perinatal CNS from Columbia University, NYC (1983) and her Doctorate in Nursing Science (PhD) at Widener University, Chester (2006) where she was awarded the Dean's Award for Excellence. She has developed and research-tested a mid-range nursing theory "Emancipated Decision-making in Women's Health Care". In addition to continuing her research about decisional science, she studies developmental outcomes of preterm infants. As Director of Nursing Research (2007–2010) for Hahnemann University Hospital, a Magnet status facility, Dr. Wittmann-Price was responsible for all evidence-based practice projects for nursing. Ruth has taught all levels of nursing students over the past 15 years (AAS, BSN, MSN and DNP) and completed an international service-learning trip (2007) to rural Mexico with undergraduate nursing and physician assistant students. She was the coordinator for the Nurse Educator track in DrNP program at Drexel University in Philadelphia (2007–2010) and sits on four dissertation committees. Ruth is co-editor and chapter contributor of three books, *Nursing Education: Foundations for Practice Excellence* (2007) Philadelphia: F. A. Davis. (AJN Book of the Year Award winner 2008) and *The Certified Nurse Examination (CNE) Review Manual* (2009), Springer Publishing, NYC, and *NCLEX-RN EXCEL Test success through unfolding case study review*, NYC: Springer Publishing. She has published three book chapters, as well as numerous articles and has presented regionally, nationally, and internationally. Ruth is a current participant in the NLN LEAD program for leader development in nursing.

Frances H. Cornelius, MSN, PhD, RN-BC, CNE is Associate Clinical Professor, Chair of the MSN Advanced Practice Role Department & Coordinator of Informatics Projects at Drexel Univ, College of Nursing and Health Professions. Fran has taught nursing since 1991, at several schools of nursing. She taught community health at Madonna University (Livonia, MI), Oakland (MI) University, Univ of Pittsburgh and Holy Family College (Phila). Fran taught Adult Health and Gerontology at Widener Univ School of Nursing until in 1997 when she began teaching at Drexel. In 2003, she was a Fellow at the Biomedical Library of Medicine. She is a certified nurse informaticist and has been the recipient of several grants. She has collaborated on the development of mobile applications as Coordinator of Informatics Projects including Patient Assessment and Care Plan Development (PACPD) tool which is a PDA tool with a Web based companion, and Gerontology Reasoning Informatics Programs (the GRIP project). She is the co-Editor of Cornelius/Gallagher-Gordon, PDA Connections (LLW), an innovative textbook designed to teach healthcare professionals how to use mobile devices for 'point-of-care' access of information. She has written 6 book chapters and has published 19 journal articles on her work. She has been invited to delivered 26 presentations and has delivered >50 peer-reviewed presentations mostly in the US, but also in Spain, Canada and Korea. She is a member of STTI, the American Informatics Association, the American Nursing Informatics Association, the International Institute of Informatics and Systemics (IIIS), NANDA, ANA and the PSNA.

Maternal-Child Nursing Test Success:
An Unfolding Case Study Review

Ruth A. Wittmann-Price, PhD, RN, CNS, CNE
Frances H. Cornelius, MSN, PhD, RN-BC, CNE

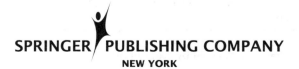

SPRINGER PUBLISHING COMPANY
NEW YORK

Copyright © 2012 Springer Publishing Company, LLC

Springer Publishing Company, LLC
11 West 42nd Street
New York, NY 10036
www.springerpub.com

Acquisitions Editor: Margaret Zuccarini
Composition: S4Carlisle Publishing Services

ISBN: 978-0-8261-4156-9
E-book ISBN: 978-0-8261-4157-6

11 12 13 14/ 5 4 3 2 1

The author and the publisher of this Work have made every effort to use sources believed to be reliable to provide information that is accurate and compatible with the standards generally accepted at the time of publication. Because medical science is continually advancing, our knowledge base continues to expand. Therefore, as new information becomes available, changes in procedures become necessary. We recommend that the reader always consult current research and specific institutional policies before performing any clinical procedure. The author and publisher shall not be liable for any special, consequential, or exemplary damages resulting, in whole or in part, from the readers' use of, or reliance on, the information contained in this book. The publisher has no responsibility for the persistence or accuracy of URLs for external or third-party Internet Web sites referred to in this publication and does not guarantee that any content on such Web sites is, or will remain, accurate or appropriate.

Library of Congress Cataloging-in-Publication Data

CIP data is available from the Library of Congress.

Special discounts on bulk quantities of our books are available to corporations, professional associations, pharmaceutical companies, health care organizations, and other qualifying groups. If you are interested in a custom book, including chapters from more than one of our titles, we can provide that service as well.

For details, please contact:
Special Sales Department, Springer Publishing Company, LLC
11 West 42nd Street, 15th Floor, New York, NY 10036-8002
Phone: 877-687-7476 or 212-431-4370; Fax: 212-941-7842
Email: sales@springerpub.com

Printed in the United States of America by Bang Printing.

*This effort, like all efforts of nurse educators,
is dedicated to our students!*

Contents

Preface   *ix*
Acknowldgments   *xi*

1. NCLEX-RN®: Preparation Tips and How We Really Feel   *1*
    A Guide FOR Students BY Students   *1*

2. Newborn Nursing Care   *13*
    Case Study 1: Jasmine and River

3. Postpartum Care   *47*
    Case Study 2: Jolene
    Case Study 3: Paula

4. Infertility, Preconception, Conception, and Preterm Labor   *73*
    Case Study 4: Isabella and Christopher

5. Hyperemesis Gravidarum (HG)   *109*
    Case Study 5: Tamiko

6. Sexually Transmitted Infections   *119*
    Case Study 6: Sonia

7. Labor and Delivery   *129*
    Case Study 7: Karen

8. First Trimester Bleeding and Previa   *149*
    Case 8: Chelsea

9. Ectopic Pregnancy   *167*
    Case Study 9: Bonita

10. Hydatidiform Mole (Gestational Trophoblastic Disease or GTD)   *173*
    Case Study 10: Lauren

11. Incompetent Cervix, Abruption, and DIC   *179*
    Case Study 11: Lillian

12. Gestational Hypertension and HELLP   *189*
    Case 12: La-Neisha

13. Gestational Diabetes (GD)   *205*
    Case Study 13: Margaret

14. ABO Incompatibility   *217*
   Case Study 14: Regina

15. Rupture of the Membranes (ROM)   *227*
   Case 15: Savannah

16. Preterm Labor (PTL)   *241*
   Case 16: Bonnie

17. Cardiac Disease   *253*
   Case Study 17: Maggie

18. Asthma   *263*
   Case Study 18: Rachel

19. Sickle Cell Anemia   *271*
   Case Study 19: Maria

20. Human Immunodeficiency Virus (HIV)   *277*
   Case Study 20: Kendall

21. Preterm Infant Care   *283*
   Case Study 21: Preterm Multiples

22. Retinopathy of Prematurity and Bronchopulmonary Dysplasia (BPD)   *307*
   Case Study 22: Robert

23. Anemia and Polycythemia   *315*
   Case Study 23: Twin-to-Twin Transfusion Syndrome (TTTS)

24. Transient Tachypnea of the Newborn (TTN)   *321*
   Case Study 24: Aaron

25. Meconium Aspiration Syndrome (MAS)   *327*
   Case Study 25: Benjamin

26. Periventricular-Interventicular Hemorrhage   *335*
   Case Study 26: Jason

27. Neonatal Abstinence Syndrome (NAS)   *345*
   Case Study 27: Michael

28. Inborn Errors of Metabolism   *355*
   Case Study 28: Frances

References   361
Index   363

Preface

To our nursing students and faculty: Dr. Fran Cornelius and I have developed this book to revolutionize studying. This book begins the second generation of *Test Success Through Unfolding Case Studies*. It contains detailed content as well as evaluative questions in a user-friendly workbook format specific to maternal-child nursing. This book is based on the very successful first *NCLEX-RN(R) Excel Test Success Through Unfolding Case Study Review* (2010), but this new version is electronically enhanced with hundreds of Web links. Now you can link directly to resources to promote thorough knowledge acquisition, critical thinking, and the development of clinical decision making.

This book is designed to help students to understand, in-depth, maternal-child nursing for classroom exams, standardized tests, and the NCLEX-RN(R). The first chapter has been written by students to give you a *bird's-eye* perspective of test preparation. Besides being a wonderful study and review book for students, nurse educators will find this book a delight for simulation experiences, classroom cases, group projects, and clinical conferences.

We know you will enjoy this format of learning and review. It is a fresh new approach that provides a break from the usual question after question review books. Each exercise has the answers with rationales in the back of the chapters, and each chapter is a separate clinical case that can stand alone. The book includes all the relevant conditions for both maternal and child health. Every case is based on a real clinical scenario—a patient condition that you may actually come across in your future clinical practice.

We hope you enjoy the adventure of imagining yourself as the professional nurse caring for and advocating for each patient as you work through the unfolding case studies. Best of luck in your nursing career, and look for the upcoming sequel books of unfolding case studies!

Ruth A. Wittmann-Price
Frances H. Cornelius

Acknowledgments

We would like to thank nursing students Kelley Moore and Stacy Wiegand for sharing their insights and test preparation tips in the first chapter. They said it better than we ever would have been able to.

Also, thank you to Margaret Zuccarini for her endless publishing support.

Maternal-Child Nursing Test Success

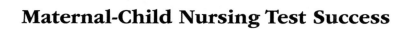

1

NCLEX-RN®: Preparation Tips and How We Really Feel

▰ A Guide FOR Students BY Students

Meet us—because we are nursing students too! We began our nursing journey just like most of you. We have had our good times and well, not so good times (we'll leave it at that). But, with our classmates' and, of course, our professors' help, we have been taught some of the best tools in order to succeed—the first time!

This chapter will include the following four topics:

1. **Study Skills and Habits**

   What we learned in our nursing school journey and how we are going to help you prevent our mishaps.

2. **Preparation for NCLEX-RN®**

   Face it, you need to know what to study, how to study, and when to study it—and we are going to tell you just that.

3. **Our Anchors and Lifesavers Section**

   Things we learned along the way that we wished someone had told us much sooner! This section will include some things that we thought anchored us down even though at times our ship almost sank. We will offer you some tips and tricks we learned that helped keep us afloat and what we think can keep you from getting hypoxic with scary reality.

4. **Leading Up to Test Day**

   All about your vacationing up until test day, because face it, you're probably tired of studying anyway.

What We Like to Call Our "Introduction"

Together we (Stacy and Kelley) have collected more than 15 books to help us prepare for nursing school tests and the most important nursing test of all, the

NCLEX-RN®. We realized in all of our reading, that we never read the "intro" chapter of any book, but why?

- Maybe because it was boring.
- Maybe because it seemed unrealistic.
- Maybe because we did not have the time or energy to read it.
- Or, maybe because we have fluids, electrolytes, cardiac, pharmacology, and other stuff on the brain.

But in skipping those introduction sections, we realized something. We should have read them—many had good tips! Then we decided to write something that is entertaining to read and what we think is realistic in study preparation. You will have to excuse us if we are a little blunt at times, it might be because we are on our last cup of coffee from Starbucks and it's 0200. Hmmm. Enjoy our roller-coaster, and excuse us if our sleep deprivation begins to affect our writing—at least you understand. Enjoy! Oh, one more thing: we will throw you a lifesaver, so hang on for dear life!

Study Skills and Habits

Bad habits need to kick the bucket. Studying material for NCLEX-RN® is really an art; it is something you must acquire over time, not something you learn overnight. By now, you should have these habits down. But, in case you don't, we are here to tell you where we messed up and what we learned along the way. Studying can be evaluated many different ways, such as by your test grades, by successfully passing the NCLEX-RN®, or by feeling prepared for the workforce by remembering most of what you learned in school. It may feel impossible to study efficiently while in nursing school. Because face it, by now you are almost completely sleep deprived. Make yourself a study schedule and be sure to include time for sleep and stick to it! You need your sleep in order to complete nursing school and your pass boards successfully.

    A time management quick fix. If you plan to stick to a time line, find a friend who is on a study schedule similar to yours, and hold each other accountable. We will admit that we have to keep tabs on each other when we study!

    Eat healthy. Trust us, your stomach will thank you later. Don't start studying or take an exam on an empty stomach. It is hard to concentrate when your stomach is yelling at you. Fresh fruits and vegetables are often recommended to reduce stress. Avoid junk food, fried foods, processed foods, carbonated drinks, and sugar. Eat small, healthy snacks during breaks to help take your mind off of your anxiety (Landsberger, 1996).

    How do you define stress? If you worry about your test too much, it will negatively impact your test performance because this is virtually the definition of testing anxiety. Anxiety can cause extreme nervousness and memory lapses among other symptoms. If you become nervous during study sessions or during the exam, the best thing to do is to take a few deep breaths to relax yourself. Do not let your mind wander; focus on the task at hand. If you begin to look beyond what you are doing at that very moment, it is easy to become overwhelmed. Always, always, remain positive and keep your eye on the prize (McDowell, 2008). "With the NCLEX-RN®, the [prize] is becoming an RN!" (McDowell, 2008).

Put your stressors aside. In order to avoid anxiety you need to understand and evaluate what triggers *your* anxiety. The best way to reduce test anxiety is to prepare and build confidence in your knowledge of the material. Approach the exam with confidence, and view the exam as an opportunity to show to yourself how much you have learned through nursing school. Think of passing the exam as a reward for all of your hard work. We know that the day we pass our boards will be our proudest day ever. So, in order to accomplish this, you need to be able to determine what stresses you out and puts you over the edge. We have already been over the edge a few times, so we will help you out for now on some stressors to avoid, such as:

- Your friends on test days
- Negative attitudes
- Cramming
- All-nighters
- Excess caffeine
- Distractions (TV, children, cell phone, Facebook)
- Prolonged study times without breaks
- Studying in your bedroom
- Procrastination

What we left out. Do not isolate yourself from your nursing friends when school is out. It is important to vent about your stressors with someone who understands exactly what you are going through. We are all in the same boat after all. It also helps to swap study tips, talk about NCLEX strategies, exchange information about job searches, and just help each other relax and unwind.

What motivates you. You need to assess what gets you excited. It is shown that diversional activities should be included in your personal wellness to reduce stress (McDowell, 2008). So, it looks like it is okay to get sidetracked every once in a while. But, don't prolong it or let it become a habit.

Where to start? You might want to begin with a time line. We know you may have put off studying for NCLEX until the last minute, but that is a bad idea. Our nursing professors tell us that discharge teaching starts when? Yes, that's right! On admission! So shouldn't our studying be done the same way? If you begin early, the material becomes more fluent and you are able to retain more (McDowell, 2008). Practice what you preach. We have created a study schedule for you, but feel free to alter it to best fit your needs. If you choose to change this up, be sure to remember that you need to make a schedule that encompasses an adequate amount of time to prepare, is flexible, and allows time to sleep!

Just a quick study blurb. When you are studying NCLEX-style questions, always be sure to read the rationales for all answers. By doing this, you will better understand why the correct answers are correct and why the incorrect answers are incorrect. Makes sense right? We thought so too!

Preparing for NCLEX-RN®

First things first—you have to register for the test. Once you've finished your classes and gotten those superior grades we know you're capable of, your institution should provide you with an application for licensure appropriate for your state board of nursing. You must submit this application to the state board to be eligible to register for NCLEX-RN®. At this point, you need to scrape together some money (post nursing school, nursing books, uniforms, and supplies) because the state board is going to want it. The price of licensure varies from state to state but the actual cost to take the NCLEX is $200 (Dunham, 2008). Whew! Our jaws just dropped, too.

Once you've applied for your license, you need to register to take the NCLEX-RN®. Be sure to provide your name *exactly* as it is printed on your identification that you will show on test day. If you offer an email address when registering, you will no longer receive snail (paper) mail about your testing. Be sure you're ready, because the $200 fee to register for NCLEX-RN® is absolutely nonrefundable (Dunham, 2008).

So you have completed your part? Now it's time for you to sit back (study a little more), and wait for your Authorization to Test (also more commonly referred to as your ATT) (Dunham, 2008). We know you are super-anxious to know exactly when you'll be taking this career-starting test, but first you have to wait for your ATT to arrive. Once your ATT arrives, go ahead and use that opportunity to call and schedule your big day. It is important to call as soon as possible, because the administrators are required to give you available test dates within 30 days of your call (Dunham, 2008).

You'll want you to be extra prepared to take this test. So, don't spread yourself thin on time when scheduling your test date unless necessary. ATT is valid only for a limited number of days; the time length varies from state to state (Dunham, 2008). Be sure to schedule your test date within that frame, but don't wait too long because you don't want to develop stress-related hypertension.

Okay, you now know where you're going to take the test and what day, but what about the time? Nursing school has tried to make us early risers, but some of us are still nocturnal. The testing center understands this and will allow you to take an afternoon test! Once you get all of the specifics, write it down! And if you're super scatter-brained like us, our research revealed that the ATT actually has a place for you to record this information (Dunham, 2008). Thank goodness! On test day, you must bring one form of identification that identically matches your registered name and what now appears on your ATT. Don't forget your ATT as well. You will not be admitted to the test without these two important things. After the test, you should receive your test scores within one month from the date you took your test (Dunham, 2008). Or you can pay to get them earlier. You can also keep trying the Web site approximately 48–72 hours after testing to see if your name comes up under the license search for your state board of nursing. The status of RN licenses is public knowledge so it will be accessible on the web.

Use your favorite highlighter (or pencil) for test days. Dress comfortably (without your PJ's—dressing down too much doesn't help your confidence).

Get plenty of sleep the night before. Take a shower before the test (to wake you up and, of course, to feel clean). Wear an article of clothing that you have been studying in (it is okay to wash it before test day). Highlight the material you think is the main point to each question (nursing diagnosis, medical diagnosis, signs and symptoms, and other valuable information).

Determine your answer before you read the answer choices. Mark out answers you know are obviously wrong (mark through the entire answer, not just the letter, so that you are not unintentionally telling yourself that that answer is still available). Make notes on your tests and next to answer choices about what you know, even if it is an incorrect answer (give yourself a reason why it is wrong) and take your time, but don't spend too long on one question.

Trust your gut! Usually your first instinct is right.

Be prepared! Wear a watch on test day. Bring ear plugs so you don't hear other students. Go to the testing site right on time to avoid listening to other students' pretest jitters. Bring a few mints with you (they can help concentration).

LISTEN! During test reviews, don't just mark what you got wrong and right. Divide your studying time into increments (e.g., 30 minutes studying with a 5-minute break, or 50 minutes studying with a 10-minute break). Create visuals when studying (e.g., posters, concept maps). Create auditory help (e.g., sayings like the ones above or make a song to help you remember). BUT the absolute most important tip to reduce test-taking anxiety is—DRUM ROLL PLEASE—that's right, you guessed it—BE PREPARED!

Sounds easy enough right? Well you have the tools to do it now. So, let's get to studying! Don't forget snack breaks and plenty of rest. Review your study time line. Make sure you check your study time line frequently before the big day so that you can keep yourself in check. Don't fall behind or lose track of what you want to cover before the exam.

YOUR PLAN: *Two to Three Months Before the Exam*

- Begin organizing your lecture notes and textbooks from classes.
- Take a comprehensive assessment using a standardized test, or whatever testing service your school has used.
- Determine your strengths and weaknesses in content areas and what you are most insecure about.
- Plan to review your weakest areas first and then save time to do a quick review of these at the end as well.
- Take practice tests that are specific to your area of weakness.
- Learn the format for NCLEX-RN® and become familiar with it.
- Even though you are still in school, try to study NCLEX-RN® for 2–3 days per week for 1–2 hours.

- Decide whether or not you want to join a study group (through standardized testing, a local test prep center, etc.).
- Determine the strategies that best help you reduce anxiety before big tests.

Four to Six Weeks Before the Exam

- Begin practice tests for all content areas.
- Organize your notes by chapter/body system or whatever makes the most sense to you.
- Continue to practice NCLEX-RN®-style questions so you are more familiar with the format.
- Be sure to continue receiving adequate amounts of sleep and exercise, eat appropriately, and balance socializing and working.
- Do not become a study hermit.
- Retake your comprehensive exam to see how well you are improving and what areas still need improvement, if any. After all, a little bit of positive reinforcement never hurt. It feels good to see your studying actually pay off.
- Once you know where you are taking the test, make your arrangements if you plan to stay the night before in a hotel room.

One Week Before the Exam

- Plan for this week to be relaxing and stress free from studying.
- Begin your final review of areas you are still insecure about.
- Retake your comprehensive assessment for the last time to evaluate how well you've prepared.
- Review all lab values and calculation formulas.
- Put all of your documents together for test day.
- Again, you need to feel your best, so get plenty of sleep, exercise, and don't over indulge in food.

Getting to know the test like your best friend. Does being around your best friend bring comfort? We thought so. So why not think of this test as your best friend? If you are prepared for what the test is like, hopefully it will kill some of those stomach butterflies that are stirring. You need to know what to expect from the moment you walk in the door to sign in, to the presentation of the actual test, and what the environment is like while you're testing. At the end, we will provide you with a checklist of what to bring to the testing center (Dunham, 2008).

Okay, so we all know what our nursing school tests look like and we are already sick of reviewing NCLEX-RN® questions. Well, guess what! There was a reason for the madness: the NCLEX-RN® is no different! By now you should be familiar with the types of questions that will be presented to you. There will be lots of multiple choice questions, some select all that apply questions, a few prioritization questions, a couple hot-spot questions, and maybe a few math fill-in-the-blank style questions thrown in as well (Dunham, 2008). Now that you know the types of questions for the NCLEX-RN®, you need to know how it will be presented to you. You will be shown one question at a time; even if you're good at multitasking, you can only answer one question at a time anyway. You must complete the question to move forward, NO SKIPPING (like class). You can't go back to change answers which is probably a good thing. I know we have been told many times in nursing school, stick to your gut answer and don't change it. Your first answer is usually right (Dunham, 2008). You will have to complete anywhere from 75–265 questions. The test is made almost specifically for you. The computer will give you a question and if you answer correctly (which we know you will), it will give you something harder. However, if you answer it incorrectly, the computer will generate an easier question. One of our favorite books says, "This dance continues, with the computer providing questions and [you] answering them and the computer deciding what question to display next until it can determine [your] skill level" (Dunham, 2008). If the computer can determine your skill level in the minimum 75 questions, it will cut off. Otherwise, it will continue to ask you questions until it is certain of your skill level (Dunham, 2008).

The key to preparing for NCLEX-RN® is finding the perfect combination of content review and practice questions. You need to be sure to balance out reviewing the mass amounts of information you learned in nursing school and, of course, using your best test-taking skills (Herman, & Johnson, 2009). That is why we are promoting this book, because it gives you both content and questions!

Anchors and Lifesavers

TIP How to approach those nasty questions. The main goal of NCLEX-RN® is to test the student's use of critical-thinking skills rather than just recall factual information. So, remember when you're studying to not focus on small details, but try and understand overall concepts (McDowell, 2008). Having a general understanding of the information will allow you to be able to think your way through an NCLEX-RN® question critically. If you start off studying every little detail in your lecture notes from nursing school, we can guarantee that you are going to become extremely overwhelmed and frustrated—and quick! It will benefit you more to have a general understanding of the information (McDowell, 2008). But, even if you get a nasty question, take a deep breath and pick out your main clues from the question. Before you look at the answers, formulate your own. Eliminate the answers you can and choose from what you have left. But, be sure you know exactly what the question is asking and read all of the answer choices before making your selection. Before starting the test, tell yourself that you are not going to panic if you are clueless about a question. Just block out everything else and focus in on that single question.

MNEMONICS and why we like 'em. We love mnemonics! We think they are one of the greatest study techniques ever. But if you keep reading we will detail it even further. Mnemonics simply take the first letter of a group of like things and put those letters together to make a work that you can remember. Here are a few of our favorites:

- Acid/Base Mnemonic—**ROME**

  R-Respiratory **O**-Opposite **M**-Metabolic **E**-Equal.

  So in other words, with Respiratory Alkalosis/Acidosis the pH and PCO2 act opposite of each other, as one increases, the other decreases and vice versa. With Metabolic Alkalosis/Acidosis the pH and PCO2 either increase together or decrease together.

- Hypertension Nursing Care Mnemonic—**DIURETIC**

  D-Daily Weight **I**-I&O's **U**-Urine Output **R**-Response of B/P **E**-Electrolytes **T**-Take Pulses **I**-Ischemic Episodes (TIA) **C**-Complications-4C's (CAD, CRF, CHF, and CVA).

So now that we have given you a few examples, take a moment to write down a few that you have memorized that have helped you study.

_____

_____

_____

_____

_____

_____

_____

_____

Great! Now we have a few other tidbits to give you while we are talking about 'em. Mnemonics are great but don't feel like you have to be told them, make some up on your own to help you study. If you have a lot of information to study, try grouping it together in the mnemonic. For example, ROY G. BIV stands for the color spectrum Red, Orange, Yellow, Green, Blue, Indigo, and Violet. Well, say you had to remember some information about each one. You could break them up into three groups of different information. ROY can be group 1, G can be group 2, and BIV can be group 3. This way you don't have just a mound of information, you have separated it so that if you forget one tiny detail , you don't lose EVERYTHING! Great idea huh?

A few other little sayings we have grown to love thanks to studying.

- You have 10 fingers total (Use them to count the following letters) C-O-U-M-A-D-I-N (affects your) P-T (and INR) = 10 total

  H-E-P-A-R-I-N (affects your) P-T-T = 10 total

- Beta One/Two Blockers

  You have one heart and two lungs so Beta 1 affects your heart and Beta 2 affects your lungs.
- Blood Sugars

  Hot and Dry = Sugar High, Cold and Clammy = Need Some Candy

You get the idea! If you need some help with fitting some information to a mnemonic to help remember it, try searching the Web, because odds are someone else has already had the same problem. We would include the 5-P's for the neurovascular assessment here but hopefully we've all heard those ENOUGH! Right? They should be second nature by now. Wait, isn't that what we are trying to accomplish anyway? Ah ha! It all makes sense now, right? Test day tricks we've learned through trial and error. We both have made plenty of mistakes on testing and have decided that the following ideas are the best ones out there. Trust us, we have used them and perfected them! If they don't work exactly right for you, try tweaking them a little bit to fit your needs.

Leading Up to Test Day

The day before the big test. If you live more than an hour away from your test site, you might want to book a hotel room the night before. This will eliminate the stress of driving a long distance, getting stuck in traffic, following the wrong directions, or getting a flat tire. It also would be wise to drive by your test site to make sure you know where you're going, to prevent getting lost. Watch television, go to a movie, go for a walk, or do anything that's not NCLEX-RN® related to help reduce anxiety and pre-test jitters. There is nothing worse than listening to a fellow student who is not prepared and has a sense of impending doom to stress you out. So, our advice: STAY AWAY. Their negativity will rub off on you and increase your anxiety.

Get your ducks in a row. To feel your absolute best about your NCLEX-RN® preparation it is important to feel a balance in your mental, physical, spiritual, and emotional wellness. Double-check that you have all the appropriate documents and identification. You would hate to miss taking your exam because you did not have the right piece of paper. Eat a good dinner and go to bed early so you can feel your best when you wake up. Our biggest goal for you the day before the test is to be relaxed and not stressed about the huge test you are about to take. Just kidding, we know you are going to be stressed and that is okay. Just try to keep it to a minimum because if you don't, it might make you restless and, in turn, make you sleepless. The most important time to take care of yourself is right before an exam, so you can be at full strength to tackle the test (Gloe, 1999).

Test Day

Don't freak out, test day is FINALLY here (breathe)...WAKE UP! WAKE UP! No matter what time your test is scheduled, get up early and get moving! You are already going to be super-anxious about the test, so let's not make it any worse.

"On the day of the test, leave sufficiently early that even a tidal wave, earthquake, and Godzilla on the loose combined would not keep you from getting to the testing center on time" (Dunham, 2008). Arrive at your scheduled center at least 30 minutes prior to your test time, but do not congregate with other test takers. This will only increase your anxiety, much like test day in nursing school. If you are more than 30 minutes late for any reason on test day, the center can choose to not let you in to take the test and keep that $200 you worked hard to give them. Once you get to the testing center, be sure to leave all personal items in your car (e.g., hats, gloves, scarves, jackets, pocketbooks, etc.). Some test centers may have a locker storage area for you, but be prepared in case they do not. Once you get to the sign-in desk, you will need to present your ATT and your photo ID. The nice lady (or man) at the desk will get your fingerprints and take your picture to make sure you haven't hired a genius to come in to take your test for you. She (or he) will make you sign some more paperwork and then give you a dry erase board or some scratch paper for use during the test. You will then get escorted to your cubicle where your entertainment for the next six hours awaits (Dunham, 2008).

If your computer decides to have a meltdown or you forget how to use it, ask someone for help (you're allowed to get help even after the test begins). To keep you from having your meltdown, here are a few things you might want to avoid. First, the test question number will be provided as the test is going on. For instance, if you are on your 34th question, it will tell you Question number 34. Try not to look at this number in anticipation of the computer cutting off after question number 75. Look at each question individually and focus on that question alone. Forget completely about the questions you have already answered and do not anticipate the future questions that will be asked. You're not a mind reader; you cannot predict what is coming up next. Second, depending on the location you take your test, you may not be completely isolated. You may notice people coming in and out of the testing room, some taking much less time than you. Understand that these testing centers may offer many more tests in addition to the NCLEX-RN®, and that other individuals may be taking a different test. You have a total of 6 hours, so relax and don't rush. But, you definitely do not need to stay too long on any one question. This is why nursing school tries to adapt us to answering about one question per 1.3 minutes (Dunham, 2008).

Awaiting your test results and where to find them. It may take several weeks, usually about four, for your test results to be mailed to you. Your state board will either send you your license because you passed or a letter stating you were not successful. Most states now offer other options to receive a quicker response. If you can fork over a little bit more moolah, you might be able to get your test scores on the Internet in a few days. Either way, it's going to seem like eternity, but if you've made it this far, what is a couple more days or weeks? (Dunham, 2008).

Once you get that license (because that is what it's going to be) the job search starts. Hopefully, you were able to network some in clinical to allow yourself to know what areas of care you like and dislike and what type of facilities you prefer. Another good thing to obtain during clinical is references. Your clinical instructors should know your abilities and hopefully will speak very highly of you. Once you get that job offer, some things you might want to consider are sign-on bonuses, health care benefits, vacation time, sick time, and patient-to-nurse ratio, to name just a few concerns.

Day of Test Checklist.

- Bring ATT.
- Bring photo identification (driver's license).
- Bring ear plugs.
- Dress comfortably (possibly something you wore studying).
- Bring your brain.
- Eat a good breakfast.
- Say a quick prayer.
- Have a talk with yourself and be proud of what you have accomplished before you walk in, and leave those jitters at the door.
- Bring any other documentation/forms necessary for your state board of nursing.
- Talk to a friend to keep you calm before the test.

As if you haven't heard enough from us already. We will keep this to a minimum because we have been talking too much already. We hope you can use some of these tips and tricks when studying for the NCLEX-RN® or even your nursing tests for that matter. We have included some humor along the way because it is much easier to retain some information if you remember laughing about it. Think about how much you learn from all of those crazy clinical stories you have accumulated thus far. The disease processes that were going on with those patients are probably the ones you understand the most. Not only do we hope that you've learned something from us, but we hope that you will also be able to apply what we taught you. You can never learn too much, so do not stop with studying for NCLEX-RN®. Try pushing your brain a little further by reading updated nursing journal articles and changes to evidence-based practices, or maybe even go back to school to further your nursing education. Whatever you do, don't be afraid! You have the tips and tricks to succeed THE FIRST TIME!

Sincerely,

Your Nursing Student Buddies, Kelley & Stacy

References

Dunham, K. S. (2008). *How to survive & maybe even love nursing school.* Philadelphia: F. A. Davis Company.

Gloe, D. (1999). Study habits and test-taking tips. *Dermatology Nurses' Association, 11(6).*

Herman, J.W., & Johnson, A.N. (2009). From beta blockers to boot camp: Preparing students for the NCLEX-RN®. *Nursing Education Perspectives, 30(6).*

Landsberger, J. (1996). Overcoming test anxiety. Retrieved from http://www.studygs.net/tstprp8.htm

McDowell, B.M. (2008). Katts: A framework for maximizing NCLEX-RN® performance. *Journal of Nursing Education, 47(4).*

Wittmann-Price, R. A., & Thompson, B. R. (2010). NCLEX-RN® EXCEL. New York, NY: Springer Publishing Company.

2

Newborn Nursing Care

Case Study 1 ▬ Jasmine and River

Welcome to orientation in the well-baby nursery! Today you, the graduate nurse, will be assigned twins with your preceptor. The twins have just been transferred from the labor and delivery (L&D) suite to the newborn nursery (NN). One of the twins is a girl, Jasmine, and the other a boy, River. They were 38 and 3/7 weeks gestation, so they are considered full-term infants. Place them under the radiant warmers to be assessed.

Exercise 2-1: *Multiple Choice Question*
The nurse understands that a consequence of hypothermia in the newborn is:

    A. Neurological shivering
    B. Kidney failure
    C. Respiratory distress
    D. Unrelieved crying

 eResource 2-1: Download and install Mobile Merck Medicus on your mobile device, a free mobile resource for health care professionals from Merck & Co. Inc. available in multiple mobile device platforms. Use the Merck Manual to learn more about the warming of neonates. [Pathway: Merck Manual → Topics → Neonate → "warming of"] *www.merckmedicus.com*

Exercise 2-2: *Fill-in*
Jasmine is 6 pounds and 14 ounces and River is 6 pounds and 7 ounces. What is the twins' weight in kilograms?

    Jasmine _____
    River _____

 eResources 2-2:
    ■ Go to *www.medcalc.com/wtmeas.html* for an online weight conversion calculator offered by MedCalc.com. [Tap on General → Weights and Measures to access the calculator.]

The answers can be found on page 33.

■ Download and install Archimedes, a free medical calculator from Skyscape, Inc. available in PC and multiple mobile device platforms. Use the Weight Conversion calculator to do the conversion. (*www.skyscape.com*) and enter "Archimedes" into the search field. [Once installed, the pathway on your device is: Archimedes → Weight Conversion]

Exercise 2-3: *Circle the Correct Answer*

    A. Does Jasmine's birth weight make her SGA (small for gestational age), AGA (appropriate for gestational age), or LGA (large for gestational age)?

    B. Does River's birth weight make him SGA (small for gestational age), AGA (appropriate for gestational age), or LGA (large for gestational age)?

 eResources 2-3:

■ Go to *www.infantchart.com* or *www.medcalc.com/growth* to utilize an interactive growth chart.

■ Go to Epocrates Online and search for Gestational Age: *www .epocrates.com/products/online/index.html*

■ Download STAT GrowthCharts™ WHO to your iPod/iPhone/iPad by going to *itunes.apple.com*. Note: You will need to download iTunes to your computer before you can search for STAT GrowthCharts™ and download the free application to your device.

The radiant warmers have been prewarmed for the twins to prevent against cold stress. River's warmer is set at 37 °C and Jasmine's is set at 36 °C.

Exercise 2-4: *Convert Temperatures to Fahrenheit*

    Jasmine's radiant warmer is _____ °F.

    River's radiant warmer is _____ °F.

 eResource 2-4: Use MedCalc or Archimedes for Weight Conversion (see Exercise 2-2)

The twins are assessed using the newborn assessment in the electronic medical records (EMR). The newborn assessment is completed from head to toe. The first part of the newborn assessment has to do with general appearance, which includes body position, color, and breathing effort. Jasmine has well-flexed extremities, is in a supine position, and is breathing at 56 breaths per minute. Also her skin is pink when blanched.

 eResources 2-5:

■ To learn more about the evaluation and care of the neonate, open Mobile Merck Medicus on your mobile device [Pathway: Merck Manual → Topics → Neonate → evaluation of . . .]

■ View video: newborn assessment *youtu.be/ijQ43e8NbZM* [no heart and lung assessment included]

The answers can be found on page 33.

■ Use MedCalc Online: (*medcalc.com*) to use the Ballard Maturational Assessment of Gestational Age tool [Pathway: Medcalc Home → Tap on Pediatrics → select Ballard to access the tool.]

Exercise 2-5: *Multiple Choice Question*
River is polycythemic due to a delay in cord clamping. The nurse would expect his general color to look:

 A. Pale

 B. Pink

 C. Mottled

 D. Plethoric

eResource 2-6: Go to The Merck Manual's Online Medical Library for more detail regarding neonatal polycythemia: [Pathway: *merckmanuals .com* → select "Healthcare Professionals" → select "Pediatrics" from the section list and enter "Neonatal polycythemia" into the search field.]

The nurse knows that normal lab values for newborns are:

 ■ Hemoglobin   17–20 g/dl

 ■ Hematocrit   52–63%

 ■ Platelets   100,000–300,000 /µL

 ■ RBCs   5.1–5.8 (1,000,000/µL)

 ■ WBCs   10–30,0000/mm³

Exercise 2-6: *Multiple Choice Question*
The nurse knows that the following value indicates polycythemia:

 A. A hemoglobin of 19 g/dl

 B. A hematocrit of 68%

 C. A platelet count of 32,000/µL

 D. RBCs of 5.7 (1,000,000/µL)

eResource 2-7: Open a browser on your mobile device and go to: *www.nlm.nih.gov* to access MedlinePlus [Pathway: nlm.nih.gov → select MedlinePlus → enter "polycythemia" into the search field → scroll down and select "Hyperviscosity—newborn."]

Exercise 2-7: *Matching*
Match the skin variations the nurse may observe on a newborn.

 _____ Thick white substance that provides protection for the fetus in utero and is seen in skinfolds of term infants.

 _____ Usually found at the nape of the neck on the eyelids and are superficial vascular, pink areas.

 _____ Unopened sebaceous glands many times found on the infant's nose.

 _____ Found on the buttocks or lower extremities and are blue or purple in color.

The answers can be found on page 34.

_____ General transient rash that looks like flea bites.

_____ Dilatation of blood vessels on one side of the infant's body.

_____ Capillary angioma located directly under the skin and purple-red color. Many times it is on the side of the face.

_____ Capillary hemangioma in the dermal or subdermal skin layers and is raised and dark red.

A. Harlequin sign

B. Vernix caseosa

C. Nevus vasculosus (strawberry hemangioma)

D. Milia

E. Stork bite

F. Mongolian spot

G. Nevus flammeus (port wine stain)

H. Erythema toxicum (newborn rash)

 eResource 2-8: Open a browser on your mobile device and go to: *nlm.nih.gov* to access MedlinePlus [Pathway: nlm.nih.gov → select MedlinePlus enter "skin variations newborn" into the search field → scroll down and select "Looking at Your Newborn: What's Normal" → click on "What's in this article?" and select "skin," "birthmarks," or "rashes" for more detail.]

Jasmine and River's vital signs (VS) are obtained every 15 minutes while they are under the radiant warmer.

Exercise 2-8: *Multiple Choice Question*

What newborn vital signs would be of concern in the first two hours after birth?

    A. Heart rate 110/minute, respiration 56/minute, and temperature 97.8 axillary

    B. Heart rate 120 / minute, respiration 66/minute, and temperature 98.0 axillary

    C. Heart rate 130/minute, respiration 60/minute, and temperature 97.0 axillary

    D. Heart rate 140/minute, respiration 70/minute, and temperature 97.8 axillary

 eResource 2-9: Open a browser on your mobile device and go to: *nlm.nih.gov* to access MedlinePlus [Pathway: nlm.nih.gov → select MedlinePlus → enter "newborn physical exam" into the search field → scroll down and select "Newborn Physical Exam" to read about normal newborn findings.]

River's axillary temperature is low (below 97.7 °F) so his assessment is continued under the warmer but his initial bath is delayed. The next area of assessment is the head.

The answers can be found on page 34.

Exercise 2-9: *Matching*

_____ River's head has an edematous soft area over the left side of the occiput that crosses over the suture lines slightly to the right side.

_____ Jasmine has a large firm bump on the left side of her occiput that does not cross over to the left side.

A. Cephalohematoma

B. Caput succidarium

e   **eResource 2-10:** Remain in the same website as eResource 2-7 (MedlinePlus)[Pathway: www.nlm.nih.gov → select MedlinePlus → enter "head shape" into the search field → scroll down and select "Baby's Head Shape: What's Normal?" to read about normal newborn findings.]

Exercise 2-10: *Multiple Choice Question*

Owing to the assessment finding about Jasmine's head in Exercise 2-8, you, the nurse, knows that she is at risk for:

A. Anemia

B. Polycythemia

C. Hyperbilirubinemia

D. Hypocalcemia

Now assess the fontanels on both infants. The nurse should feel the anterior and posterior.

Exercise 2-11: *Fill-in*

When describing normal fontanels on infants they should be described as _____ and _____.

Exercise 2-12: *Matching*

_____ Anterior fontanel shape

_____ Posterior fontanel shape

A. Δ

B. ◊

The nurse measures the infants' heads and Jasmine's head is 32 cm.

e   **eResource 2-11:** To view the World Health Organization's (WHO) Head Circumference Standards, go to: *www.who.int* [Pathway: WHO International → enter "Child Growth Standards" into the search field → scroll down to locate "Head Circumference for Age" and click on link.]

Exercise 2-13: *Multiple Choice Question*

If River's chest is 28 cms around, the nurse would expect his head to measure:

A. 26 cms

B. 28 cms

C. 30 cms

D. 32 cms

The answers can be found on page 35.

Erythromycin ointment 0.5% is instilled in both infants' eye (instilled inner to outer lower canthus of each eye) prophylactically to prevent against ophthalmia neonatorum, which can cause blindness if an infant contracts chlamydial eyes disease during the birth process.

Next you check ear placement on both infants.

Exercise 2-14: *Multiple Choice Question*
Which ear placement is correct?

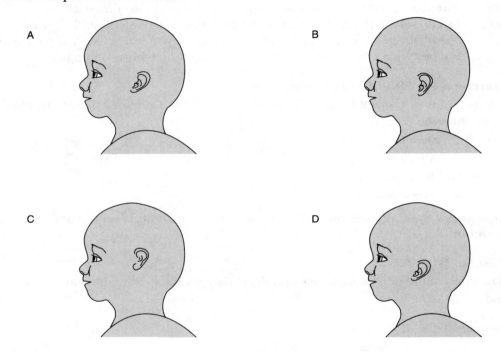

A good oral assessment is also necessary for both infants.

Exercise 2-15: *Multiple Choice Question*
A thorough oral assessment is necessary to visualize and record newborn findings. Which of the following are normal newborn findings?

    A. Pernicious teeth, Epstein pearls, intact soft palate

    B. Epstein pearls, thrush, cleft hard palate

    C. Pernicious teeth, intact hard palate, Epstein pearls

    D. Intact hard palate, Epstein pearls, intact soft palate

Next you examine each infant's neck.

The answers can be found on page 36.

Exercise 2-16: *Multiple Choice Question*

Jasmine's neck is examined closely for a low hair line because of a genetic mutation that is specific to females, called:

    A. Down syndrome

    B. Turner syndrome

    C. Patau syndrome

    D. Edwards syndrome

After the neck assessment, you stop to take vital signs (VS) again! Both infants have VS that are within normal limits (WNL) and the assessment continues.

Exercise 2-17: *Multiple Choice Question*

The nurse understands that it is important to keep a neutral thermal environment (NTE) for infants in order to prevent:

    A. Hypothyroidism

    B. Hypocalcemia

    C. Hypoglycemia

    D. Hypogalactosemia

Another important assessment done on all infants is palpation of the clavicle. The clavicle is the most commonly fractured bone for an infant.

Exercise 2-18: *Select All That Apply*

The nurse understands that the incidence of birth trauma is increased when which of the following conditions exist:

    ❑ Large for gestational age infants

    ❑ Breech presentations

    ❑ Infants of diabetic mothers

    ❑ Shoulder dystocia

    ❑ Prolapsed cord

    ❑ Small for gestational age infants

Exercise 2-19: *Fill-in*

What finding would the nurse expect to feel on palpation if the infant had a fractured clavicle? _____

Both infants' clavicles are intact. Next you assess their respiratory status. You count both infants' respiratory rates.

Exercise 2-20: *Fill-in*

You expect the normal respiratory rate (RR) for an infant to be between _____ and _____ breaths per minute.

The respiratory effort of both infants is assessed using the Silverman–Anderson Index.

The answers can be found on page 37.

eResource 2-12: To learn more about the Silverman-Anderson Scoring System, go to: *www.ceu.org/cecourses/981117/ch11b.htm*

Jasmine is a 0 on the scale, meaning there is no respiratory distress.
River has minimal nasal flaring and minimal grunting. His Silverman–Anderson Index score would be a 3.

Exercise 2-21: *Multiple Choice Question*
Because River has slight nasal flaring and grunting, the next priority for the nurse would be to:

     A. Call the pediatrician and report the finding.
     B. Observe to see if the nasal flaring and grunting increases.
     C. Wrap the infant and give him to his mother to breastfeed.
     D. Obtain a pulse oximeter reading.

The nasal flaring and grunting exhibited by River subsides within an hour, and both infants' lung fields are clear on auscultation. Both infants' point of maximum impact (PMI) is at the fourth intercostals space, in the midclavicular line.

Exercise 2-22: *Hot Spot*
Put an X on the fourth intercostals space in the midclavicular line.

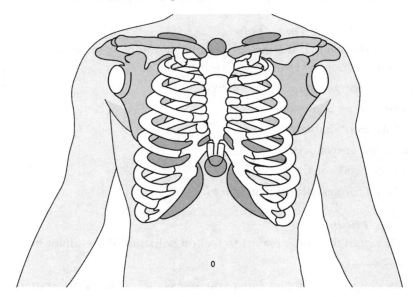

When you perform auscultation on River's heart, you hear a murmur.

Exercise 2-23: *Ordering*
Place the interventions in order that the nurse would take after assessing an infant patient with a murmur.

     _____ Call the pediatrician to inform him/her of the finding.
     _____ Record pre and post ductal blood pressures.

The answers can be found on page 38.

——————— Receive an order and have a 12-lead EKG (electrocardiogram) performed.

——————— Consult a pediatric cardiologist after the order was received from the primary practitioner.

——————— Assess pre and post ductal pulse oximeter readings.

It is time to take the infants' VS again! Jasmine's heart rate (HR) is 156 beats per minute (bpm).

Exercise 2-24: *Multiple Choice Question*

The nurse understands that the following finding warrants further assessment on an infant:

A. RR—66; HR 156
B. RR—56; HR 146
C. RR—60; HR 160
D. RR—46; HR 148

Next you auscultate bowel sounds. Bowel sounds are present in all four quadrants for both infants. You move on to observing their umbilical cords to make sure the clamp is secure and the proper numbers of vessels are present in the cord.

Exercise 2-25: *Fill-in*

How many arteries are present in an umbilical cord normally? ———————

How many veins are present in an umbilical cord normally? ———————

Both umbilical cords look normal. Next you assess the infants' genitalia. Jasmine has labia minora that are covered by her majora which denotes that she is a term infant. Jasmine also has some **pseudomenstrual** discharge.

Exercise 2-26: *Multiple Choice Question*

The nurse understands that further parental teaching is needed when Jasmine's mother states:

A. "I know it is normal for babies to have **pseudomenstruation** for one year."
B. "I understand that **pseudomenstruation** is from my hormones."
C. "I know that **pseudomenstruation** is not a concern."
D. "I understand that **pseudomenstruation** does not need treatment."

You inspect the genitalia of River to make sure that the meatus opening is on the tip of the penis and that both testes are in the scrotum, which they are.

The answers can be found on page 39.

Exercise 2-27: *Matching*

Match the description and abnormal male genital condition.

_____ Opening of the meatus is on the ventral side of the penis.

_____ Undescended testes.

_____ The opening of the meatus is on the dorsal side of the penis.

A. Epispadias

B. Hypospadias

C. Cryptorchidism

Time to check VS!

The twins' parents ask about a circumcision for River. The nurse explains the two types of circumcision most often performed in nurseries: surgical removal of the foreskin and bell circumcisions that tie off the foreskin using a plastic ring. You explain the procedures to the parents and review the analgesia provided, EMLA cream is applied to the penis before the procedure, dorsal penile nerve block, and concentrated glucose orally. You know as a nurse that circumcision is a surgical procedure and, like any surgical procedure, you must call for a TIME OUT. Both infants' rectal areas are checked to determine if they have a patent anus. Both have had a meconium stool, which is a sign that their gastrointestinal tract (GI) is patent. An imperforate anus or one that does not connect to the outside of the body would be a surgical emergency in the newborn. Usually, the majority of infants pass meconium in the first 24 hours after birth. Next you check the extremities of both infants. The upper extremities should be examined for movement and finger placement.

Exercise 2-28: *Matching*

Match the descriptions and conditions the nurse may observe in the newborn.

_____ Extra digits

_____ Single palmer crease

_____ Arm hangs limp at the infant's side

_____ Fused fingers

A. Simian crease

B. Polydactyly

C. Syndactyly

D. Brachial plexus injury (Erb's palsy)

Upon examining both infants' legs, you turn them on their abdomens to check that gluteal folds are equal and there is no developmental dysplasia of the hips (DDH). It is also important to check their spines to make sure they are straight without any pilonidal dimples at the base, tufts of hair, cysts or masses, all of which can indicate a spinal cord problem. At this point you stop and administer to both infants a dose of vitamin K, IM 0.5–1.0 mg in the vastus lateralis muscles.

The answers can be found on page 39.

Exercise 2-29: *Hot Spot*

Circle the spot to administer vitamin K.

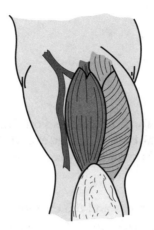

Exercise 2-30: *Multiple Choice Question*

The nurse understands that the patient needs further teaching when she states:

    A. "My babies need vitamin K because I was anemic during my pregnancy."

    B. "My babies need vitamin K because their gastrointestinal tract is sterile."

    C. "My babies need vitamin K because it will help them produce clotting factor."

    D. "My babies need vitamin K in their leg because it may not be effective by mouth."

Next you assess the neurological status of the infants by checking their reflexes.

Exercise 2-31: *Matching*

Match the reflex and finding.

    _____ Stroke the lateral sole of the foot and the toes fan out.

    _____ The infant closes his/her hand if you place your finger in the palm.

    _____ Stimulated by touching the infant's lips.

    _____ The newborn will curl his/her toes around a finger placed just below them.

    _____ Stimulated by touching the infant's check.

    _____ Hold the infant upright and have the soles of the feet touch a flat surface.

    _____ When the infant is startled he/she throws his/her hands out, flexes knee, and places hands in a C-position.

    _____ This is also called a fencing reflex; if the infant's head is turned he/she will extend the arm on that side.

The answers can be found on page 40.

    A. Sucking
    B. Moro
    C. Stepping
    D. Tonic neck
    E. Rooting
    F. Babinski
    G. Palmer grasp
    H. Planter grasp

After the neurological exam for both infants you can take their VS again, and it is time to give them their initial bath! You get everything ready for their baths and review the modes of heat loss with your preceptor in order to maintain a NTE.

Exercise 2-32: *Matching*
Match the method of body heat loss and the example.

_____ The nurse places the infant on a cold counter in order to provide a bath.

_____ The nurse does not dry the infant well.

_____ The nurse carries the infant past a closed outside window during subtemperatures.

_____ The nurse examines the infant in an open crib that is next to a swinging door.

    A. Convection
    B. Evaporation
    C. Radiation
    D. Conduction

After the infants are bathed you double-wrap them and place a stocking cap on their heads. They are ready to be transported to their parent's postpartum hospital room. You recruit another nurse to help you transport them and when you enter the room you think about any safety issues.

Exercise 2-33: *Select All That Apply*
Appropriate identifiers used to match mothers and infants are:

❑ Ask the father to read the infants' band and confirm.

❑ Ask the mother her full name.

❑ Ask the mother her infant's date of birth (DOB).

❑ Ask the mother what time the infant was born.

❑ Ask the mother for her DOB.

❑ Compare the armbands of mother and infant.

The answers can be found on page 41.

After identifying the infants, you assist Kerry (the twins' mother) to place the infants to breast. First you help River since he is awake in his second period of reactivity, which is the third behavioral pattern seen in the newborn after birth and lasts from 2 to 8 hours. First newborns have a period of reactivity for approximately 30 minutes after birth in which they are wide awake and alert. This is followed by a period of decreased responsiveness from approximately 30 to 120 minutes of age, and during this phase the infant is usually in a sleep state and is difficult to arouse. Quality of breast-feeding is assessed using the LATCH score method which can be found at: *www.adhb.govt.nz/newborn/Guidelines/LatchScore.htm*

River does well breast-feeding and his LATCH score is 8. He needs some assistance latching on and Kerry needs assistance positioning him. River sucks for 8 minutes on the left breast and 5 on the right and dozes off. Jasmine is sleepier. Jasmine takes a few, nonaudible sucks from the right everted nipple when she is stimulated. Kerry positions her well and is comfortable. Jasmine's LATCH score is 7.

Exercise 2-34: *Matching*

The nurse understands that breast-feeding is important for immunoglobulin protection. Match the immunolglobin and its characteristics.

_____ Normally found only with an intrauterine infection.

_____ This is transferred in breast milk.

_____ This immunoglobulin crosses the placenta.

A. IgA
B. IgG
C. IgM

River is placed to sleep in his open crib on his back. Jasmine is taken to the nursery for a glucose check.

Exercise 2-35: *Ordering*

Place in order the following steps for obtaining a glucose sample:

_____ Wipe the first drop of blood off.

_____ Identify the patient with two identifiers.

_____ Check the glucometer to make sure the controls have been completed in the past 24 hours.

_____ Don clean gloves.

_____ Wipe off the area with alcohol.

_____ Clean the area and place a clean bandage on it.

The answers can be found on page 42.

Exercise 2-36: *Hot Spot*

Draw an X on a spot on which it is safe to obtain a blood specimen:

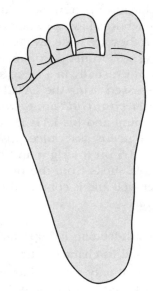

Exercise 2-37: *Multiple Choice Question*

The nurse understands that the reason for drawing blood from the correct spot is important because:

    A. The proper areas produce less pain for the patient.

    B. The proper areas bleed more and the nurse is more likely to obtain enough blood.

    C. The proper areas are easier to access.

    D. The proper areas are free of transecting nerves that may be damaged.

Jasmine's glucose level is 35 mg/dl which is low since in utero a fetus's glucose level is 70–80% of the maternal glucose. Normal maternal glucose is 80–120 mg/dl.

Exercise 2-38: *Calculation*

Calculate what the low limit of glucose would be (70% of 80 mg/dl) = _____ mg/dl and; calculate what the high limit of glucose would be (80% of 120 mg/dl) = _____ mg/dl.

Exercise 2-39: *Select All That Apply*

The nurse understands that infants may demonstrate the following symptoms when hypoglycemic:

    ❏ Lethargy

    ❏ Hypertonicity

    ❏ Hypotonicity

The answers can be found on page 43.

❑ Muscle twitching

❑ Excessive sleepiness

❑ Well-coordinated suck

❑ Diaphoresis

Exercise 2-40: *Calculation*

If an infant needs intravenous (IV) glucose infusion it is given in the following dose: Dextrose 10% at 5–8 mg/kg/min

If Jasmine is 6 pounds and 14 ounces, what would be her hourly dose in mL/hr?

 eResource 2-13: Go to *www.medcalc.com/wtmeas.html* to do the weight conversion and then to *www.medcalc.com/ivrate.html* to use the IV Rate calculator offered by MedCalc.com.

Jasmine is fed 15 mL of 20 cal/oz formula and her blood glucose is rechecked in 30 minutes and is 55 mg/dl. In 2 hours, breast-feeding will be attempted again.

Both twins room-in with their parents and are breast-fed every 2–3 hours around the clock for the first day. Each baby is weighed every 24 hours and diapers are counted to keep accurate intake and output (I&O). Below is the nurses' notes for both infants' I&O.

Day One	Jasmine	River
No. of breast-feedings	10	8
Meconium	1	1
Wet diapers	1	2
24-hour weight	6 lbs and 2 oz	6 lbs and 2 oz

The following day (day 2 of life), the twins appeared fussier and Kerry became increasingly concerned. Kerry and Terrell (the twins' father) were both told that this is normal, and Kerry was encouraged to continue to feed both infants on demand. As the evening approached Kerry and Terrell decided to send the infants to the nursery and have them brought out on demand in order to get some sleep before their discharge in the AM. The second day I&O chart was reviewed.

Day Two	Jasmine	River
No. of breast-feedings	12	11
Meconium	2	2
Wet diapers	4	5
24-hour weight	6 lbs and 0 oz	6 lbs and 1 oz

Infants' weight is calculated daily in order to prevent excessive weight loss or more than 10% of their birth weight.

The answer can be found on page 43.

Exercise 2-41: *Calculation*

What would each infant weigh if they lost 10% of their birth weight?

(Jasmine was 6 pounds and 14 ounces and River was 6 pounds and 7 ounces.)

During the second night both infants nurse three times well, and the following day Kerry and Terrell are prepared for discharge. Two screening tests are completed on the infants before they are discharged: universal newborn hearing screen (UNHS) and genetic and inborn errors of metabolism screening. States differ in the number of genetic and inborn error of metabolic diseases that are screened. The more common conditions included in screenings are Phenylketonuria (PKU), hypothyroidism, sickle cell disease, and galactosemia. The tests are done by placing drops of blood from an infant's heel stick onto specially treated paper and sending the specimen to a state-approved lab.

 eResource 2-14:
- For more information regarding screening guidelines, go to the National Guideline Clearinghouse (NGC) to view Practice Guidelines: *guideline.gov* [Pathway: NGC → enter "newborn screening" into the search field → enter each of the following terms into the search field to find relevant practice guidelines: PKU, congenital hypothyroidism, sickle cell disease, and galactosemia.
- Additional information regarding screening guidelines can be obtained from the CDC *www.cdc.gov* [Pathway: CDC.gov → enter "newborn screening" into the search field → select "Newborn Screening" → scroll down to view selected screening guidelines]

Exercise 2-42: *Fill-in*

The nurse knows that in order for the screening tests for some metabolic disorders and inborn errors of metabolism to be accurate, the infant needs to be taking oral nutrition for at least _____ hours in order for detectable levels of phenylalanine (PKU) to be present in the blood.

The UNHS need to be completed in a quiet area while the infants are quiet or asleep. All infants are screened, but infants that are high risk for hearing deficits that are:
- Born preterm
- Have a family history of hearing deficits
- Have anomalies of the ears
- Have perinatal asphyxia
- Have prenatal or post natal infections
- Have been receiving ototoxic drugs

Also during the infants' assessment on the third morning, the nurse notices that River is slightly jaundiced at 48 hours. The nurse draws a bilirubin test by heel stick and sends it to the lab for a total bilirubin level. River's total bilirubin is 6.2 mg/dl.

The answers can be found on page 43.

eResources 2-15:

■ Use BiliTool™, either the online tool or download the mobile app, to assess risks. (*bilitool.org*)

■ Review the American Academy of Pediatrics Subcommittee on Hyperbilirubinemia issued Clinical Practice Guideline: *www.aap .org/qualityimprovement/quiin/SHB/Hyperbili.pdf*

■ Go to the National Guideline Clearinghouse (NGC) to view Practice Guidelines: *guideline.gov* [Pathway: NGC → enter "newborn" into the search field → review "Guidelines for management of jaundice in the breastfeeding infant equal to or greater than 35 weeks' gestation" guideline.

Exercise 2-43: *Exhibit Question*

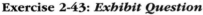

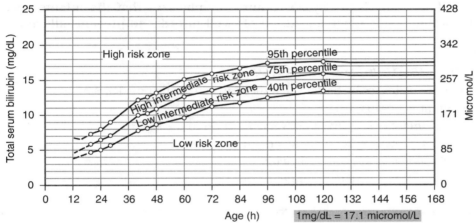

Using the bilirubin graph pictures shown on the Web, River's total bilirubin level falls into which category?

    A. Low risk zone

    B. Low intermittent risk zone

    C. High intermittent risk zone

    D. High risk zone

Kerry and Terrell are overwhelmed by the amount of information they need to know in order to care for the twins safely. Another safety issue to be addressed is their infant car seats.

The answer can be found on page 44.

Exercise 2-44: *Multiple Choice Question*

The nurse knows that additional teaching is needed about safety when the patient states:

    A. "Both infant car seats need to be in the back seat."

    B. "The infant car seats should be balanced using the mechanism built into the seat that shows the correct position."

    C. "The infant car seat has a 5-point restraining system."

    D. "We can use a homemade head roll that is inserted behind the infants' back."

Another teaching session reviews changing and bathing the infants. The nurse shows Kerry and Terrell how to sponge bath their infants until the umbilical stumps fall off in 7–10 days. The nurse emphasizes that the infants need to be bathed in a safe place and dried off well in order to prevent falls and cold stress.

Exercise 2-45: *Multiple Choice Question*

The nurse explains to the parents that the reason that talc powder is not recommended for an infant is because:

    A. Infants may have an adverse reaction to the scent.

    B. Infants may have an adverse skin reaction.

    C. Talc is a respiratory irritant.

    D. Talc can irritate the infants' eyes.

Kerry and Terrell are also asked to sign a voluntary commitment statement (VCS) that discusses the effects of shaking baby syndrome (SBS) and requests that the parents understand they can never shake the infants regardless of their level of frustration.

 eResource 2-16: To supplement your patient teaching, show this March of Dimes Baby Care 101 video: *bcove.me/3pmbiw18*

Exercise 2-46: *Select All That Apply*

Some of the suggestions provided for parents who become frustrated with infant crying are to:

    ❑ Place the infant in another room.

    ❑ Give the infant a pacifier.

    ❑ Medicate the infant.

    ❑ Call a helpline.

    ❑ Place the infant in a prone position.

    ❑ Provide the infant with cereal fortified formula.

The answers can be found on page 45.

Elimination is another concern for parents. The nurse explains to Kerry and Terrell that infants should, as a rule of thumb, wet at least one diaper on the first day of life, two diapers on the second day of life, three diapers on the third day of life, and so on, until they are up to 7–10 wet diapers a day. The nurse provides them with a chart to write down the number of times that each infant is voiding. They also ask about the infants stool patterns.

Exercise 2-47: *Multiple Choice Question*
The nurse correctly explains that breast-fed infants should:

    A. Have yellow seedy stool by one week of age

    B. Continue to have meconium stools for the first week

    C. Not stool every day

    D. Have brown, formed, pasty stools by one week of age

 eResource 2-17: To obtain the Input/Output Tracker chart to give to the parents, go to The Bump (*pregnant.thebump.com*) [Pathway: The Bump → enter "input/output" into the search field → select "Tool: Input/Output Tracker."]

How to place the infants to sleep is also discussed.

Exercise 2-48: *Fill-in*
The nurse teaches the parents to place the infants in a _____ position for the best prevention against sudden infant death syndrome (SIDS).

 eResources 2-18:
- ■ To supplement new parent teaching regarding SIDS, you can show them this brief tutorial developed by South Carolina's Healthy Start Program. To view, go to *youtu.be/t-Q9qfOKUNE*
- ■ Listen to this brief audio clip about "Back to Sleep" initiative from the American Academy of Pediatrics *www.aap.org/audio/mfk/011408.mp3*
- ■ For more teaching material regarding a safe sleeping environment for the infant, go to: *www.cdc.gov/SIDS*

The nurse continues with the discharge teaching and explains that Kerry and Terrell should bring the infants back to the pediatrician or primary care practitioner (PCP) as ordered, which is in two days. This appointment is important in order to check the infants' weight and bilirubin status.

    The nurse instructs them to record their baby's weight and date of visits as well as any immunization in order to keep accurate health records. Kerry and Terrell acknowledge that they understand the discharge education and sign the discharge instruction sheet. One infant identification (ID) band is removed from each infant and placed on the hospital identification sheet and the numbers are checked to make sure they match with the initial numbers.

The answers can be found on page 45.

eResources 2-19:

■ Go to the National Guideline Clearinghouse (NGC) to view Practice Guidelines: *guideline.gov* [Pathway: NGC → enter "newborn" into the search field → review "Postpartum maternal and newborn discharge" and other available newborn discharge guidelines.

■ Go to the National Guideline Clearinghouse (NGC) to view Practice Guidelines: *guideline.gov* [Pathway: NGC → enter "routine preventable services infants" into the search field → select and review the "Routine preventive services for infants and children (birth–24 months)" guideline.

Answers

Exercise 2-1: *Multiple Choice Question*

The nurse understands that a consequence of hypothermia in the newborn is:

A. Neurological shivering—NO, infants do not have the capability to shiver.

B. Kidney failure—NO, this is usually not the direct consequence of cold stress.

C. **Respiratory distress—YES, infants will increase their metabolism to keep warm and breathe faster. Eventually they will tire and it will cause respiratory distress.**

D. Unrelieved crying—NO, even though they may cry because they are uncomfortable it is not a definitive consequence of cold stress.

Exercise 2-2: *Fill-in*

What is the twins' weight in kilograms?

Jasmine __3.12__

River __2.92__

Exercise 2-3: *Circle the Correct Answer*

A. Does Jasmine's birth weight make her SGA (small for gestational age), **AGA (appropriate for gestational age),** or LGA (large for gestational age)?

B. Does River's birth weight make him SGA (small for gestational age), **AGA (appropriate for gestational age),** or LGA (large for gestational age)?

*Both infants are within the 10th to 90th percentile and are therefore AGA.

Exercise 2-4: *Fill-in*

Convert the temperatures to Fahrenheit.

Jasmine's radiant warmer is __99__ °F

River's radiant warmer is __97__ °F

Exercise 2-5: *Multiple Choice Question*

River is polycythemic due to a delay in cord clamping. The nurse would expect his general color to look:

A. Pale—NO, polycythemic is an excess of RBCs (red blood cells).

B. Pink—NO, pink is the normal color of infants with RBCs within normal limits (WNLs).

C. Mottled—NO, this is a color variation that usually happens when infants are cold.

D. **Plethoric—YES, this is a ruddy color produced form too many RBCs.**

Exercise 2-6: *Multiple Choice Question*

The nurse knows that the following value indicates polycythemia:

A. A hemoglobin of 19 g/dl—NO, this is not an indicator, it is WNL.

B. **A hematocrit of 68%—YES, this is high and warrants investigation, over 70% may warrant a transfusion to prevent cerebral clots.**

C. A platelet count of 32,000/μL—NO, this is not an indicator, but it is very low.

D. RBCs of 5.7 (1,000,000/μL)—NO, this is not an indicator, it is WNL.

Exercise 2-7: *Matching*

Match the skin variations a nurse may observe on a newborn.

___**B**___ Thick white substance that provides protection for the fetus in utero and is seen in skin folds of term infants.

___**E**___ Usually found at the nape of the neck on the eyelids and are superficial vascular, pink areas.

___**D**___ Unopened sebaceous glands many times found on the infant's nose.

___**F**___ Found on the buttocks or lower extremities and are blue or purple in color.

___**H**___ General transient rash that looks like flea bites.

___**A**___ Dilatation of blood vessels on one side of the infant's body.

___**G**___ Capillary angioma located directly under the skin and purple-red color. Many times it is on the side of the face.

___**C**___ Capillary hemangioma in the dermal or subdermal skin layers and is raised and dark red.

    A. Harlequin sign

    B. Vernix caseosa

    C. Nevus vasculosus (strawberry hemangioma)

    D. Milia

    E. Stork bite

    F. Mongolian spot

    G. Nevus flammeus (port wine stain)

    H. Erythema toxicum (newborn rash)

Exercise 2-8: *Multiple Choice Question*

What newborn vital signs would be of concern in the first two hours after birth?

A. Heart rate 110/minute, respiration 56/minute, and temperature 97.8 axillary—NO, these are WNLs.

B. Heart rate 120/minute, respiration 66/minute, and temperature 98.0 axillary—NO, these are WNLs.

C. **Heart rate 130/minute, respiration 60/minute, and temperature 97.0 axillary— YES, the low temperature is a concern.**

D. Heart rate 140/minute, respiration 70/minute, and temperature 97.8 axillary—NO, these are WNLs, respirations may be at a rate of up to 70 in the initial hours after birth.

Exercise 2-9: *Matching*

__B__ River's head has an edematous soft area over the left side of the occiput that crosses over the suture lines slightly to the right side.

__A__ Jasmine has a large firm bump on the left side of her occiput that does not cross over to the left side.

    A. Cephalohematoma

    B. Caput succidarium

Exercise 2-10: *Multiple Choice Question*

Due to the assessment finding about Jasmine's head in Exercise 2-8, you, the nurse knows that she is at risk for:

A. Anemia—NO, this is not a consequence of the collection of blood under the periosteum of the skull.

B. Polycythemia—NO, this is not a consequence of the collection of blood under the periosteum of the skull.

C. **Hyperbilirubinemia—YES, the accumulation of RBCs will break down and form heme.**

D. Hypocalcemia— NO, this is not a consequence of the collection of blood under the periosteum of the skull.

Exercise 2-11: *Fill-in*

When describing normal fontanels on infants they should be described as __soft__ and __flat__.

Exercise 2-12: *Matching*

__A__ Anterior fontanel shape

__B__ Posterior fontanel shape

    A. Δ

    B. ◊

Exercise 2-13: *Multiple Choice Question*

If River's chest is 28 cms around, the nurse would expect his head to measure:

A. 26 cms—NO, the head should be 1–2 cms larger than the chest circumference.

B. 28 cms—NO, the head should be 1–2 cms larger than the chest circumference.

C. **30 cms—YES, the head should be 1–2 cms larger than the chest circumference.**

D. 32 cms—NO, the head should be 1–2 cms larger than the chest circumference.

Exercise 2-14: *Multiple Choice Question*

Which ear placement is correct?

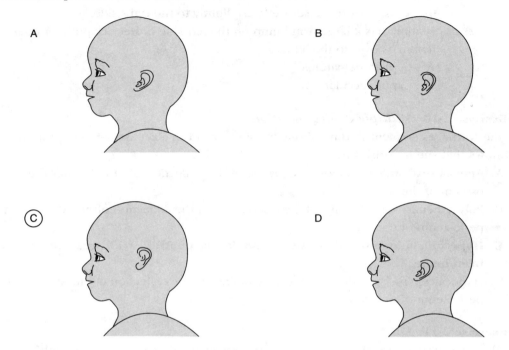

A. NO, the picture of the ear in A is at too much of an angle.

B. NO, the picture of the ear in B is slightly low.

C. **YES, C is the correct placement. When a line is drawn from the inner to outer eye canthus, it touches the ear and the ear is at a 20 degree angle.**

D. NO, the ear in D is slightly low and is too angled.

Exercise 2-15: *Multiple Choice Question*

A thorough oral assessment is necessary to visualize and record newborn findings. Which of the following are normal newborn findings?

A. Pernicious teeth, Epstein pearls, intact soft palate—NO, pernicious teeth are not normally present and need to be removed to prevent chocking.

B. Epstein pearls, thrush, cleft hard palate—NO, clefts and thrush are both abnormal conditions.

C. Pernicious teeth, intact hard palate, Epstein pearls—NO, see answer to A.

D. **Intact hard palate, Epstein pearls, intact soft palate—YES, the palates should be intact and Epstein pearls are a normal occurrence and are found in 80% of infants. They are fluid-filled cysts found on the roof of the mouth and gums.**

Exercise 2-16: *Multiple Choice Question*

Jasmine's neck is examined closely for a low hair line because of a genetic mutation that is specific to females, called:

A. Down syndrome—NO, trisomy 21 can occur in both male and females.

B. **Turner syndrome—YES, this condition is sex-linked in which a female is missing an X chromosome.**

C. Patau syndrome—NO, trisomy 13 can occur in both male and females.

D. Edwards syndrome—NO, trisomy 18 can occur in both male and females.

Exercise 2-17: *Multiple Choice Question*

The nurse understands that it is important to keep a neutral thermal environment (NTE) for infants in order to prevent:

A. Hypothyroidism—NO, this occurs from a malfunctioning thyroid.

B. Hypocalcemia—NO, this is directly related to poor prenatal stores of Ca.

C. **Hypoglycemia—YES, the infant uses glucose to increase metabolism to keep warm.**

D. Hypogalactosemia—NO, this is related to an inborn error of metabolism.

Exercise 2-18: *Select All That Apply*

The nurse understands that the incidence of birth trauma is increased when which of the following conditions exist.

❑ **Large for gestational age infants—YES, due to difficult deliveries.**

❑ **Breech presentations—YES, due to difficult deliveries.**

❑ **Infants of diabetic mothers—YES, due to difficult deliveries.**

❑ **Shoulder dystocia—YES, due to difficult deliveries.**

❑ Prolapsed cord—NO, this usually calls for an emergency Cesarean birth.

❑ Small for gestational age infants—NO, smaller infants do not usually cause difficult deliveries.

Exercise 2-19: *Fill-in*

What finding would the nurse expect to feel on palpation if the infant had a fractured clavicle? **Crepitus (A feeling of bone rubbing against bone)**

Exercise 2-20: *Fill-in*

You expect the normal respiratory rate (RR) for an infant to be between __**30**__ and __**60**__ breaths per minute. **(During the first hours of life respirations may occur between 30 and 70 breaths per minute normally).**

Exercise 2-21: *Multiple Choice Question*

Because River has slight nasal flaring and grunting, the next priority for the nurse would be to:

A. Call the pediatrician and report the finding—NO, assess peripheral oxygenation first.

B. Observe to see if the nasal flaring and grunting increases—NO, further assessment should be done right away.

C. Wrap the infant and give him to his mom to breast-feed—NO, this will increase the infant's oxygen needs which may already be compromised.

D. **Obtain a pulse oximeter reading—YES, this will provide the nurse with more assessment information in order to make an accurate clinical decision.**

Exercise 2-22: *Hot Spot*

Put an X on the fourth intercostals space in the midclavicular line.

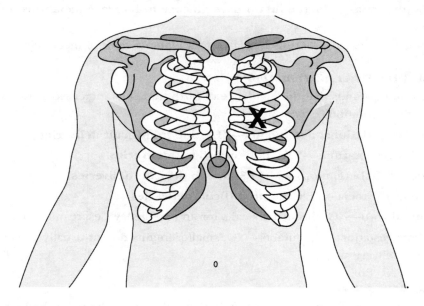

Exercise 2-23: *Ordering*

Place the interventions in the order that the nurse would take after assessing an infant patient with a murmur.

    4   Call the pediatrician to inform him/her of the finding.

    1   Record pre and post ductal blood pressures.

    3   Receive an order and have a 12-lead EKG (electrocardiogram) performed. **(For most nurseries this is a standing order for an infant with a murmur.)**

    5   Consult a pediatric cardiologist after the order was received from the primary practitioner.

    2   Assess pre and post ductal pulse oximeter readings.

Exercise 2-24: *I*

The nurse understands that the following finding warrants further assessment on an infant:

A. **RR—66; HR 156—YES, this is an elevated respiratory rate for infants more than a few hours old.**

B. RR—56; HR 146—NO, these VS are WNL.

C. RR—60; HR 160—NO, these VS are WNL.

D. RR—46; HR 148—NO, these VS are WNL.

Exercise 2-25: *Fill-in*

How many arteries are present in an umbilical cord normally? __2__

How many veins are present in an umbilical cord normally? __1__

Remember AVA (Artery, vein, artery)

Exercise 2-26: *Multiple Choice Question*

The nurse understands that further parental teaching is needed when Jasmine's mother states:

A. **"I know it is normal for babies to have pseudomenstruation for one year."— YES, this condition only lasts for approximately one week.**

B. "I understand that **pseudomenstruation** is from my hormones."—NO, this is correct.

C. "I know that **pseudomenstruation** is not a concern."—NO, this is correct.

D. "I understand that **pseudomenstruation** does not need treatment."—NO, this is correct.

Exercise 2-27: *Matching*

Match the description and abnormal male genital condition.

__B__ Opening of the meatus is on the ventral side of the penis.

__C__ Undescended testes.

__A__ The opening o the meatus is on the dorsal side of the penis.

    A. Epispadias

    B. Hypospadias

    C. Cryptorchidism

Exercise 2-28: *Matching*

Match the descriptions and conditions the nurse may observe in the newborn.

__B__ Extra digits

__A__ Single palmer crease

__D__ Arm hangs limp at the infant's side

__C__ Fused fingers

    A. Simian crease

    B. Polydactyly

    C. Syndactyly

    D. Brachial plexus injury (Erb's palsy)

Exercise 2-29: *Hot Spot*

Circle the spot to administer vitamin K.

Infant thigh

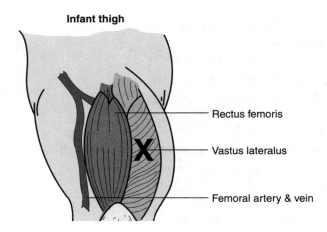

— Rectus femoris

— Vastus lateralus

— Femoral artery & vein

Exercise 2-30: *Multiple Choice Question*

The nurse understands that the patient needs further teaching when she states:

A. "My babies need vitamin K because I was anemic during my pregnancy."—NO, this is not the reason.

B. "My babies need vitamin K because their gastrointestinal tract is sterile."—NO, this is not the reason.

C. **"My babies need vitamin K because it will help them produce clotting factor."—YES, infants have sterile guts, and bacteria are needed in the gastrointestinal tract to synthesize vitamin K.**

D. "My babies need vitamin K in their leg because it may not be effective by mouth."—NO, this is not the reason.

Exercise 2-31: *Matching*

Match the reflex and finding.

___**F**___ Stock the lateral sole of the foot and the toes fan out.

___**G**___ The infant closes his/her hand if you place your finger in the palm.

___**A**___ Stimulated by touching the infant's lips.

___**H**___ The newborn will curl his/her toes around a finger placed just below them.

___**E**___ Stimulated by touching the infant's check.

___**C**___ Hold the infant upright and have the soles of the feet touch a flat surface.

___**B**___ When the infant is startled, he/she may throw his/her hands out, flexes knee, and places hands in a C-position.

___**D**___ This is also called a fencing reflex; if the infant's head is turned, he/she will extend the arm on that side.

A. Sucking

B. Moro

C. Stepping

D. Tonic neck

E. Rooting

F. Babinski

G. Palmer grasp

H. Planter grasp

Exercise 2-32: *Matching*

Match the method of body heat loss and the example.

   D   The nurse places the infant on a cold counter in order to provide a bath.

   B   The nurse does not dry the infant well.

   C   The nurse carries the infant past a closed outside window during subtemperatures.

   A   The nurse examines the infant in an open crib that is next to a swinging door.

A. Convection

B. Evaporation

C. Radiation

D. Conduction

Exercise 2-33: *Select All That Apply*

Appropriate identifiers used to match mothers and infants are:

❑ Ask the father to read the infant's band and confirm.—NO, the nurse should read the band.

❑ **Ask the mother her full name.—YES, this should match with the infant's name band.**

❑ Ask the mother her infant's date of birth (DOB).—NO, this is not a good identifier for infants since many are born on the same day.

❑ **Ask the mother what time the infant was born.—YES, this is better than the day.**

❑ Ask the mother for her DOB.—NO, this may not be on the infant band.

❑ **Scan the armbands of mother and infant.—YES, this is good if the nursery has the capability.**

Exercise 2-34: *Matching*

The nurse understands that breast-feeding is important for immunoglobulin protection. Match the immunolglobin and its characteristics.

   C   Normally found only with an intrauterine infection.

   A   This is transferred in breast milk.

   B   This immunoglobulin crosses the placenta.

A. IgA

B. IgG

C. IgM

Exercise 2-35: *Ordering*

Place the following steps for obtaining a glucose in order:

   5   Wipe the first drop of blood off.

   1   Identify the patient with two identifiers.

   2   Check the glucometer to make sure the controls have been completed in the past 24 hours.

   3   Don clean gloves.

   4   Wipe off the area with alcohol.

   6   Clean the area and place a clean bandage on it.

Exercise 2-36: *Hot Spot*

Draw an X on a spot on which it is safe to obtain a blood specimen:

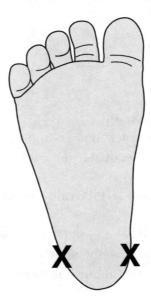

Exercise 2-37: *Multiple Choice Question*

The nurse understands that the reason for drawing blood from the correct spot is important because:

A. The proper areas produce less pain for the patient.—NO, this is not the reason.

B. The proper areas bleed more and the nurse is more likely to obtain enough blood. —NO, this is not the reason.

C. The proper areas are easier to access.—NO, this is not the reason.

D. **The proper areas are free of transecting nerves that may be damaged.—YES, this is the physiological reason.**

Exercise 2-38: *Calculation*

Calculate what the low limit of glucose would be (70% of 80 mg/dl) = __**56**__ mg/dl and; calculate what the high limit of glucose would be (80% of 120 mg/dl) = __**96**__ mg/dl.

Exercise 2-39: *Select All That Apply*

The nurse understands that infants may demonstrate the following symptoms when hypoglycemic:

❑ **Lethargy—YES, this has been a recorded symptom in some infants.**

❑ **Hypertonicity—YES, this has been a recorded symptom in some infants.**

❑ **Hypotonicity—YES, this has been a recorded symptom in some infants.**

❑ **Muscle twitching—YES, this has been a recorded symptom in some infants.**

❑ Excessive sleepiness—NO, this is usually not a symptom.

❑ Well-coordinated suck—NO, this is usually not a symptom.

❑ Diaphoresis—NO, this is usually not a symptom.

Exercise 2-40: *Calculation*

If an infant needs intravenous (IV) glucose infusion it is given in the following dose: Dextrose 10% at 5–8 mg/kg/min

If Jasmine is 6 pounds and 14 ounces what would be her hourly dose in mL/hr?

Jasmine weighs 3.12 kg.

5 mg × 3.12 = 15.60 mg/min or 936 mg/hr

Dextrose 10% means there is 10 grams in every 100 mL or 1 gram in 10 mL which equals 1,000 mg/10 mL or 100 mg/mL therefore you want 9.36 mL/hr for the lower limit of 5 mg/kg/min

For 8 mg/kg/hr (the upper limit)

8 mg × 3.12 kg = 24.96 mg/min or 1497.6 mg/hr

14.98 mL/hr for the upper limit of 8 mg/kg/hr

Exercise 2-41: *Calculation*

What would each infant weigh if they lost 10% of their birth weight?

(Jasmine was 6 pounds and 14 ounces and River was 6 pounds and 7 ounces.)

Jasmine is 110 ounces (6 pounds × 16 ounces + 14 ounces), therefore 11 ounces weight loss would be 10% (6 pounds and 14 ounces − 11 ounces = 6 pounds and 3 ounces). River is 103 ounces so 10% weight loss = 10 ounces or 5 pounds and 13 ounces.

Exercise 2-42: *Fill-in*

The nurse knows that in order for the screening tests for some metabolic disorders and inborn errors of metabolism to be accurate, the infant needs to be taking oral nutrition for at least __**24**__ hours in order for detectable levels of phenylalanine (PKU) to be present in the blood.

Exercise 2-43: *Exhibit Question*

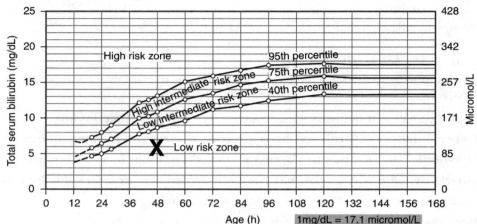

Using the bilirubin graph, River's total bilirubin level falls into which category?

A. **Low risk zone—YES, in this zone the bilirubin should be watched.**

B. Low intermittent risk zone—NO, further assessment should be done.

C. High intermittent risk zone—NO, further assessment should be done.

D. High risk zone—NO, further treatment should be done.

Exercise 2-44: *Multiple Choice Question*

The nurse knows that additional teaching is needed about safety when the patient states:

A. Both infant car seats need to be in the back seat—NO, this is correct.

B. The infant car seats should be balanced using the mechanism built into the seat that shows the correct position—NO, this is correct.

C. The infant car seat has a 5-point restraining system—NO, this is correct.

D. We can use a homemade head roll that is inserted behind the infant's back—**YES, homemade head roles should not be used because car seats are tested for safety with the manufacturer's material only.**

Exercise 2-45: *Multiple Choice Question*

The nurse explains to the parents that the reason that talc powder is not recommended for infants is because:

A. Infants may have an adverse reaction to the scent—NO, this is not the reason.

B. Infants may have an adverse skin reaction—NO, this is not the reason.

C. **Talc is a respiratory irritant—YES, the talc can obstruct respiratory passages.**

D. Talc can irritate the infant's eyes—NO, this is not the reason.

Exercise 2-46: *Select All That Apply*

Some of the suggestions provided for parents who become frustrated with infant crying are to:

❏ **Place the infant in another room—YES.**

❏ **Give the infant a pacifier—YES.**

❏ Medicate the infant—NO, this is not recommended.

❏ **Call a helpline—YES.**

❏ Place the infant in a prone position—NO, this is not recommended.

❏ Prove the infant with cereal fortified formula—NO, this is not recommended.

Exercise 2-47: *Multiple Choice Question*

The nurse correctly explains that breast-fed infants should:

A. **Have yellow seedy stool by one week of age—YES, this is correct.**

B. Continue to have meconium stools for the first week—NO, breast-fed infants usually have frequent, seedy yellow stools.

C. Not stool every day—NO, breast-fed infants usually have frequent, seedy yellow stools.

D. Have brown, formed, pasty stools by one week of age—NO, breast fed infants usually have frequent, seedy yellow stools.

Exercise 2-48: *Fill-in*

The nurse teaches the parents to place the infants in a __supine__ position for the best prevention against sudden infant death syndrome (SIDS).

3

Postpartum Care

Case Study 2 — Jolene

Jolene and Tom are thrilled about the birth of their son. Because it is two hours since her delivery, Jolene is moved from the labor and delivery suite to her post-partum bed. The infant is taken to the nursery to be assessed and washed. The nurse orientates Jolene and Tom to the postpartum unit and describes the basic routine. The nurse does a complete physical examination on Jolene at this time. The nurse uses the B-U-B-B-L-E-H-E format that was taught in her nursing school.

Exercise 3-1: *Matching*
Match the letter and the assessment.

B _____ This assessment uses palpation to assess urinary retention.

U _____ This assessment visualizes the amount and type of endometrial sloughing.

B _____ This assessment notes the height and consistency of the fundus.

B _____ This assessment checks for the signs of deep vein thrombosis.

L _____ This assessment is done to check for any engorgement or lumps on the mammary glands.

E _____ This assessment checks for emotional status or some use it to assess edema.

H _____ This assessment looks at the healing of the perineal-abdominal incision.

E _____ This assessment auscultates sounds in all four quadrants.

 eResource 3-1: Go to: *youtu.be/PJvK7Xbs0DQ* to view Post-Partum Assessment by Donna Badowski and Theresa Bucy which provides an overview of assessment utilizing the B-U-B-B-L-E-H-E format.

Since Jolene had a vaginal delivery, she received a right medial lateral episiotomy. In order to check the episiotomy the nurse uses another acronym that is commonly used to check incisions: R (red) - E (ecchymotic) - E (edema) - D (drainage) - A (approximated). Jolene's episiotomy looks intact and clean.

The answer can be found on page 63.

Exercise 3-2: *Multiple Choice Question*

The nurse knows that a right or left mediolateral episiotomy is often done rather than a median episiotomy because:

    A. There is less chance it will extend to the rectal sphincter.

    B. It heals better.

    C. It preserves the musculature.

    D. It bleeds less.

 eResources 3-2:

    ■ Go to the National Guideline Clearinghouse (NGC) to view Practice Guidelines: *www.guideline.gov* [Pathway: NGC → enter "episiotomy" into the search field → review practice guideline for episiotomy from the American College of Obstetricians and Gynecologists.

    ■ For Patient Education material regarding episiotomy, go to the Agency for Health and Research Quality *ahrq.gov* (AHRQ) [Pathway: AHRQ Home → Priority Populations → Women's Health → scroll down and select "What you need to know about episiotomy"

The nurse assists Jolene OOB (out of bed) for the first time.

Exercise 3-3: *Multiple Choice Question*

Patients should be assessed to a sitting position first and then slowly raised to a standing position in order to prevent against what possible condition?

    A. Hypotension

    B. Hypoglycemia

    C. Deep vein thrombosis

    D. Transient ischemia

The nurse measures Jolene's output in order to determine if she is voiding adequately.

Exercise 3-4: *Fill-in*

A urinary residual of _____ mL indicates urinary retention.

Jolene voids 500 mL and the nurse provides peri care instructions. Jolene complains of perineal discomfort. One a scale of 1–10, she rates it as a 5.

 eResources 3-3:

    ■ Go to NIH Pain Consortium to view available pain scales to utilize when assessing patient pain *painconsortium.nih.gov/pain_scales*

    ■ Go to the National Guideline Clearinghouse (NGC) to view Practice Guidelines: *guideline.gov* [Pathway: NGC → enter "postpartum pain" into the search field → select and review the practice guideline for "Analgesia and anesthesia for the breast-feeding mother."

The answers can be found on page 64.

Exercise 3-5: *Select All That Apply*

Appropriate nursing measures to decrease perineal discomfort from an episiotomy are:

❑ Provide a sitz bath.

❑ Provide ice packs in the first 24 hours.

❑ Medicate with analgesia as ordered.

❑ Provide a heating pad.

❑ Provide topical ointment or sprays as ordered.

❑ Provide a donut ring.

❑ Keep on bed rest.

The nurse medicates Jolene with ibuprofen 800 mg po.

Exercise 3-6: *Calculation*

Ibuprofen comes in 200 mg tablets. How many tablets should the nurse give to Jolene?

Exercise 3-7: *Multiple Choice Question*

The nurse knows that the patient understands her teaching when the patient states:

  A. "I should take two ibuprofen tablets and see if they work; if not take the other two."

  B. "I should take the ibuprofen every four hours."

  C. "I should take the ibuprofen a half an hour before I eat."

  D. "I should take the ibuprofen after I eat."

 eResource 3-4: Check RxDrugs™, a free drug resource from Skyscape .com, to learn more about this drug [Pathway: → enter "ibuprofen" into the search field→ select "ID" or "C" to view information about Indications and Dosage or Warnings/Precautions.]

After an hour Jolene rates her discomfort as a 3 and her son is brought to her room. Jolene breast-feeds her baby and her LATCH score is 8. Jolene has visitors in the evening and rooms-in with her husband and baby throughout the night. The following day (postpartum day 1), Jolene is feeling well, voiding q. s. (quantity sufficient), and ambulating back and forth to the kitchen and nursery ad lib. She joins the newborn feeding class at 10 AM in the unit's lounge.

Exercise 3-8: *Fill-in*

The nurse teaches the patients that both mature breast milk and newborn formula have _____ kcal/ounce.

The nurse explains the pros and cons of both feeding methods.

Exercise 3-9: *Matching*

Match the assets of each different type of infant feeding:

      A. Breast-feeding

      B. Bottle-feeding

The answers can be found on page 65.

_____ IgA is acquired.

_____ Reported easier by working mothers.

_____ Decreased ear infections.

_____ Some are more comfortable in public feeding this way.

_____ This method costs more money.

_____ This method allows fathers more active involvement.

The nurse educator demonstrates proper positioning of infants for both types of feedings and reviews the proper method to mix formula. The patients who have had other children discuss their past experiences with infant feeding methods.

 eResources 3-5:
- Go to *bcove.me/hom3i5mi* to view the March of Dimes video regarding the benefits of breast-feeding
- Go to *vimeo.com/9309036* to view the MedlinePlus video regarding the benefits of breast-feeding.

Jolene finds the class and the discussion very helpful. The following day Jolene and Tom are planning for discharge. The nurse observes Jolene bathing and dressing her infant herself.

Exercise 3-10: *Multiple Choice Question*
The nurse understands that the maternal phase exhibited when a mother begins to participate in infant care independently is the:
- A. Taking-in phase
- B. Taking-hold phase
- C. Letting-in phase
- D. Letting-go phase

After the infant is dressed the nurse observes the father leaning over the infant and talking.

Exercise 3-11: *Select All That Apply*
The nurse understands that the following paternal behavior is typical of "engrossment":
- ❏ The father comments on how good-looking the infant is.
- ❏ The father protects himself by pretending to watch TV.
- ❏ The father is cautious in touching the infant.
- ❏ The father feels let down because his expectations were not met.
- ❏ The father believes the infant is perfect.

The nurse reviews all the discharge instructions verbally and in writing with Jolene and Tom, including the following topics:
- Feeding
- Changing

The answers can be found on page 65.

- Bathing
- Sudden Infant Death Syndrome (SIDS)
- Shaking Baby Syndrome (SBS)
- Car seat safety
- Immunizations
- Hand washing
- Kegel exercises

Exercise 3-12: *Select All That Apply*

The following danger signs warrant a call to the pediatrician or primary care practitioner (PCP):

- ❏ Temperature rectally of 101 °F
- ❏ Waking up three times or more a night
- ❏ Wetting less than three diapers a day
- ❏ Excessive drooling
- ❏ Excessive crying
- ❏ Vomiting
- ❏ No stool in 24 hours

Jolene is also interested in family planning.

Exercise 3-13: *Multiple Choice Question*

The nurse understands that the patient needs further teaching when she states:

- A. "I cannot get pregnant while I am breast-feeding."
- B. "I need to use an alternative birth control (BC) method."
- C. "I cannot use any hormones while I am breast-feeding or it will dry up my milk."
- D. "I cannot use condoms because I will be too dry."

e **eResource 3-6:** Go to the National Guideline Clearinghouse (NGC) to view Practice Guidelines related to postpartum birth control: *guideline.gov* [Pathway: NGC → enter "birth control" into the search field → select and review practice guideline for "Contraception during breast-feeding."]

The nurse discusses many different BC options with Jolene and Tom.

Exercise 3-14: *Matching*

Match the type of BC to its description.

_____ Implanted under the skin and lasts 3 years.

_____ Refrain from sex during fertile period.

_____ A sheath placed over the penis to block sperm.

_____ Polyurethane sheath placed into vagina to bock sperm.

_____ Injectable progesterone given every 12 weeks.

The answers can be found on page 66.

_____ A plastic ring with estrogen and progesterone that is inserted into the vagina for 3 weeks each month.

_____ Progestin only pills taken within 72 hours of unprotected intercourse.

_____ T-shaped device that is inserted into the uterus that lasts 10 years and releases copper.

_____ T-shaped device inserted into the uterus lasts 5 years and releases synthetic progesterone.

_____ Fallopian tubes are blocked.

_____ Vas deferens are cut surgically.

_____ Transdermal patch that releases estrogen and progesterone into the circulation.

_____ Monthly injections of progesterone and estrogen.

_____ Pills that suppress ovulation can be progesterone only or estrogen and progesterone.

_____ Disk-shaped contraceptive device that covers the cervix, was temporarily taken off the market but is now available OTC (over-the-counter).

_____ Shallow latex cup that has to be fitted to each woman so the rim fits well into the vagina.

_____ Latex device that just covers the cervix.

A. Male condom
B. Depo-Provera®
C. Implanon
D. ParaGard IUD
E. Mirena IUD
F. Fertility awareness
G. Female surgical sterilization
H. Ortho Evra patch
I. Female condom
J. Sponge
K. Postcoital emergency contraceptive (EC)
L. Oral contraceptives
M. NuvaRing®
N. Cervical cap
O. Diaphragm
P. Lunelle injectable
Q. Male sterilization

eResources 3-7:
■ Go to CDC Web site for more information about Unintended Pregnancy Prevention *www.cdc.gov/reproductivehealth/ UnintendedPregnancy/Contraception.htm*

The answer can be found on page 67.

- Open the Merck Manual on your mobile device to review a considerations for postpartum contraceptive methods [Pathway: Merck Manual → select "Topics" → in the search field enter "contraception" → scroll down and select "postpartum".]
- Continue your patient teaching by reviewing a pamphlet on birth control from ACOG [Pathway: www.acog.org -> Publications -> Patient Education Pamphlets -> select "Birth Control"] *www.acog .org/publications/patient_education/ab020.cfm*

Exercise 3-15: *Fill-in*

Using the list of contraceptive methods listed in Exercise 3-14 to fill in the following statements:

1. Which BC method should not be used in women who weigh over 200 lbs? _____
2. Which BC method may be rendered ineffective in a few cases if the patient uses antibiotics, especially rifampin? _____
3. Which BC method protects against ovarian cancer? _____
4. Which BC method is associated with pelvic inflammatory disease? _____
5. Which BC method has the side effects of nausea and diarrhea? _____

Jolene chooses Medroxyprogesterone acetate (Depo-Provera) and the nurse receives the dose from the pharmacy.

Exercise 3-16: *Hot Spot*

The nurse receives 150 mg of Depo-Provera from the pharmacy and the instructions are to give it IM. Place an X on the spot where it should be administered.

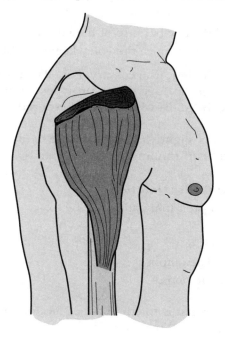

The answer can be found on page 68.

As Jolene and Tom are walking down the hall carrying the infant in the infant seat, other nurses are pushing a stretcher to the nursery window in order for Paula, a new patient, can see her infant daughter being bathed. Paula delivered her infant just two hours ago by Cesarean birth.

Case Study 3 ▬ Paula

Paula has a PCA (patient-controlled analgesia) pump for the incision discomfort.

Exercise 3-17: *Calculation*
The PCA order reads 50 mg Morphine in 50 mL/Normal Saline to run by PCA pump at 1 mg every 10 min for a total of 6 mg/hr. If the patient was able to access the medication on each attempt, how many hours and minutes would it take to exhaust the supply of morphine in the bag?

The nurse assesses Paula using the B-U-B-B-L-E-H-E assessment and finds that her initial abdominal dressing is dry and intact. Paula's bowels sounds are hypoactive in all four quadrants and her lochia is scant rubra.

Exercise 3-18: *Multiple Choice Question*
The nurse understands that a postoperative Cesarean birth patient's lochia has the following characteristics:
    A. It is initially less than that of a patient with a vaginal birth.
    B. It is basically serosa right after the birth.
    C. It is increased initially because of the uterine manipulation.
    D. It has a steadier flow since the Foley keeps the bladder deflated.

 eResource 3-8: Review, if necessary, Post-Partum Assessment by Donna Badowski and Theresa Bucy which provides an overview of assessment utilizing the B-U-B-B-L-E-H-E format (eResource 3-1).

Paula's blood pressure was slightly elevated before delivery and is still 130/84 but her pulse is 74 and had been running 80–84 prenatally.

Exercise 3-19: *Multiple Choice Question*
A decrease in pulse in a postpartum patient is due to:
    A. Dieresis
    B. Excessive blood loss
    C. Decreased cardiac output
    D. Increased cardiac output

Paula has a Foley catheter that is to come out 12 hours postoperative. She is tolerating fluids and moving around well in bed.

The answers can be found on page 69.

Exercise 3-20: *Calculation*

Paula has received the following fluids during the last 24 hours:

3 liters of IV fluids during labor.

One 240 mL cup of ice chips preoperatively.

2 liters of fluid post operatively.

2 4-ounce glasses of juice.

What is her 24-hour intake _____ mL?

 eResource 3-9: Go to *www.medcalc.com/wtmeas.html* to do the volume conversion.

The nurse discontinues the Foley catheter which has 1030 mL in it and advises Paula to increase her fluids.

Exercise 3-21: *Multiple Choice Question*

The nurse understands that the patient does not need further teaching when she states:

A. "I need to restrict my fluids because I am bottle-feeding."

B. "I need to drink at least 8–10 glasses of water a day."

C. "I need to urinate on my own before I drink fluids."

D. "I need to stick to ice chips for the first 24 hours after the delivery."

The nurse also checks Paula's IV. The site is clean and intact and the flow is maintained.

Exercise 3-22: *Calculation*

The order for the IV is maintain at 125 mL/hr for 24 hours.

Paula has 1000 mL NS (Normal Saline) hanging for her IV.

The drip factor is a macrodrip at 10 gtts/mL

If you did not have a pump, how many gtts/min would you set the rate at?

 eResource 3-10: Go to *www.medcalc.com/ivrate.html* IV Rate calculator offered by MedCalc.com.

The lab calls the nurse to notify her that Paula's infant's is Rh + and Paula is Rh negative. The nurse sends the slip to pharmacy to obtain the Rh_o (D) Immune Globulin (RhoGAM) to give to Paula IM or IV.

Exercise 3-23: *Multiple Choice Question*

Rh_o(D) Immune Globulin works by:

A. Attacking Rh negative blood cells and destroying them.

B. Attacking Rh positive blood cells and destroying them.

C. Developing antigens that "trick" the body into making different antibodies.

D. Developing antibodies that are nonspecific and attack all antigens present.

 eResource 3-11: Go to: *youtu.be/7OWp8d8WKkg* to learn about Rh negative blood type effects upon the fetus.

The answers can be found on page 70.

Exercise 3-24: *Fill-in*

The nurse knows that RhoGAM should be given within _____ hours of delivery.

Later that evening the nurse discontinues Paula's IV fluids.

Exercise 3-25: *Multiple Choice Question*

The nurse assesses a recovering surgical Cesarean patient and should question the discontinuation of IV fluids if the following assessment findings exist:

  A. The IV site is red and tender to the touch.
  B. The normotensive patient's blood pressure is 110/70.
  C. The patient indicates she would like her IV to stay in so she doesn't have to eat hospital food.
  D. The patient has a temperature orally of 100.4 °F

Paula is doing well for her first postoperative day and the nurse explains that getting in and out of bed is fine but not to overdo it because her body also needs rest for healing. The following day Paula is "sore" and rates her pain as a 4 out of 10. The nurse administers 2 tabs of Tylenol #3 and a half hour later checks for its effectiveness. At this time Paula rates her pain as a 2.

 eResources 3-12: Go to MedCalc on your mobile device to use the Pain Visual Scale.

The obstetrical surgeon comes in to see Paula and removes the initial dressing. Her incision is a Pfannenstiel incision that is closed by surgical staples, and it is dry and intact. The nurses R-E-E-D-A assessment of the incision is as follows:

R	No redness
E	Slightly ecchymosed over the mons pubis
E	No edema
D	No drainage noted
A	Well approximated with skin staple closures

Paula is also concerned about not having a bowel movement.

Exercise 3-26: *Multiple Choice Question*

An appropriate intervention for a patient concerned about having a bowel movement postpartum would be to:

  A. Call the PCP for an enema.
  B. Keep the patient NPO until she is more comfortable.
  C. Encourage a diet of cheese and eggs.
  D. Administer Colace as ordered prn.

Once Paula's gastrointestinal issues are resolved, you discuss other concerns she has. You teach her infant bathing and cord care. She is doing well feeding her

The answers can be found on page 70.

infant. During the second night Paula complains of pain in her left leg. You assess her leg by observation and light palpation and the findings are as follows:

- Slightly paler than the right leg
- Slightly edematous
- + pedal pulse
- Left calf is tender to touch

Since you suspect a deep vein thrombosis (DVT) you do not do a Homan's sign; in case there is a clot you do not want to dislodge it.

Exercise 3-27: *Multiple Choice Question*

The appropriate priority nursing diagnosis for the assessment stated above is:

 A. Self-care deficit toileting

 B. Interrupted family processes

 C. Pain acute

 D. Ineffective tissue perfusion

You tell Paula to stay in bed while you call the PCP. You use the SBAR communication tool to relay the situations to the PCP as follows:

S (Situation)	Hello I am calling to inform you that patient Paula is complaining of pain in her left calf.
B (Background)	She is a two-day postoperative cesarean birth patient who is a Gravida 1, now Para 1 with no relevant health history.
A (Assessment)	Paula's left calf is tender to touch, pale, warm, and slightly edematous. She has pedal pulses on both feet and I did not do a Homan's sign check.
R (Recommendation)	I am concerned about her and would like to call the radiology department for a stat Doppler flow study of her left leg.

The PCP agrees with the recommendation and orders a Doppler flow study. The Doppler flow study of the leg shows a DVT and orders are received from the PCP.

 eResource 3-13: For Patient Educational Material regarding the Doppler flow study, go to: *merckmedicus.com* [Pathway: Select "Patient Education" tab → "Searchable Patient Handouts" → enter "Doppler" into the search field.]

Exercise 3-28: *Select All That Apply*

Appropriate interventions for DVT treatment include:

 ❑ Analgesic

 ❑ Bed rest

The answers can be found on page 70.

❑ Cold packs to area

❑ Elevate hips

❑ Elastic support stockings

❑ Warfarin therapy for breast-feeding mothers

eResources 3-14:

■ To learn more about DVT go to the Merck Manual Online *merckmedicus .com* [Pathway: enter "DVT" into the search field in the upper right corner of the screen.]

■ For Patient Educational Material regarding DVT, go to: *merckmedicus .com* [Pathway: Select "Patient Education" tab → "Searchable Patient Handouts" → enter "DVT" into the search field.]

Heparin therapy IV is started for Paula. She is given an initial dose of 7,500 units and then placed on continuous IV.

Exercise 3-29: *Calculation*

Heparin is ordered continuous IV at 20 units/kg/hr. Paula is 150 pounds. The pharmacy sends the routine dosage of 20,000 units in 500 mL of D5W. At how many mL/hr should you set the pump?

eResource 3-15: Go to *medcalc.com* to do the weight conversion and then to use the IV Rate calculator.

Paula's activated partial thromboplastin time (aPTT) is monitored closely and a sliding heparin scale is used to keep it in therapeutic range of 35–45 seconds. The scale is:

aPTT in Seconds	Action	Labs to Be Done
Less than or equal to 49.9 seconds	Increase by 240 units per hour	Repeat aPTT in 6 hours
20.0–64.9 seconds	Increase by 120 units per hour	Repeat aPTT in 6 hours
65–100 seconds	Maintain current rate	Not needed
110.1–124.9 seconds	Decrease by 120 units per hour	Repeat aPTT in 6 hours
125 seconds or over	Hold for one hour and then decrease rate by 240 units per hour	Repeat aPTT in 6 hours after infusion is restarted

Paula is maintained on bed rest and heparin for 5 days and then she is given heparin subq.

eResource 3-16:

■ To learn more about this medication, refer to RxDrugs™, a free drug resource from Skyscape.com, on your mobile device [Pathway: RxDrugs™ → enter "heparin" into the search field → select "ID" to

The answers can be found on page 71.

locate information about Indications and Dosage, then tap on "C," to locate information about "Warnings and Precautions."]
■ To learn more about blood clotting, view this brief video: *youtu.be/ QqUEjYMXBNw*

During that time she continues to breast-feed her infant. On day 5 she is very uncomfortable due to engorgement.

Exercise 3-30: *Multiple Choice Question*
The nurse understands that a therapeutic intervention for breast engorgement is:

    A. Instruct the patient to stop breast-feeding.
    B. Instruct the patient to go without a bra.
    C. Instruct the patient to use ice constantly.
    D. Instruct the patient to feed frequently.

 eResource 3-17: For Patient Educational Material regarding DVT, go to: *merckmedicus.com* [Pathway: Select "Patient Education" tab → "Searchable Patient Handouts" → enter "engorgement" into the search field.]

Sore nipples are a common discomfort for women.

Exercise 3-31: *Select All That Apply*
The nurse knows that the following interventions are appropriate for sore nipples:

    ❏ Use body lotion.
    ❏ Bottle-feed every other feeding.
    ❏ Start feedings on the least sore nipple.
    ❏ Use your finger to break suction.
    ❏ Use a plastic bra liner.

Home care is arranged for her to continue to receive subq. heparin at home. The pain in Paula's leg is resolved and the Doppler study is now negative. Paula is upset that she had a complication and keeps asking questions about why it happened.

Exercise 3-32: *Multiple Choice Question*
The nurse understands that pregnancy is a hypercoagulable state due to:

    A. Increased fibrin
    B. Decreased clotting factors 1–5
    C. Increased clotting factors 7–10
    D. Decreased platelets

Paula is discharged to home with her infant and home care will follow up and give her the daily subq. heparin injections for another week.

The answers can be found on page 72.

eResources 3-18:
- For Patient Educational Material regarding heparin, go to: *merckmedicus.com* [Pathway: Select "Patient Education" tab → "Searchable Patient Handouts" → enter "heparin" into the search field → select "Anticoagulants and Antiplatelets."]
- For Patient Education Material regarding infant care and positive parenting during the first year, go to: *www.cdc.gov/ncbddd/child/infants.htm*

When Paula's infant is approximately two weeks old, Paula calls back to the postpartum unit "hotline," which is set up for moms to access if they are having specific questions or a problem while they are in the six-week postpartum period. You, her postpartum primary nurse, happen to pick up the phone when she calls and she is happy that it is you. She tells you that she has this nagging feeling of doubt that she is going to be a good mother to her baby, yet doesn't want to ask anyone for help.

Exercise 3-33: *Select All That Apply*
The flowing risk factors increase a mother's chance of developing postpartum depression:
- ❑ History of previous depression.
- ❑ No evidence of depressive symptoms during pregnancy.
- ❑ Family history of depression.
- ❑ Child care stress.
- ❑ Overbearing family trying to help.
- ❑ Uncomplicated pregnancy.

eResources 3-19:
- To learn more about postpartum depression and obtain patient education material for Paula, go to: *www.womenshealth.gov/faq/depression-pregnancy.cfm* and *www.cdc.gov/reproductivehealth/Depression*
- To view the National Institute of Mental Health's (NIMH) video regarding Postpartum Depression, go to: *youtu.be/QqUEjYMXBNw*
- Go to the National Guideline Clearinghouse (NGC) to view Practice Guidelines: *guideline.gov* [Pathway: NGC → enter "postpartum depression" in the search field → review "Use of antidepressants in nursing mothers" guideline.
- To learn more about incidence and practice guidelines, review the Agency for Healthcare Research and Quality's (AHRQ) summary report regarding Perinatal Depression: Prevalence, Screening Accuracy, and Screening Outcomes: *www.ahrq.gov/clinic/tp/perideptp.htm.*
- For more information regarding postpartum depression, open Merck Manual on your mobile device [Pathway: Merck Manual → select "Topics" → enter "pregnancy" into the search field → enter "depression after . . ." → select "Postpartum Care."]

You ask Paula to expand on how she feels.

The answer can be found on page 72.

Exercise 3-34: *Multiple Choice Question*

The nurse understands that patients who self-report the following symptoms may have postpartum depression:

    A. Loss of appetite, focused concentration on issues, sleep difficulties.
    B. Increased appetite, loss of concentration, excessive sleepiness.
    C. Increased libido, focused concentration, excessive sleepiness.
    D. Decreased libido, loss of concentration, sleep difficulties.

Paula reports a loss of confidence and is still tearful even though her infant is eating and growing well.

 eResources 3-20:

   ■ To use the use a depression screening questionnaire, go to the Agency for Healthcare Research and Quality's (AHRQ) Electronic Preventive Services Selector (ePSS) *epss.ahrq.gov/ePSS/index.jsp* [Pathway: select "Tools" → choose from the list the available depression screening tools and guidelines].

   ■ To learn more about the screening questions to ask Paula, go to: *www.womenshealth.gov/faq/depression-pregnancy.cfm#c.*

   ■ You can download "Sad Scale," a free depression inventory for iPod/iPhone/iPad (iOS operating system) by going to: *www .deeppocketseries.com/Sad_Scale.html/Sad_Scale.html* or go directly to iTunes: *itunes.apple.com.*

   ■ You can also download STAT Depression Screener, another free depression inventory for your iOS device by Austin Physician Productivity, LLC by going to: *statcoder.com* and searching for the tool or you can go directly to iTunes: *itunes.apple.com.*

Exercise 3-35: *Multiple Choice Question*

The best nursing diagnosis for the patient self-reporting loss of confidence and tearfulness at two weeks postpartum is:

    A. Hopelessness
    B. Fear
    C. Stress overload
    D. Dysfunctional family processes

You call Paula's PCP with her permission and receive a referral for the counseling group who services the postpartum patients from your institution. A counselor calls Paula and sets up an appointment. You follow up the next day to ensure the appointment is established and thank Paula for reaching out. You also reassure her that she should use the hot line again should she need it.

 eResources 3-21:

   ■ To locate AHRQ recommended information to share with your patient on Depression go to *healthfinder.gov* [Pathway: HealthFinder.gov → enter "Depression" into search field and select "Depression: Quick Guide to Healthy Living."

The answers can be found on page 72.

■ For more information regarding available supports for Postpartum Depression, go to Postpartum Education for Parents (PEP.org) *www.sbpep.org* or Postpartum Support International *postpartum.net.*

■ To supplement patient education re: postpartum depression you may show Paula a video highlighting Mary Codey, wife of former New Jersey Governor Richard Codey, describing her experience with postpartum depression go to: Part 1: *youtu.be/cibKJToxHlU* and Part 2: *youtu.be/mQpbDKtsdR8*

Answers

Exercise 3-1: *Matching*

Match the letter and the assessment.

B	**(BREASTS)**	This assessment is done to check for any engorgement or lumps on the mammary glands.
U	**(UTERUS)**	This assessment notes the height and consistency of the fundus.
B	**(BOWEL)**	This assessment auscultates sounds in all four quadrants.
B	**(BLADDER)**	This assessment uses palpation to assess urinary retention.
L	**(LOCHIA)**	This assessment visualizes the amount and type of endometrial sloughing.
E	**(EPISIOTOMY AND/ OR INCISION)**	This assessment looks at the healing of the perineal or abdominal incision.
H	**(HOMANS SIGN)**	This assessment checks for the signs of deep vein thrombosis.
E	**(EMOTIONAL OR EDEMA)**	This assessment checks for emotional status or some use it to assess edema.

Exercise 3-2: *Multiple Choice Question*

The nurse knows that a right or left mediolateral episiotomy is often done rather than a median episiotomy because:

A. **There is less chance it will extend to the rectal sphincter—YES, a median or midline episiotomy has more of a chance of extending through the rectal mucosa.**

B. It heals better—NO, actually a median or midline episiotomy heals better because it is made along a natural muscles junction.

C. It preserves the musculature—NO, a median or midline episiotomy better preserves the muscles.

D. It bleeds less—NO, there is more blood loss with a mediolateral episiotomy.

Exercise 3-3: *Multiple Choice Question*

Patients should be assessed to a sitting position first and then slowly raised to a standing position in order to prevent against what possible condition:

A. **Hypotension—YES, this maneuver prevents orthostatic hypotension.**

B. Hypoglycemia—NO, this is not the reason.

  C. Deep vein thrombosis—NO, this is not the reason.

  D. Transient ischemia—NO, this is not the reason.

Exercise 3-4: *Fill-in*

A urinary residual of __250__ mL indicates urinary retention.

Exercise 3-5: *Select All That Apply*

Appropriate nursing measures to decrease perineal discomfort from an episiotomy are:

☑ **Provide a sitz bath—YES, this is usually done after the first 24 hours.**

☑ **Provide ice packs in the first 24 hours—YES.**

☑ **Medicate with analgesia as ordered—YES.**

☐ Provide a heating pad—NO, direct heat is usually not indicated.

☑ **Provide topical ointment or sprays as ordered—YES, many time topical analgesics are ordered.**

☐ Provide a donut ring—NO, this is no longer indicated in most cases because the rim of the donut ring may decrease circulation to the healing area.

☐ Keep on bed rest—NO, this is too risky in relation to deep vein thrombosis (DVTs).

Exercise 3-6: *Calculation*

Ibuprofen comes in 200 mg tables. How many tablets should the nurse give to Jolene?

Desired = 800 mg

On hand = 200 mg

800 divided by 200 = **4 tabs.**

Exercise 3-7: *Multiple Choice Question*

The nurse knows that the patient understands her teaching when the patient states:

  A. "I should take two ibuprofen tablets and see if they work and if not take the other two."—NO, a full dose as ordered should always be taken to ensure a therapeutic effect.

  B. "I should take the ibuprofen every four hours."—NO, it is taken every 6 hours.

  C. "I should take the ibuprofen a half an hour before I eat."—NO, it should be taken with food.

  D. **"I should take the ibuprofen after I eat."—YES, this would decrease stomach irritation.**

Exercise 3-8: *Fill-in*

The nurse teaches the patients that both mature breast milk and newborn formula have __20__ kcal/ounce.

Exercise 3-9: *Matching*

Match the assets of each different type of infant feeding:

___A___ IgA is acquired.

___B___ Reported easier by working mothers.

___A___ Decreased ear infections.

___B___ Some are more comfortable in public feeding this way.

___B___ This method costs more money.

___B___ This method allows fathers more active involvement.

    A. Breast-feeding

    B. Bottle-feeding

Exercise 3-10: *Multiple Choice Question*

The nurse understands that the maternal phase exhibited when a mother begins to participate in infant care independently is the:

A. Taking-in phase—NO, this is the first phase that lasts one to two days and the woman is usually preoccupied with herself and the delivery.

B. **Taking-hold phase—YES, in this phase the mom begins to show independence in caring for the infant.**

C. Letting-in phase—NO, this is not one of Dr. Reva Rubin's stages of postpartum adjustment.

D. Letting-go phase—NO, in this phase the mom is assimilating the role of mother and is adjusting to the new family structure.

Exercise 3-11: *Select All That Apply*

The nurse understands that the following paternal behavior is typical of "engrossment":

☑ **The father comments on how good-looking the infant is—YES, this is typical behavior.**

❑ The father protects himself by pretending to watch TV—NO, this is not typical behavior.

❑ The father is cautious in touching the infant—NO, this is not typical behavior.

❑ The father feels let down because his expectations were not met—NO, this is not typical behavior.

☑ **The father believes the infant is perfect—YES, this is typical behavior.**

Exercise 3-12: *Select All That Apply*

The following danger signs warrant a call to the pediatrician or primary care practitioner (PCP):

☑ **Temperature rectally of 101 °F—YES, this indicates an infectious process**.

❑ Waking up three times or more a night—NO, many infants wake up during the night.

☑ **Wetting less than three diapers a day—YES, this is a concern for possible dehydration. Infants should wet one diaper at least on the first day of birth, two on the second, three on the third, and so on until they are wetting 8–10 diapers each day.**

❑ Excessive drooling—NO, infants drool and it increases when they are teething.

☑ **Excessive crying—YES, infants should be able to be comforted.**

☑ **Vomiting—YES, spitting up is normal but vomiting is not.**

❑ No stool in 24 hours—NO, not all infants stool every day.

Exercise 3-13: *Multiple Choice Question*

The nurse understands that the patient needs further teaching when she states:

A. "I cannot get pregnant while I am breast-feeding."—NO, this is not true; some women ovulate while they are breast-feeding.

B. **"I need to use an alternative birth control (BC) method."—YES, this is the recommendation.**

C. "I cannot use any hormones while I am breast-feeding or it will dry up my milk."—NO, once breast-feeding is established, this should not be a problem.

D. "I cannot use condoms because I will be too dry."—NO, condoms can be used with vaginal lubricant if needed.

Exercise 3-14: *Matching*

Match the type of BC to its description.

C	Implanted under the skin and lasts 3 years.
F	Refrain from sex during fertile period.
A	A sheath placed over the penis to block sperm.
I	Polyurethane sheath placed into vagina to bock sperm.
B	Injectable progesterone given every 12 weeks.
M	A plastic ring with estrogen and progesterone that is inserted into the vagina for 3 weeks each month.
K	Progestin only pills taken within 72 hours of unprotected intercourse.
D	T-shaped device that is inserted into the uterus that lasts 10 years and releases copper.
E	T-shaped device inserted into the uterus lasts 5 years and releases synthetic progesterone.
G	Fallopian tubes are blocked.
Q	Vas deferens are cut surgically.
H	Transdermal patch that releases estrogen and progesterone into the circulation.
P	Monthly injections of progesterone and estrogen.

   L   Pills that suppress ovulation can be progesterone only or estrogen and progesterone.

   J   Disk shaped contraceptive device that covers the cervix, was temporarily taken off the market but is now available OTC (over-the-counter).

   O   Shallow latex cup that has to be fitted to each women so the rim fits well into the vagina.

   N   Latex device that just covers the cervix.

A. Male condom
B. Depo-Provera®
C. Implanon
D. ParaGard IUD
E. Mirena IUD
F. Fertility awareness
G. Female surgical sterilization
H. Ortho Evra patch
I. Female condom
J. Sponge
K. Postcoital emergency contraceptive (EC)
L. Oral contraceptives
M. NuvaRing®
N. Cervical cap
O. Diaphragm
P. Lunelle injectable
Q. Male sterilization

Exercise 3-15: *Fill-in*

Using the list of contraceptive methods listed in Exercise 3-14 to fill in the following statements:

1. Which BC method should not be used in women who weigh over 200 lbs? **Ortho Evra Patch**
2. Which BC method may be rendered ineffective in a few cases if the patient uses antibiotics, especially rifampin? **Oral contraceptives**
3. Which BC method protects against ovarian cancer? **Oral contraceptives**
4. Which BC method is associated with pelvic inflammatory disease? **IUDs**
5. Which BC method has the side effects of nausea and diarrhea? **Postcoital emergency contraceptive (EC)**

Exercise 3-16: *Hot Spot*

The nurse receives 150 mg of Depo-Provera from the pharmacy and the instructions are to give it IM. Place an X on the spot where it should be administered.

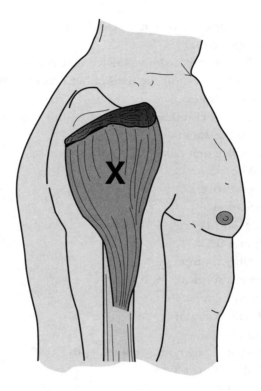

Exercise 3-17: *Calculation*

The PCA order reads 50 mg Morphine in 50 mL/Normal Saline to run by PCA pump at 1 mg every 10 min for a total of 6 mg/hr. If the patient was able to access the medication on each attempt, how many hours and minutes would it take to exhaust the supply of morphine in the bag?

6 mg/hr = 6 mL/hr

50 mL divided by 6 mL/hr = **8.3 hours or 8 hours and 20 minutes**

Exercise 3-18: *Multiple Choice Question*

The nurse understands that a postoperative Cesarean birth patient's lochia has the following characteristics:

A. **It is initially less than that of a patient with a vaginal birth—YES, it is less initially because the uterus is manually cleaned out, but then the sloughing off continues as it would in a vaginal delivery.**

B. It is basically serosa right after the birth—NO, it goes through the normal stages of rubra, serosa, and alba.

C. It is increased initially because of the uterine manipulation—NO, it is less initially.

D. It has a steadier flow since the Foley keeps the bladder deflated—NO, the flow is not altered by the bladder unless a bladder is overdistended and obstructing involution. The primary cause of a boggy uterus or one that is not contracting is a distended bladder.

Exercise 3-19: *Multiple Choice Question*

A decrease in pulse in a postpartum patient is due to:

A. Dieresis—NO, fluid loss does not decrease heart rate and may actually increase it if the loss is excessive.

B. Excessive blood loss—NO, blood loss causes an increased heart rate due to the heart trying to compensate and move the blood around the body faster.

C. Decreased cardiac output—NO, this would increase the heart rate due to decreased volume.

D. **Increased cardiac output—YES, a large volume of blood is reverted back into the general circulation and therefore the heart is more efficient and increases stroke volume and decreases rate.**

Exercise 3-20: *Calculation*

Paula has received the following fluids during the last 24 hours:

3 liters of IV fluids during labor = **3,000 mL**

One 240 mL cup of ice chips preoperatively = **240 mL**

2 liters of fluid post operatively = **2,000 mL**

2 4-ounce glasses of juice = **240 mL**

What is her 24 hour intake? **5,480 mL**

Exercise 3-21: *Multiple Choice Question*

The nurse understands that the patient does not need further teaching when she states:

A. "I need to restrict my fluids because I am bottle-feeding."—NO, this indicates that she does need further teaching because fluids should not be restricted.

B. **"I need to drink at least 8–10 glasses of water a day."—YES, this indicates that she understands the education about fluid intake.**

C. "I need to urinate on my own before I drink fluids."—NO, this indicates that she does need further teaching because she may need to drink in order to void.

D. "I need to stick to ice chips for the first 24 hours after the delivery."—NO, this indicates that she does need further teaching because she should be able to drink as much as she would like as long as she is not nauseous.

Exercise 3-22: *Calculation*

The order for the IV is maintain at 125 mL/hr for 24 hours.

Paula has 1000 mL NS (Normal Saline) hanging for her IV.

The drip factor is a macrodrip at 10 gtts/mL.

If you did not have a pump, for how many gtts/min would you set the rate?

125 mL/hr = 1,250 gtts/hr

Divide 1,250 by 60 = 20.83 gtts/min or **21 gtts/min**

Exercise 3-23: *Multiple Choice Question*

Rh$_o$(D) Immune Globulin works by:

A. Attacking Rh negative blood cells and destroying them—NO, this is not the action of immunoglobulins.

B. **Attacking Rh positive blood cells and destroying them—YES, they will seek out and attack the Rh positive cells therefore the woman will not build up immunity to them.**

C. Developing antigens that "trick" the body into making different antibodies—NO, this is not the action of immunoglobulin.

D. Developing antibodies that are nonspecific and attack all antigens present—NO, this is not the action of immunoglobulins.

Exercise 3-24: *Fill-in*

The nurse knows that RhoGAM should be given within <u>72</u> hours of delivery.

Exercise 3-25: *Multiple Choice Question*

The nurse assesses a recovering surgical Cesarean patient and should question the discontinuation of IV fluids if the following assessment findings exist:

A. The IV site is red and tender to the touch—NO, this is an indication to discontinue the IV.

B. The normotensive patient's blood pressure is 110/70—NO, this is a normal finding in a postpartum patient.

C. The patient indicates she would like her IV to stay in so she doesn't have to eat hospital food—NO, this is a situation that needs dietary referral not intravenous fluids.

D. **The patient has a temperature orally of 100.4 °F—YES, this may indicate an infection and it would be prudent to leave the IV in case she needs antibiotics.**

Exercise 3-26: *Multiple Choice Question*

An appropriate intervention for a patient concerned about having a bowel movement postpartum would be:

A. Call the PCP for an enema—NO, this is not the first intervention that should be done.

B. Keep the patient NPO until she is more comfortable—NO, postpartum patients need nutrition for healing.

C. Encourage a diet of cheese and eggs—NO, these are not especially high in fiber.

D. **Administer Colace as ordered prn.—YES, this is a common order and many times corrects the problem.**

Exercise 3-27: *Multiple Choice Question*

The appropriate priority nursing diagnosis for the assessment stated above is:

A. Self-care deficit toileting—NO, this is not the priority, but a later concern.

B. Interrupted family processes—NO, this is not the priority but a later concern.

C. Pain acute—NO, this is not the priority but a later concern.

D. **Ineffective tissue perfusion—YES, this is a concern if a possible blood clot is blocking venous return.**

Exercise 3-28: *Select All That Apply*

Appropriate interventions for DVT treatment include:

☑ **Analgesic—YES, it is painful.**

☑ **Bed rest—YES, it is painful and until anticoagulant therapy is effective, movement may dislodge the clot into the general circulation.**

☐ Cold packs to area—NO, this causes vasoconstriction.

☐ Elevate hips—NO, the legs should be elevated to increase venous return.

☑ **Elastic support stockings—YES, this will assist venous return.**

☐ Warfarin therapy for breast-feeding mothers—NO, breast-feeders should not use oral anticoagulants because they are expressed in the breast milk and can cause hemorrhaging in the newborn.

Exercise 3-29: *Calculation*

Heparin is ordered continuous IV at 20 units/kg/hr. Paula is 150 pounds. The pharmacy sends the routine dosage of 20,000 units in 500 mL of D5W. At how many mL/hr should you set the pump?

150 lbs = 68.2 kg

20 units × 68.2 = 1,364 units/hr

Each mL has 40 units

1,364 units/hr divided by 40 units/mL = 34.1 mL/hr

Exercise 3-30: *Multiple Choice Question*

The nurse understands that a therapeutic intervention for breast engorgement is:

A. Instruct the patient to stop breast-feeding—NO, this will increase engorgement.

B. Instruct the patient to go without a bra—NO, the support is needed.

C. Instruct the patient to use ice constantly—NO, this will "dry up" the milk supply.

D. **Instruct the patient to feed frequently—YES, feeding the baby will help relieve the engorgement and eventually supply will meet demand.**

Exercise 3-31: *Select All That Apply*

The nurse knows that the following interventions are appropriate for sore nipples:

☐ Use body lotion—NO, this will further irritate them.

☐ Bottle-feed every other feeding—NO, this may disrupt the breast-feeding pattern being established.

☑ **Start feedings on the least sore nipple—YES, this will be less painful.**

☑ **Use your finger to break suction—YES, this will be less painful.**

☐ Use a plastic bra liner—NO, plastic will promote skin breakdown by containing moisture.

Exercise 3-32: *Multiple Choice Question*

The nurse understands that pregnancy is a hypercoagulable state due to:

A. Increased fibrin—NO, this is not the mechanism that occurs.

B. Decreased clotting factors 1–5—NO, this is not the mechanism that occurs.

C. **Increased clotting factors 7–10—YES, there is an increase naturally in Factors VII, VIII, IX, and X to protect postpartum women from hemorrhaging.**

D. Decreased platelets—NO, this is not the mechanism that occurs.

Exercise 3-33: *Select All That Apply*

The flowing risk factors increase a mother's chance of developing postpartum depression:

☑ **History of previous depression—YES, this is a known risk factor.**

☐ No evidence of depressive symptoms during pregnancy—NO, this is not a risk factor.

☑ **Family history of depression—YES, this is a known risk factor.**

☑ **Child care stress—YES, this is a known risk factor.**

☐ Overbearing family trying to help—NO, social support is good.

☐ Uncomplicated pregnancy—NO, women with complicated pregnancies are at risk.

Exercise 3-34: *Multiple Choice Question*

The nurse understands that patients who self-report the following symptoms may have postpartum depression:

A. Loss of appetite, focused concentration on issues, sleep difficulties—NO, there is less focus.

B. Increased appetite, loss of concentration, excessive sleepiness—NO, there is usually a loss of appetite.

C. Increased libido, focused concentration, excessive sleepiness—NO, there is usually a decreased libido.

D. **Decreased libido, loss of concentration, sleep difficulties—YES, these are the symptoms.**

Exercise 3-35: *Multiple Choice Question*

The best nursing diagnosis for the patient self-reporting loss of confidence and tearfulness at two weeks postpartum is:

A. Hopelessness—NO, hopelessness is usually from a longer standing depressive state.

B. Fear—NO, usually they are not afraid of anything specific.

C. Stress overload—NO, this is usually not the case but may be a secondary diagnosis.

D. **Dysfunctional family processes—YES, the entire family is affected.**

4

Infertility, Preconception, Conception, and Preterm Labor

Case Study 4 ▪ Isabella and Christopher

Isabella and Christopher are a young couple, ages 26 and 28, who have been married for two years and have not been using birth control for the past year. They are concerned and have come to the infertility clinic where you are working as a graduate nurse. You explain to them that infertility is not uncommon and occurs in 10–15% of couples. During the extensive history of both partners you review not only sexual history but nutrition and exercise.

Exercise 4-1: *Calculation*
Isabella is 5′ 4″ and weighs 133 lbs. Is her body mass index (BMI) within normal limits (WNL)? Christopher is 6′ 3″ and weighs 220 lbs. Is his BMI WNL?

eResource 4-1:
- Use MedCalc online to calculate BMI. Go to *medcalc.com*. [Pathway: Tap on "General" → "Body Mass Index" and enter height and weight.]
- Download and install MedCalc on your mobile device *www.med-ia.ch/medcalc*. [Pathway: MedCalc → Body Mass Index and enter height and weight → tap on "*i*" to interpret results.]
- Use Archimedes on your mobile device [Pathway: Archimedes → Body Mass Index (Adult) and enter height and weight.] *www.skyscape.com*

You discuss the menstrual cycle with them so they understand that the chance of conceiving is increased at the time of ovulation. Isabella's cycle is 28–30 days. The menstrual phase occurs in days 1 through 6 of the cycle.

eResource 4-2:
- Supplement your patient teaching by educational materials offered by WomensHealth.gov: *www.womenshealth.gov/faq/menstruation.cfm*

■ Continue your patient teaching by showing the couple a MedlinePlus video about Ovulation: *www.nlm.nih.gov* [Pathway: *nlm.nih.gov* → select MedlinePlus from the menu → enter "Ovulation video" into the search field → click on the link to video to view.]

Exercise 4-2: *Multiple Choice Question*

The menstrual phase of the menstrual cycle is caused by:

    A. Increased progesterone and estrogen

    B. Decreased progesterone and estrogen

    C. Increased follicle stimulating hormone and luteinizing hormone

    D. Decreased follicle stimulating hormone and luteinizing hormone

Isabella also reports painful menses for which she takes ibuprofen. You take a detailed history of her menses.

Exercise 4-3: *Matching*

Match the term to its definition.

    _____ Lack of menstrual periods

    _____ Painful menstrual periods

    _____ Very little menstrual flow

    _____ Frequent but irregular menses

    _____ Heavy but frequent and irregular menses

    _____ Heavy menses

    _____ Cycles fewer than 21 days

    _____ Cycles longer than 35 days

    A. Hypomenorrhea

    B. Menometrorrhea

    C. Menorrhagia

    D. Amenorrhea

    E. Polymenorrhea

    F. Menometrorrhagia

    G. Oligomenorrhea

    H. Dysmenorrhea

You explain the hormonal influence of the menstrual cycle to Isabella and Christopher.

 eResource 4-3: Supplement your patient teaching by educational materials offered by the Merck Manuals Online Medical Library: *www.merckmanuals.com/home.* [Pathway: Select section "Women's Health Issues" → "Biology of the Female Reproductive System" → "Menstrual Cycle"]

The answers can be found on page 95.

Exercise 4-4: *Multiple Choice Question*

The nurse knows that the patient understands the teaching about the menstrual cycle when she states:

A. "The pituitary gland responds to luteinizing hormone input from the hypothalamus."

B. "The pituitary gland responds to follicle stimulating hormone input from the hypothalamus."

C. "The pituitary gland responds to estrogen input from the hypothalamus."

D. "The pituitary gland responds to gonadotropin-releasing hormone input from the hypothalamus."

During the secretory phase of the menstrual cycle (days 15–26), the uterus prepares for implantation. During the proliferative phase (days 5–14) the follicular stimulating hormone (FSH) and the leutinizing hormone (LH) mature the ovum for fertilization.

Exercise 4-5: *Fill-in*

FSH and LH are produced by the _____ pituitary gland.

A surge in LH on or around the 14th day of the cycle causes ovulation.

Exercise 4-6: *Matching*

Match the term with its definition.

_____ Absence of ovulation

_____ Infrequent and irregular ovulation

A. Oligoovulation

B. Anovulation

The nurse explains there are other symptoms that indicate when a woman is ovulating.

Exercise 4-7: *Select All That Apply*

Select the other symptoms that indicate a woman is ovulating:

❏ Thick nonstretchable vaginal mucus

❏ Decrease in body temperature by 1 °F

❏ Cervical mucosa ferns

❏ Mittelschmerz

Isabella questions how they will know if she is ovulating normally. You describe the four diagnostic tests that are most often done.

■ **FSH blood level**—Measures FSH in a woman's blood and this will tell if she are is actually in an early menopause state.

■ **Progesterone blood level**—Measures progesterone in a woman's blood to tell if ovulation has occurred.

■ **Ultrasound**—visualizes if follicles are developing in the ovaries.

■ **Endometrial biopsy**—Takes a sample of a woman's endometrial tissue for examination to determine if it is reacting appropriately to hormonal stimulation.

The answers can be found on page 96.

eResource 4-4: Ovulation calendars

■ To supplement patient teaching regarding ovulation, you may choose to show Isabella this video clip demonstrating how to create an Ovulation Calendar: *youtu.be/t72Al74ML7o*

■ To use an interactive online ovulation calendar provided by the March of Dimes, open a browser on your mobile device and go to the March of Dimes Web site [Pathway: *marchofdimes.com* → and enter "ovulation calendar" into the search field.]

Exercise 4-8: *Multiple Choice Question*

The nurse understands that the patient needs further teaching when she states:

    A. "At-home ovulation predictor kits should be used mid-cycle."

    B. "At-home ovulation predictor kits test your blood from a finder stick."

    C. "At-home ovulation predictor kits use urine for the test."

    D. "At-home ovulation predictor kits test for the surge in LH."

You explain to Isabella that the first infertility tests will be completed on Christopher to ensure his sperm count is not contributing to the problem. The sperm will be collected and tested for number, size, shape, and motility.

 eResource 4-5:

■ Supplement your patient teaching by educational materials offered by Merck Manuals Online Medical Library: *www.merckmanuals .com/home* [Pathway: select section "Women's Health Issues" → "Infertility" → "Problems with Sperm."]

■ For more information on assistive reproductive technology, go to the Center for Disease Control's (CDC) Web site: *www.cdc.gov/art.*

■ In addition, you can supplement your patient teaching by playing the Center for Disease Control's podcast on Assistive Reproductive Technology (ART) by going to *www.cdc.gov/podcast* [pathway: *www.cdc.gov/podcast* → scroll down to the bottom of the screen to locate and select the podcast "Search" tab → enter "Assisted Reproductive Technology" and tap "Start Search" → select the 6:23 min. version of the podcast.]

Exercise 4-9: *Select All That Apply*

Risk factors for men that may lower their sperm count are:

❑ Active contact sports

❑ Inactivity

❑ Smoking

❑ Chewing tobacco

❑ Tight clothing

❑ Scrotal varicosities

❑ Specific autoimmune diseases

The answers can be found on page 96.

Christopher's sperm count was adequate, so on the next visit you take the couple's detailed social and sexual history. Isabella and Christopher discuss the timing and duration of intercourse, and you ask them to record Isabella's basal body temperature every morning at the same time in order to see if there is a surge during mid-cycle. Three other tests are also done on Isabella for a baseline health examination. These include:

- Complete blood count (CBC)
- Urinalysis
- Pap smear

 eResource 4-6: Go to WomensHealth.gov to locate a basal temperature chart for Isabella and Christopher. *www.womenshealth.gov* [Pathway: Enter "basal temperature chart" into the search field and click on link.]

Exercise 4-10: *Fill-in*

An important social and safety issue to determine is the couple's intimate partner violence (IPV) risk because it is the number _____ cause of pregnancy-related deaths in the United States.

You use the HITS screening tool to assess for risk of IPV (Sherin et al., 1998). This tool contains four questions that ask the client how often their partner has physically Hurt, Insulted, Threatened with harm, and Screamed at them (HITS).

 eResource 4-7:
- To use the online HITS risk assessment tool, go to *healthyplace.com* [Pathway: HealthyPlace.com → select "Psychological Tests" from the menu → scroll down and select "Domestic Violence Screening Test."
- Go to the National Guidelines Clearinghouse (NGC) to view established practice guidelines for routine prenatal screening [*guideline.gov* → enter "prenatal care" into the search field → scroll down to select the guideline "Routine prenatal care." Note: screening for domestic violence is recommended.]

A month later the couple returns to the clinic with their chart. There seems to have been no change in basal body temperature throughout the entire month. All Isabella's other diagnostic tests come back normal so a hysterosalpingography is scheduled. This is scheduled during the follicular phase of her menstrual cycle. In this procedure, dye is instilled thorough the cervix and enters the uterus and fallopian tubes for visualization via X-ray. Nonsteroidal anti-inflammatory drugs (NSAID) are provided 30 minutes before the procedure, because it often produces cramping.

 eResource 4-8: Hysterosalpingography
- Go to: *youtu.be/Hbvbq-oXNfM* to view a brief overview of this procedure.

The answer can be found on page 97.

■ Go to the National Guideline Clearinghouse (NGC) to view Practice Guidelines: *guideline.gov* [Pathway: NGC → enter "hysterosalpingography" into the search field → review available guidelines for standards of care.

Exercise 4-11: *Select All That Apply*
Select all the NSAIDS:

❑ Diclofenac

❑ Ibuprofen

❑ Indomethacin

❑ Naproxen

❑ Acetaminophen

e **eResource 4-9:** To learn more about nonsteroidal anti-inflammatory drugs, open the Merck Manual on your mobile device (eResource 2-1) [Pathway: Merck Manual → select "Topics" → enter "Nonsteroidal anti-inflammatory" into the search field.]

At this time, preconceptually, you discuss teratogens and their effect on fetal development. You discuss the known detrimental effects of the following substances and teach Isabella to avoid them. These effects include:

■ Alcohol
■ Tobacco
■ Caffeine
■ Cocaine
■ Opiates
■ Sedatives
■ Amphetamines
■ Marijuana
■ Radiation
■ Lead

e **eResource 4-10:**
■ For more information regarding the effects of teratogens on fetal development, go to the online Merck Manual: *www.merckmanuals .com/home* [Pathway: Merck Manual → scroll down and select "Women's Health Issues" → scroll down and select "Drug Use During Pregnancy."
■ Another source for more information regarding drug use during pregnancy is the Merck Manual on your mobile device (eResource 2-1) [Pathway: Merck Manual → select "Topics" → enter "pregnancy" into the search field → and enter "drug use during . . ."]

The answers can be found on page 97.

Exercise 4-12: *Multiple Choice Question*

The patient states, "I have heard that one small glass of wine a day is fine when you are pregnant and helps you to relax so you can get a good night's sleep." The nurse should respond:

   A. "Whoever told you that is wrong."

   B. "I have heard that also but do not think it is true."

   C. "Let's think of other ways to have you relax."

   D. "It is unknown how much causes damage so you should not have any."

 eResource 4-11: For more information regarding alcohol use during pregnancy, open the Merck Manual on your mobile device [Pathway: Merck Manual → select "Topics" → enter "pregnancy" into the search field → and enter "alcohol use during . . ."]

Exercise 4-13: *Matching*

Match the following FDA pregnancy categories for drugs.

   _____ Animal studies have shown no harm to the fetus.

   _____ Adequate, well-controlled studies have shown a risk to the fetus.

   _____ Adequate, well-controlled studies have shown positive evidence of fetal abnormalities.

   _____ Animal studies have shown an adverse effect, but there are no adequate, well-controlled studies of pregnant women.

   _____ Adequate, well-controlled studies of pregnant women have not shown an increased risk to the fetus in any trimester.

   A. A

   B. B

   C. C

   D. D

   E. X

After a normal hysterosalpingography, Isabella is placed on Clomiphene citrate (Clomid) 50 mg/day for five days to induce ovulation. Isabella conceives during the first month taking Clomid, and during the luteal phase of the cycle she is given IM progesterone to assist in the preparation of the uterine lining.

 eResource 4-12: Go to Epocrates to look up information regarding infertility treatments [Pathway: *www.epocrates.com* → select "Epocrates Online" → enter "infertility" and select "infertility in women" → select "Treatment" and review "Follow-Up" focusing on potential complications.]

The answers can be found on page 97.

Exercise 4-14: *Multiple Choice Question*

Typical side effects of Progesterone injections include:

    A. Weight loss, nausea, fluid retention

    B. Weight gain, excessive urination, nausea

    C. Increased appetite, weight gain, fluid retention

    D. Nausea, weight gain, fluid retention

 eResource 4-13: Go to *MerckMedicus.com* to read more about Clomophene and Progesterone. [Pathway: *MerckMedicus.com* → select "Clinical Resources" tab → select "Harrison's Practice Online" → select "Drugs" tab → enter drug name into search field.]

Isabella and Christopher are very excited and relieved to hear they do not need further assistance or advanced reproductive technology (ART) to conceive.

Exercise 4-15: *Matching*

Match the artificial reproductive therapy with its description.

    _____ Three to five oocytes are harvested from the ovary and placed in a catheter with a mobile donor or a partner sperm and returned to the fallopian tube.

    _____ Retrieved oocytes are fertilized outside the woman's body and then placed back in the tubes.

    _____ Oocytes are retrieved from the ovary and fertilized in the lab until one develops into an embryo which is then placed back into the woman's uterus.

    _____ Oocytes are retrieved from the ovary and fertilized in the lab until one develops into an embryo which is placed back into the woman's fallopian tubes.

    _____ Freezing of ovarian tissue, sperm, or embryos for future use.

    A. Zygote intrafallopian transfer (ZIFT)

    B. In vitro fertilization (IVF)

    C. Cryopreservation

    D. Gamete intrafallopian transfer (GIFT)

    E. Tubal embryo transfer (TET)

 eResource 4-14: Refer to the Merck Manual on your mobile device to learn more about assistive reproductive techniques. [Pathway: Merck Manual → select "Topics" → enter "reproduction" into the search field → select "assisted."]

At their eight-week visit, Isabella and Christopher are doing well with the confirmation of the pregnancy. Infertility is stressful for couples due to loss of spontaneity in intimacy and lack of privacy. Many times counseling is recommended in order to open discussion about the stressfulness of the infertility treatments and the repeated disappointments over not conceiving.

The answers can be found on page 98.

Exercise 4-16: *Multiple Choice Question*
A priority diagnosis for a couple that confides they are often arguing about the infertility treatments and process would be:

    A. Ineffective coping related to infertility
    B. Posttraumatic response related to infertility
    C. Spiritual distress related to infertility
    D. Situational low self-esteem related to infertility

Exercise 4-17: *Fill-in*
You explain to Isabella the word for implantation is _____.

Exercise 4-18: *Matching*
Match the terminology for the endometrial lining layers (deciduas) and its function.

    _____ External layer of the endometrium
    _____ Endometrium below the implanted blastocyst
    _____ Endometrium that covers the embryo
    A. Decidua basalis
    B. Decidua capsularis
    C. Decidua vera

An internal exam is done on Isabella to look for cervical changes. Two cervical changes are noted on assessment.

Exercise 4-19: *Fill-in*
Isabella's cervix looks vascular and blue and this is called _____ sign; and her cervix is softer than normal and this is called _____ sign.

Isabella is concerned about having sex while she is pregnant so you explain to her that the mucus plug (operculum) protects the fetus from the external environment. Your patients are very interested in knowing about the growth and development of their fetus. You review other terminology with them and explain the purpose of the structures.

eResource 4-15:
    ■ To supplement your teaching, you use your mobile device to access MedlinePlus (*nlm.nih.gov*) to provide more information regarding fetal development during the first trimester [Pathway: MedlinePlus → enter "fetal development" into the search field → scroll down and select "Fetal Development" → scroll down to show the couple week-to-week development, video, and images.]
    ■ In addition, you can show the couple a video about fetal development: *youtu.be/J_knnENhzwg*

The answers can be found on page 99.

Exercise 4-20: *Matching*

Match the structure with its term.

_____ The thick layer that forms the sac that is closest to the fetus.

_____ Specialized connective tissue that surrounds the umbilical cord for protection.

_____ The formation of blood cells that first begin in the yoke sac.

_____ The outer membrane that surrounds the fetus.

A. Wharton's jelly

B. Hematopoiesis

C. Chorion

D. Amnion

Isabella and Christopher ask how the infant can breathe in the uterus. You explain about fetal circulation and how oxygen is carried to the fetus.

 eResource 4-16: To supplement your patient teaching, you may want to show Isabella and Christopher this brief video describing the function of the placenta: *youtu.be/gHnFoWEVs7o*

Exercise 4-21: *Multiple Choice Question*

After blood from the maternal circulation enters the umbilical cord of the fetus, it takes a path of:

A. Foramen ovale, ductus venosus, ductus arteriosis

B. Foremen ovale, ductus arteriosis, ductus venosus

C. Ductus venosus, foramen ovale, ductus arteriosis

D. Ductus venosus, ductus arteriosis, foramen ovale

Exercise 4-22: *Multiple Choice Question*

The nurse understands that fetal circulation enables:

A. Most of the blood to bypass the liver and lungs.

B. Most of the blood to bypass the liver and gastrointestinal tract.

C. Most of the blood to bypass the gastrointestinal tract and lungs.

D. Most of the blood to bypass the lower pancreas and lungs.

You teach the couple about embryology and the importance of good health during the entire pregnancy. During week 3 of development, the embryo differentiates into germ layers.

Exercise 4-23: *Matching*

Match the germ layer development and the correct body systems.

_____ Skin, teeth, and glands or the mouth and nervous system

_____ Epithelium of the respiratory and gastrointestinal tract

_____ Connective tissue, skeletal muscles, and skeleton

A. Mesoderm

B. Ectoderm

C. Endoderm

The answers can be found on page 100.

Exercise 4-24: *Multiple Choice Question*

When an infant is born with an abnormality of the ears, careful assessment of which other organ from the same germ layer is warranted?

    A. Spinal cord

    B. Muscles

    C. Optical

    D. Kidneys

During week 4 the neural tube develops.

Exercise 4-25: *Multiple choice questions*

What dietary vitamin is linked to adequate neural tube development?

    A. Vitamin A

    B. Niacin

    C. Folic Acid

    D. Pantothenic acid

 eResource 4-17:

    ■ Open Medscape on your mobile device to:

        ■ read about neural tube defects and to see images [Pathway: Medscape → enter "neural tube" into the search field at the top of the screen → select "Neural Tube Defects in the Neonatal Period."]

        ■ learn more about these supplements [Pathway: Medscape → enter supplement name into the search at the top of the screen, one at a time.]

    ■ Go to the National Guidelines Clearinghouse (NGC) to view established practice guidelines for the prevention of neural tube defects [*guideline.gov* → enter "neural tube defects" into the search field → tap to select the guidelines to review.]

By week 8 the fetus has well-distinguished upper and lower limbs and most of the organ systems are rudimentarily developed. By the end of week 8 the embryonic phase is ended and the fetal phase is begun. In this phase there is rapid body growth and differentiation of tissue. Isabella and Christopher would like to know when they can tell if their baby will be a boy or a girl. The external genitalia are recognizable by 12–14 weeks. At their 12-week visit, Isabella's uterus is well above the symphysis pubis level.

Exercise 4-26: *Fill-in*

At 20-week's gestation, the uterine fundus should be at the level of _____.

You check her dates using Naegele's rule.

Exercise 4-27: *Multiple Choice Question*

The patient's last menstrual period (LMP) was August 5; therefore her expected date of delivery (EDD) would be:

    A. April 5
    B. April 12
    C. May 5
    D. May 12

 eResource 4-18:
   ■ Using MedCalc's pregnancy calculator on your mobile device, calculate Isabella's EDD [Pathway: MedCalc → Main Index → tap on "P" and scroll down to "Pregnancy Wheel"]
   ■ Or go to Skyscape's Archimedes on your mobile device [pathway: Archimedes → enter "pregnancy" scroll down to select "Pregnancy calculator (1st day of LMP)."]

Another ultrasound is done on Isabella and three fetuses are visualized, which is not uncommon in pregnancies induced by Clomiphene citrate (Clomid). This places her at a higher risk for complications and she will need to be seen more often. Another alternative is selective reduction, thereby providing one or two fetus(es) a better chance of being carried to term. Isabella and

 eResource 4-19: Open Medscape on your mobile device to read about Clomid [Pathway: Medscape → enter "clomid" into the search field at the top of the screen → select "Clomid."]

Christopher admit that they wanted only two children but they ask to "sleep on it" until their next visit in 2 weeks. Before they leave the office you review the danger signs of pregnancy with the couple so they can call if anything abnormal is experienced.

Exercise 4-28: *Matching*

Match the danger sign and the possible cause (causes can be used more than once).

    _____ Painful vaginal bleeding
    _____ Abdominal cramping
    _____ Painless vaginal bleeding
    _____ Prolonged vomiting
    _____ Burning upon urination
    _____ Fever and increased pulse
    _____ Decreased or absent fetal movement
    _____ Swelling of hands and feet
    _____ Epigastric or right upper quadrant (RUQ) discomfort
    _____ Gush or constant leak of vaginal fluid
    _____ Headache

The answer can be found on page 101.

A. Previa

B. Infection

C. Preterm premature rupture of membranes (PPROM)

D. Fetal demise

E. Abruption

F. Pregnancy induced hypertension

G. Urinary tract infection (UTI)

H. Preterm labor

I. Hyperemesis gravidarum

 eResource 4-20:

■ You can supplement your patient teaching by playing two Center for Disease Control's podcasts "Have a Healthy Pregnancy" and "Folic Acid: Helping to Ensure a Healthy Pregnancy" [Pathway: *www.cdc.gov/podcast* → scroll down to the bottom of the screen to locate and select the podcast "Search" tab → enter "Healthy Pregnancy" and tap "Start Search."]

■ To see a list of routine tests conducted during pregnancy, open a browser on your mobile device and go to the March of Dimes Web site [Pathway: *marchofdimes.com* → enter "routine prenatal tests" into the search field.]

At 14 weeks Isabella and Christopher return to the office and announce their decision to carry all three infants to term.

They have enlisted family members who do not work to stay with Isabella so she can remain on her left side in bed for longer periods on time and Isabella will stop working as a cashier. Fetal Heart Tones (FHT) are obtained via Doppler on all three infants. Each has a distinct rate so you are assured that you are hearing three different heart rates.

Exercise 4-29: *Multiple Choice Question*

Which of the following findings warrant further investigation?

   A. FHTs: Infant A—155, Infant B—145, Infant C—160

   B. FHTs: Infant A—145, Infant B—135, Infant C—160

   C. FHTs: Infant A—155, Infant B—125, Infant C—160

   D. FHTs: Infant A—155, Infant B—115, Infant C—160

At 14 weeks, gestation of a quad screen is also done. This is a blood sample taken from the mother to identify four biomarkers. An abnormal range of these biomarkers may indicate a fetus with Down syndrome or a Trisomy.

 eResource 4-21: To learn more about this go to:

■ Merck Manual on your mobile device [Pathway: Merck Manual → scroll down and select "Congenital anomalies" → select "Screening for . . ." → Select " Genetic Evaluation."]

■ Access Medscape on your mobile device to read about these genetic disorders [Pathway: Medscape → enter "down" into search field at the top of the screen → select "Down Syndrome."]

The answers can be found on page 101.

Exercise 4-30: *Multiple Choice Question*

The biomarker specific to Down syndrome is:

    A. Human chorionic gonadotrophin (hCG)
    B. Alpha fetal protein (AFP)
    C. Inhibin A
    D. Unconjugated Estriol

Exercise 4-31: *Hot Spot*

Place an X on the spot on which you would most likely hear the FHTs for Infant A, who is right occipital posterior (ROP).

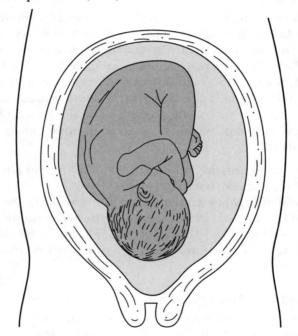

At the 16-week visit, Isabella tells you that her hands are often itchy and tingling. Some of the other complaints that affect integumentary system changes are reviewed with Isabella.

Exercise 4-32: *Matching*

Match the condition to the description.

_____ Increased whitish vaginal discharge

_____ Sebaceous gland enlargement around nipples

_____ Stretch marks around the breasts and abdomen

_____ Leakage of creamy whitish-yellowish liquid from nipples

_____ Darkened line from umbilicus to mons pubis

_____ Mask of pregnancy or melasma gravidarum

_____ Vascular spiders due to increased estrogen levels

_____ Vascular spiders on the palms of the hands

The answers can be found on page 102.

    A. Montgomery tubercles

    B. Colostrum

    C. Angiomas

    D. Palmer erythema

    E. Chloasma

    F. Striae gravidarum

    G. Linea nigra

    H. Leukorrhea

Another complaint that Isabella is having is cheesy white vaginal discharge that is often irritating.

Exercise 4-33: *Multiple Choice Question*

Many pregnant women are susceptible to monilia or vaginal yeast infections due to:

    A. The increase glycogen levels, which make them more susceptible to Candida albicans.

    B. The decreased glycogen levels, which make them more susceptible to Candida albicans.

    C. The increase alkalinity, which makes them more susceptible to Candida albicans.

    D. The decreased leukorrhea, which makes them more susceptible to Candida albicans.

Isabella asks when she will be able to feel the babies kick.

Exercise 4-34: *Fill-in*

Quickening occurs normally at _____ weeks gestation.

Exercise 4-35: *Matching*

Match the fetal term to the somatic process.

    _____ Protects fetal skin from amniotic fluid

    _____ Decreases surface tension in the alveoli

    _____ Fine hair covering

    _____ Subcutaneous deposits used for heat

    A. Vernix

    B. Lanugo

    C. Brown fat

    D. Surfactant

The answers can be found on page 103.

Exercise 4-36: *Multiple Choice Question*

The normal recommended weight gain for a pregnant women with a BMI within the normal range is:

        A. 10–15 pounds

        B. 20–25 pounds

        C. 30–35 pounds

        D. 40–45 pounds

eResource 4-22: To calculate BMI:
- Go to MedCalc.com for an online BMI calculator [Pathway: *medcalc .com* → Tap on "General" → "Body Mass Index" to access the calculator.]
- On your mobile device, use Skyscape's Archimedes to calculate BMI [pathway: Archimedes → select "Main Index" → enter "BMI" into the Main Index → scroll down to select "BMI (Adult)."]

You explain to Isabella that she will have to gain an extra 10 pounds (5 pounds for each extra fetus). At 20-week's gestation, Isabella on examination has a systolic murmur but is asymptomatic for shortness of breath (SOB) and palpitations.

Exercise 4-37: *Multiple Choice Question*

Systolic murmurs during pregnancy are due to cardiac:

        A. Hypertrophy due to increased blood volume.

        B. Decompensation due to load excess.

        C. Overstimulation due to hormonal influences.

        D. Mitral valve stress.

At 22 weeks, Isabella is becoming fairly uncomfortable with the size of her uterus which measures 30 weeks. She is encouraged to take rest periods often. Isabella complains of carpal tunnel syndrome and you explain to her that the condition is common in pregnancy.

Exercise 4-38: *Multiple Choice Question*

Carpal tunnel syndrome in pregnancy is related to:

        A. Nerve compression due to weight gain.

        B. Decreased oxygenation due to compressed vessels.

        C. Edema from increased vascular permeability.

        D. Muscle strain from more use of arms than abdominal muscles.

At 24 weeks, repeat laboratory tests show that Isabella's Hgb is 11.1 g/dL, but you explain that this is due to the physiological anemia of pregnancy.

The answers can be found on page 104.

Exercise 4-39: *Multiple Choice Question*

Physiological anemia of pregnancy is due to:

    A. Blood being shunted to the fetus.

    B. Excessive red blood cells (RBCs) being used by the fetus.

    C. Lack of iron intake.

    D. Increase in plasma content of blood.

 eResource 4-23: Open a browser on your mobile device and go to the Trip Database [Pathway: *tripdatabase.com* → enter "Physiological Changes in Pregnancy" into the search field → scroll down and select topic to view (note that the content may take you to outside resources).]

During labor, Isabella's white blood cell (WBC) may go as high as 24,000/ mm³

Exercise 4-40: *Multiple Choice Question*

During labor you would expect WBCs to increase because the body is:

    A. Responding to stress and exercise.

    B. Responding to an infection.

    C. Shunting WBCs to the fetus for protection.

    D. Misreading the fetus as a foreign body.

At 26 weeks, fetal locations are also attempted by Leopold maneuvers.

Exercise 4-41: *Multiple Choice Question*

The second step in Leopold's maneuvers attempts to locate:

    A. Fetal head position.

    B. Presenting part.

    C. Fetal small parts.

    D. Degree of engagement.

 eResource 4-24:

    ■ To learn more about the Leopold maneuvers use your mobile device, open MerckMedicus and go to the Merck Manual [Merck Manual → Topics → enter "Leopold Maneuvers" into the search field → scroll down and select "Leopold Maneuvers" → scroll down to read the procedure. Note: be sure to tap on "image" to view the diagram depicting the maneuver.]

    ■ To view a short video presented by East Caroline University College of Nursing on assessing the pregnant abdomen and demonstrating the Leopold maneuver, go to: *youtu.be/nIog3oizP8A*

At 28 weeks, a nonstress test (NST) is ordered for Isabella and each of the fetuses is externally monitored electronically by Doppler for their fetal heart rate (FHR). A reactive (good) NST shows two accelerations of is beats per minute for at least 15 seconds in FHR with fetal movement in a 10-minute period.

The answers can be found on page 104.

eResource 4-25: To supplement patient education regarding NST, view a short video presented by Edward Hospital and Health Services. Go to: *youtu.be/DvcDXvlCXAE*

Exercise 4-42: *Either/Or*

This is baby A's FHR. Is the NST reactive or nonreactive? (circle one)

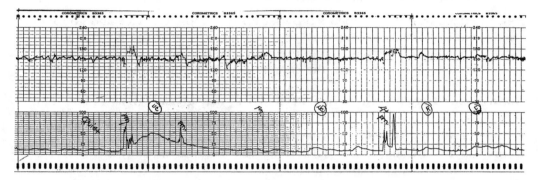

Exercise 4-43: *Either/Or*

This is baby B's FHR. Is the NST reactive or nonreactive? (circle one)

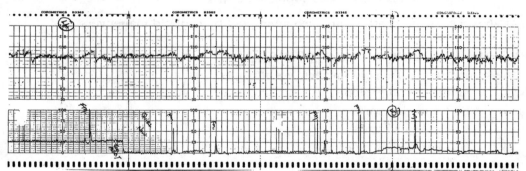

Exercise 4-44: *Either/Or*

This is baby C's FHR. Is the NST reactive or nonreactive? (circle one)

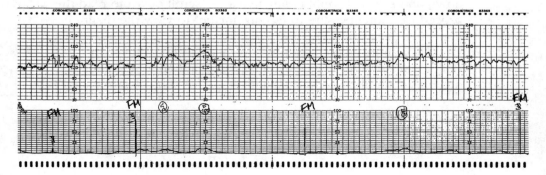

The answers can be found on page 105.

Infant A is vertex, infant B is breech, and infant C is transverse lie. The primary care practitioner (PCP) measures Isabella's pelvis for adequacy.

Exercise 4-45: *Multiple Choice Question*
The true conjugata or conjugata vera is an estimated measurement
> A. Between the anterior surface of the sacral prominence and the posterior surface of the inferior margin of the symphysis pubis.
> B. Between the ischial tuberosities.
> C. Between the anterior surface of the sacral prominence and the anterior surface of the inferior margin of the symphysis pubis.
> D. Between the coccyx and the anterior surface of the inferior margin of the symphysis pubis.

Isabella's true conjugata is estimated at 11.0 cms which is adequate.
At 30 weeks, Isabella and Christopher ask about prenatal classes.

Exercise 4-46: *Multiple Choice Question*
What type of childbirth preparation classes should the nurse recommend for couples who want the father of the baby to be the birth coach?
> A. Dick-Read method
> B. Doula experience
> C. Lamaze method
> D. Bradley method

At 32-week's gestation, before they can finish their classes, Isabella experiences uterine contractions and goes directly to the emergency department (ED). When they arrive Isabella is visibly upset because she is worried about the infants being born so early. The nurses in the ED call the labor and delivery (L&D) suite and have Isabella immediately transferred. Once she is in L&D, Isabella begins to calm down enough to answer questions.

Exercise 4-47: *Multiple Choice Question*
A priority nursing diagnosis for Isabella at this point would be:
> A. Moral distress
> B. Ineffective coping
> C. Acute discomfort
> D. Moderate anxiety

The answers can be found on page 106.

Exercise 4-48: *Multiple Choice Question*

In order to distinguish true labor from false labor or Braxton Hicks contractions, the nurse understands that for true labor:

    A. Eating will produce nausea with contractions.

    B. Walking will increase contractions.

    C. Time will decrease contractions.

    D. Sleeping will increase contractions.

A sterile vaginal exam (SVE) is done on Isabella to find out the condition of her cervix. Isabella's cervix is 80% effaced and 3 cms dilated. The decision to try to stop labor is discussed and terbutaline (Brethine) is ordered 0.25 mg subq. stat and q 20 minutes × 2.

Exercise 4-49: *Calculation*

Terbutaline comes in 0.5 mg/mL units. How many mL should the nurse administer?

 eResource 4-26: On your mobile device, open Medscape [Pathway: Medscape → enter "Terbutaline" into the search field at the top of the screen → select "Terbutaline" to review drug information. Note: this is an off-label use for Preterm Labor.]

An IV is started with an 18-gauge 1¼″ angio catheter, and Isabella is hooked up to the external fetal monitor for all three infants and to the toco transducer to monitor uterine contractions.

Exercise 4-50: *Fill-in*

This is Isabella's initial fetal monitor strip. How often are her contractions?

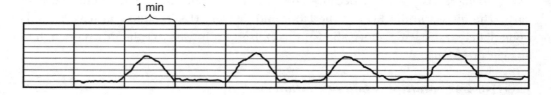

Exercise 4-51: *Multiple Choice Question*

The nurse is about to administer the second dose of terbutaline (Brethine) and Isabella's pulse rate is 120/min. The nurse should:

    A. Give the medication as ordered.

    B. Hold the medication and try in 10 minutes.

    C. Hold the medication and call the PCP.

    D. Give half the dose.

Exercise 4-52: *Calculation*

Isabella's IV is ordered to run at 200 mL/hour. There is a 1,000 mL IV bag hanging and the drop factor is 15 gtts/mL. At what level should you set the pump? At how many gtts/min?

The answers can be found on page 107.

eResource 4-27:
- Go to MedCalc.com to use the online IV Rate calculator [Pathway: *medcalc.com* → select "Fluids/Electrolytes" → select "IV Rate."]
- On your mobile device, use Skyscape's Archimedes to calculate the infusion rate [pathway: Archimedes → enter "IV" into the Main Index → and scroll down to "IV Calc: Infusion rate mL/hr."]

Exercise 4-53: *Multiple Choice Question*

The nurse knows that the IV is important in Isabella's case because:

    A. Extra fluid may be needed if there is a hemorrhage.

    B. Preterm labor is often caused by dehydration.

    C. It will keep Isabella's kidneys functioning well.

    D. It will aid her to make more amniotic fluid.

Suddenly Isabella puts her call light on and Isabella states, "I don't know if I wet myself but everything is wet; I didn't feel like I had to urinate."

Exercise 4-54: *Multiple Choice Question*

The first action the nurse should take when spontaneous rupture of membranes is suspected is:

    A. Observe the color of the fluid.

    B. Use litmus paper to check that it is not urine.

    C. Weigh the bed pad to see how much came out.

    D. Check the fetal heart tones.

eResource 4-28: Go to the National Guidelines Clearinghouse (NGC) to view established practice guidelines for Premature Rupture of Membranes [*guideline.gov* → enter "premature rupture of membranes" into the search field → tap to select the guideline "Premature Rupture of Membranes."]

Although there are three amnions present in Isabella's uterus, it is difficult to determine how many sacs ruptured; so labor is allowed to continue naturally and the neonatal intensive care unit (NICU) is notified that triplets will be born in the near future.

The answers can be found on page 107.

Answers

Exercise 4-1: *Calculation*

Isabella is 5′ 4″ and weighs 133 lbs. Is her body mass index (BMI) within normal limits (WNL)? **YES, it is 22.8**.

Christopher is 6′ 3″ and weighs 220 lbs. Is his BMI WNL? **NO, it is 27.5—overweight**.

Exercise 4-2: *Multiple Choice Question*

The menstrual phase of the menstrual cycle is caused by:

A. Increased progesterone and estrogen—NO, there is a lack of hormones to sustain the endometrium.

B. **Decreased progesterone and estrogen—YES.**

C. Increased follicle stimulating hormone and luteinizing hormone—NO, there is a lack of hormones to sustain the endometrium.

D. Decreased follicle stimulating hormone and luteinizing hormone—NO, it is estrogen and progesterone, progesterone is responsible for maintaining pregnancies.

Exercise 4-3: *Matching*

Match the term with the definition.

    D   Lack of menstrual periods

    H   Painful menstrual periods

    A   Very little menstrual flow

    F   Frequent but irregular menses

    E   Heavy but frequent and irregular menses

    C   Heavy menses

    B   Cycles fewer than 21 days

    G   Cycles longer than 35 days

A. Hypomenorrhea

B. Menometrorrhea

C. Menorrhagia

D. Amenorrhea

E. Polymenorrhea

F. Menometrorrhagia

G. Oligomenorrhea

H. Dysmenorrhea

Exercise 4-4: *Multiple Choice Question*

The nurse knows that the patient understands the teaching about the menstrual cycle when she states:

A. "The pituitary gland responds to luteinizing hormone input from the hypothalamus."—NO, the hypothalamus secretes gonadatropin-releasing hormone.

B. "The pituitary gland responds to follicle stimulating hormone input from the hypothalamus."—NO, the hypothalamus secretes gonadatropin-releasing hormone.

C. "The pituitary gland responds to estrogen input from the hypothalamus."—NO, the hypothalamus secretes gonadatropin-releasing hormone.

D. **"The pituitary gland responds to gonadatropin-releasing hormone input from the hypothalamus."—YES.**

Exercise 4-5: *Fill-in*

FSH and LH are produced by the <u>**anterior**</u> pituitary gland.

Exercise 4-6: *Matching*

Match the term with its definition.

__**B**__ Absence of ovulation

__**A**__ Infrequent and irregular ovulation

A. Oligoovulation

B. Anovulation

Exercise 4-7: *Select All That Apply*

Select the other symptoms that indicate a woman is ovulating:

❏ Thick nonstretchable vaginal mucus—NO, it is thin and stretchable.

❏ Decrease in body temperature by 1 °F—NO, it is an increase in body temperature.

☑ **Cervical mucosa ferns—YES, this is a sign.**

☑ **Mittelschmerz—YES, this is felt by some women.**

Exercise 4-8: *Multiple Choice Question*

The nurse understands that the patient needs further teaching when she states:

A. "At home ovulation predictor kits should be used mid-cycle."—NO, this is true.

B. **"At home ovulation predictor kits test your blood from a finder stick."—YES, it uses a urine sample.**

C. "At home ovulation predicator kits use urine for the test."—NO, this is true.

D. "At home ovulation predictor kits test for the surge in LH."—NO, this is true.

Exercise 4-9: *Select All That Apply*

Risk factors for men that may lower their sperm count are:

☑ **Active contact sports—YES.**

❏ Inactivity—NO.

☑ **Smoking—YES.**

❏ Chewing tobacco—NO.

☑ **Tight clothing—YES**.

☑ **Scrotal varicosities—YES**.

☑ **Specific autoimmune diseases—YES**.

Exercise 4-10: *Fill-in*

An important social and safety issue to determine is the couple's intimate partner violence (IPV) risk because it is the number ___**1**___ cause of pregnancy-related deaths in the United States.

Exercise 4-11: *Select All That Apply*

Select all the NSAIDS:

☑ **Diclofenac—YES**.

☑ **Ibuprofen—YES**.

☑ **Indomethacin—YES**.

☑ **Naproxen—YES**.

❏ Acetaminophen—NO.

Exercise 4-12: *Multiple Choice Question*

The patient states that, "I have heard that one small glass of wine a day is fine when you are pregnant and helps you to relax so you can get a good night's sleep." The nurse should respond:

A. "Whoever told you that is wrong."—NO, this is very judgmental.

B. "I have heard that also but do not think it is true."—NO, this does not address the dangerous behavior.

C. "Let's think of other ways to have you relax."—NO, this does not address the dangerous behavior.

D. **"It is unknown how much causes damage, so you should not have any."—YES, this is the best answer—it stops the behavior nonjudgmentally**.

Exercise 4-13: *Matching*

Match the following FDA pregnancy categories for drugs.

___**B**___ Animal studies have shown no harm to the fetus.

___**D**___ Adequate, well-controlled studies have shown a risk to the fetus.

___**X**___ Adequate, well-controlled studies have shown positive evidence of fetal abnormalities .

___**C**___ Animal studies have shown an adverse effect but there are no adequate, well-controlled studies in pregnant women.

___**A**___ Adequate, well-controlled studies in pregnant women have not shown an increased risk to the fetus in any trimester.

Exercise 4-14: *Multiple Choice Question*

Typical side effects of progesterone injections include:

A. Weight loss, nausea, fluid retention—NO, fluid retention would produce weight gain.

B. Weight gain, excessive urination, nausea—NO, fluid retention decreases urination.

C. Increased appetite, weight gain, fluid retention—NO, women are often nauseous.

D. **Nausea, weight gain, fluid retention—YES, this is common.**

Exercise 4-15: *Matching*

Match the artificial reproductive therapy with its description.

___D___ Three to five oocytes are harvested from the ovary and placed in a catheter with mobile donor or partner sperm and returned to the fallopian tube.

___B___ Retrieved oocytes are fertilized outside the woman's body and then are placed back in the tubes.

___A___ Oocytes are retrieved from the ovary and fertilized in the lab until it is an embryo and then placed back into the woman's uterus.

___E___ Oocytes are retrieved from the ovary and fertilized in the lab until it is an embryo and then placed back into the woman's fallopian tubes.

___C___ Freezing of ovarian tissue, sperm or embryos for future use.

A. Zygote intrafallopian transfer (ZIFT)

B. In vitro fertilization (IVF)

C. Cryopreservation

D. Gamete intrafallopian transfer (GIFT)

E. Tubal embryo transfer (TET)

Exercise 4-16: *Multiple Choice Question*

A priority diagnosis for a couple that confides they argue often about the infertility treatments and process would be:

A. **Ineffective coping related to infertility—YES, they are having trouble coping with the health situation.**

B. Posttraumatic response related to infertility—NO, this is not the criteria for post-traumatic stress syndrome.

C. Spiritual distress related to infertility—NO, they have not verbalized a loss or questioning of faith.

D. Situational low self-esteem related to infertility—NO, they have not verbalized feelings of inadequacy about themselves.

Exercise 4-17: *Fill-in*

You explain to Isabella the word for implantation is __**Nidation**__.

Exercise 4-18: *Matching*

Match the terminology for the endometrial lining layers (deciduas) and its function.

___**C**___ External layer of the endometrium

___**A**___ Endometrium below the implanted blastocyst

___**B**___ Endometrium that covers the embryo

A. Decidua basalis

B. Decidua capsularis

C. Decidua vera

Exercise 4-19: *Fill-in*

Isabella's cervix looks vascular and blue and this is called **Chadwick's** sign; and her cervix is softer than normal and this is called **Hegar's** sign.

Exercise 4-20: *Matching*

Match the structure and with its term.

___**D**___ Thick layer that forms the sac that is closest to the fetus

___**A**___ Specialized connective tissue that surrounds the umbilical cord for protection

___**B**___ The formation of blood cells that first begins in the yoke sac

___**C**___ The outer membrane that surrounds the fetus

A. Wharton's jelly

B. Hematopoiesis

C. Chorion

D. Amnion

Exercise 4-21: *Multiple Choice Question*

After the blood from the maternal circulation enters the umbilical cord of the fetus it takes a path of:

A. Foramen ovale, ductus venoses, ductus arteriosis—NO, this is not the pathway.

B. Foremen ovale, ductus arteriosis, ductus venosus—NO, this is not the pathway.

C. **Ductus venosus, foramen ovale, ductus arteriosis—YES, this is the path it takes first thorough the ductus venosus up to the heart and through the foremen ovale to bypass the pulmonary circulation. Then it goes through the left side of the heart to the ascending aorta and goes to the brain and upper body. Blood from the superior vena cava flows into the right side of the heart and is pumped to the pulmonary artery, which gets shunted to the ductus arteriosis to the descending aorta again to bypass the lungs.**

D. Ductus venosus, ductus arteriosis, foramen ovale—NO, this is not the pathway.

Exercise 4-22: *Multiple Choice Question*

The nurse understands that fetal circulation enables:

A. **Most of the blood to bypass the liver and lungs—YES, this is the rationale, because the placenta takes over these functions**.

B. Most of the blood to bypass the liver and gastrointestinal tract—NO.

C. Most of the blood to bypass the gastrointestinal tract and lungs—NO.

D. Most of the blood to bypass the lower pancreas and lungs—NO.

Exercise 4-23: *Matching*

Match the germ layer development and the correct body systems.

   B   Skin, teeth, and glands or the mouth and nervous system.

   C   Epithelium of the respiratory and gastrointestinal tract.

   A   Connective tissue, skeletal muscles, and skeleton.

A. Mesoderm

B. Ectoderm

C. Endoderm

Exercise 4-24: *Multiple Choice Question*

When an infant is born with an abnormality of the ears, careful assessment of which other organ from the same germ layer is warranted?:

A. Spinal cord—NO, this is the ectoderm.

B. Muscles—NO, this is the mesoderm.

C. Optical—NO, this is the mesoderm.

D. **Kidneys—YES, this is also the ectoderm, epithelial cell lined**.

Exercise 4-25: *Multiple choice questions*

What dietary vitamin is linked to adequate neural tube development?

A. Vitamin A—NO.

B. Niacin—NO.

C. **Folic acid—YES.**

D. Pantothenic acid—NO.

Exercise 4-26: *Fill-in*

At 20-week's gestation, the uterine fundus should be at the level of **umbilicus**.

Exercise 4-27: *Multiple Choice Question*

The patient's last menstrual period (LMP) was August 5; therefore her expected date of delivery (EDD) would be:

A. April 5—NO.

B. April 12—NO.

C. May 5—NO.

D. **May 12—YES, this is counted back 3 months and adding 7 days**.

Exercise 4-28: *Matching*

Match the danger sign and the possible cause (causes can be used more than once).

____**E**____ Painful vaginal bleeding

____**H**____ Abdominal cramping

____**A**____ Painless vaginal bleeding

____**I**____ Prolonged vomiting

____**G**____ Burning on urination

____**B**____ Fever and increased pulse

____**D**____ Decreased or absent fetal movement

____**F**____ Swelling of hands and feet

____**F**____ Epigastric or right upper quadrant (RUQ) discomfort

____**C**____ Gush or constant leak of vaginal fluid

____**F**____ Headache

A. Previa

B. Infection

C. Preterm premature rupture of membranes (PPROM)

D. Fetal demise

E. Abruption

F. Pregnancy induced hypertension

G. Urinary tract infection (UTI)

H. Preterm labor

I. Hyperemesis gravidarum

Exercise 4-29: *Multiple Choice Question*

Which of the following findings warrant further investigation?

A. FHTs: Infant A—155, Infant B—145, Infant C—160., NO, these are WNL.

B. FHTs: Infant A—145, Infant B—135, Infant C—160., NO, these are WNL.

C. FHTs: Infant A—155, Infant B—125, Infant C—160. NO, these are WNL.

D. **FHTs: Infant A—155, Infant B—115, Infant C—160. YES, Infant B has a low FHR**.

Exercise 4-30: *Multiple Choice Question*

The biomarker specific to Down syndrome is:

A. Human chorionic gonadotropin (hCG)—NO.

B. **Alpha fetal protein (AFP)—YES**.

C. Inhibin A—NO.

D. Unconjugated Estriol—NO.

Exercise 4-31: *Hot Spot*
Place an X on the spot on which you would most likely hear the FHTs for Infant A, who is right occipital posterior (ROP).

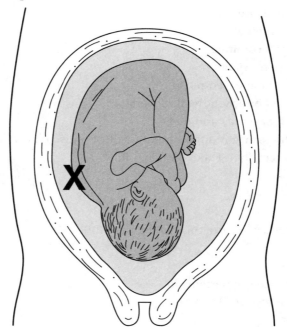

YES, the FHTs are heard loudest through the infant's back because small parts cover the chest.

Exercise 4-32: *Matching*
Match the condition to the description.

   H   Increased whitish vaginal discharge

   A   Sebaceous gland enlargement around nipples

   F   Stretch marks around the breasts and abdomen

   B   Leakage of creamy whitish-yellowish liquid from nipples

   G   Darkened line from umbilicus to mons pubis

   E   Mask of pregnancy or melasma gravidarum

   C   Vascular spiders due to increased estrogen levels

   D   Vascular spiders on the palms of the hands

A. Montgomery tubercles

B. Colostrum

C. Angiomas

D. Palmer erythema

E. Chloasma

F. Striae gravidarum

G. Linea Nigra

H. Leukorrhea

Exercise 4-33: *Multiple Choice Question*
Many pregnant women are susceptible to monilia or vaginal yeast infections due to:

A. **The increase glycogen levels make it more susceptible to Candida albicans—YES**.
B. The decreased glycogen levels make it more susceptible to Candida albicans—NO, it is the increased level that increases susceptibility.
C. The increase alkalinity makes it more susceptible to Candida albicans—NO, it is increased in acidity.
D. The decreased leukorrhea makes it more susceptible to Candida albicans—NO, this is increased and makes a better medium for Candida.

Exercise 4-34: *Fill-in*
Quickening occurs normally at __18–20__ weeks gestation.

Exercise 4-35: *Matching*
Match the fetal term to the somatic process.
___A___ Protects fetal skin from amniotic fluid
___D___ Decreases surface tension in the alveoli
___B___ Fine hair covering
___C___ Subcutaneous deposits used for heat
A. Vernix
B. Lanugo
C. Brown fat
D. Surfactant

Exercise 4-36: *Multiple Choice Question*
The normal recommended weight gain for a pregnant women with a BMI within the normal range is:
A. 10–15 pounds—NO, this is not enough.
B. 20–25 pounds—NO, this is not enough.
C. **30–35 pounds—YES, this is what is recommended**.
D. 40–45 pounds—NO, this is too much.

Exercise 4-37: *Multiple Choice Question*
Systolic murmurs during pregnancy are due to cardiac:
A. **Hypertrophy due to increased blood volume—YES, this is the reason.**
B. Decompensation due to load excess—NO, this is not what happens in pregnancy normally.
C. Overstimulation due to hormonal influences—NO, this is not what happens in pregnancy normally.
D. Mitral valve stress—NO, this is not what happens in pregnancy normally.

Exercise 4-38: *Multiple Choice Question*

Carpal tunnel syndrome in pregnancy is related to:

A. Nerve compression due to weight gain—NO, this is not the physiology.

B. Decreased oxygenation due to compressed vessels—NO, this is not the physiology.

C. **Edema from increased vascular permeability—YES, this is the reason it is so common in pregnancy**.

D. Muscle strain from more use of arms than abdominal muscles—NO, this is not the physiology.

Exercise 4-39: *Multiple Choice Question*

Physiological anemia of pregnancy is due to:

A. Blood being shunted to the fetus—NO, this is not the reason.

B. Excessive RBC's being used by the fetus—NO, this is not the reason.

C. Lack of iron intake—NO, this is not the reason.

D. **Increase in plasma content of blood—YES, there is a larger proportion of increased plasma (40–50%) than cellular content (30%)**.

Exercise 4-40: *Multiple Choice Question*

During labor you would expect WBCs to increase because the body is:

A. **Responding to stress and exercise—YES, this is the reason**.

B. Responding to an infection—NO, this is not necessarily true.

C. Shunting WBCs to the fetus for protection—NO, this is not true.

D. Misreading the fetus as a foreign body—NO, this is not true.

Exercise 4-41: *Multiple Choice Question*

The second step in Leopold maneuvers attempts to locate:

A. Fetal head position—NO, this is the first maneuver in the fundal region.

B. Presenting part—NO, this is the third maneuver.

C. **Fetal small parts—YES, this is the reason for the second maneuver**.

D. Degree of engagement—NO, this is the fourth maneuver.

Exercise 4-42: *Either/Or*

This is baby A's FHR. Is the NST **reactive** or nonreactive? (circle one).

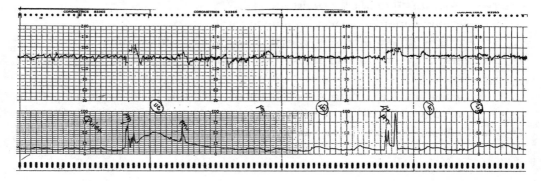

YES, it is reactive because there are four fetal movements (FMs) marked on the fetal monitor strip, and the fetal heart rate increases at least 15 BPM for 15 seconds with each one.

Exercise 4-43: *Either/Or*

This is baby B's FHR. Is the NST **reactive** or nonreactive? (circle one).

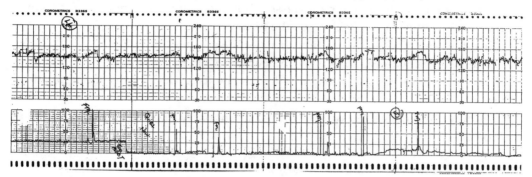

YES, there are six fetal movements marked on the strip, and five correspond with fetal heart rate accelerations that are at least 15 seconds long.

Exercise 4-44: *Either/Or*

This is baby C's FHR. Is the NST **reactive** or nonreactive? (circle one).

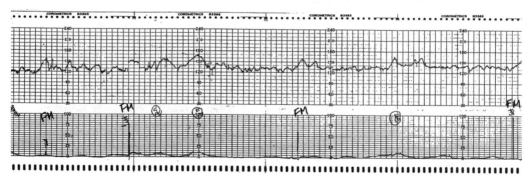

YES, there are three fetal heart rate accelerations with fetal movements that last at least 15 seconds each.

Exercise 4-45: *Multiple Choice Question*

The true conjugate or conjugate vera is an estimated measurement:

A. **Between the anterior surface of the sacral prominence and the posterior surface of the inferior margin of the symphysis pubis—YES, the posterior surface cannot be reached so it is an estimate.**

B. Between the ischial tuberosities—NO, this can be measured.

C. Between the anterior surface of the sacral prominence and the anterior surface of the inferior margin of the symphysis pubis—NO, this can be measured.

D. Between the coccyx and the anterior surface of the inferior margin of the symphysis pubis—NO, this can be measured.

Exercise 4-46: *Multiple Choice Question*
What type of childbirth preparation classes should the nurse recommend for couples who want the father of the baby to be the birth coach?
A. Dick-Read method—NO, this does not use the partner as coach.
B. Doula experience—NO, this is having another woman present.
C. Lamaze method—NO, this may use the partner as a coach but is about breathing properly.
D. **Bradley method—YES, this is founded on participation of the partner as coach**.

Exercise 4-47: *Multiple Choice Question*
A priority nursing diagnosis for Isabella at this point would be:
A. Moral distress—NO, she has not verbalized a questioning of faith at this point.
B. Ineffective coping—NO, this is not a priority diagnosis at this time.
C. Acute discomfort—NO, this contractions are not that strong yet.
D. **Moderate anxiety—YES, she is demonstrating justifiable worry and anxiety about the welfare of her infants**.

Exercise 4-48: *Multiple Choice Question*
In order to distinguish true labor from false labor or Braxton Hicks contractions, the nurse understands that for true labor:
A. Eating will produce nausea with contractions—NO, this is not always true.
B. **Walking will increase contractions—YES, this is true if it is true labor**.
C. Time will decrease contractions—NO, this is not true for true labor.
D. Sleeping will increase contractions—NO, this is not a way that can be done practically.

Exercise 4-49: *Calculation*
Terbutaline comes in 0.5 mg/mL how many mL should the nurse administer?
Desired = 0.25 mg
On hand = 0.5 mg/mL
$$\frac{0.25}{0.5} = .5 \text{ mL}$$

Exercise 4-50: *Fill-in*

This is Isabella's initial fetal monitor strip. How often are her contractions? <u>**Every**</u>
<u>**2 minutes**</u>

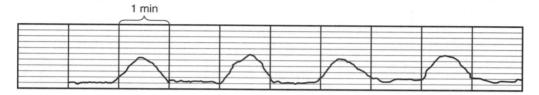

Exercise 4-51: *Multiple Choice Question*

The nurse is about to administer the second dose of terbutaline (Brethine) and Isabella's
pulse rate is 120/min. The nurse should:

  A. Give the medication as ordered—NO, her pulse rate is too high.

  B. Hold the medication and try in 10 minutes—NO, this is not how it is ordered.

  C. **Hold the medication and call the PCP—YES, you need further orders.**

  D. Give half the dose.—NO, this is not how it is ordered;, you would be prescribing.

Exercise 4-52: *Calculation*

Isabella's IV is ordered to run at 200 mL/hour. There is a 1,000 mL IV bag hanging
and the drop factor is 15 gtts/mL. At What level should you set the pump? How many
gtts/min?

  200 mL/hr × 15 gtts/mL = 3,000 gtts/hr divided by 60 = 50 gtts/min.

Exercise 4-53: *Multiple Choice Question*

The nurse knows that the IV is important in Isabella's case because:

  A. Extra fluid may be needed if there is a hemorrhage—NO, this may be true but is
     not the priority answer.

  B. **Preterm labor is often caused by dehydration—YES.**

  C. It will keep Isabella's kidneys functioning well—NO, this may be true but is not
     the priority answer.

  D. It will help her to make more amniotic fluid—NO, this is not true.

Exercise 4-54: *Multiple Choice Question*

The first action the nurse should take when spontaneous rupture of membranes is
suspected is:

  A. Observe the color of the fluid—NO, this is not the first priority.

  B. Use litmus paper to check that it is not urine—NO, this is not the first priority.

  C. Weigh the bed pad to see how much came out—NO, this is not the first priority.

  D. **Check the fetal heart tones—YES, you must make sure there is not a cord
     prolapsed that cannot be seen.**

Reference

Sherin, K. M., Sinacore, J. M., Li, X. Q., Zitter, R. E., & Shakil, A. (1998). HITS: A short domestic violence screening tool for use in a family practice setting. *Family Medicine, 30*(7), 508–512.

5

Hyperemesis Gravidarum (HG)

Case Study 5 ▰ Tamiko

Tamiko is 10 weeks gestation and has been experiencing nausea and vomiting for the past 3 weeks. Recently she has not been able to keep any food down and has not been able to feel well enough even to get to work. She is seen in the prenatal clinic where you are now working as a graduate nurse (GN). Tamiko appears listless and less responsive compared to the last time you saw her. She states that she has been nauseous and vomiting everything for a week and is unable to keep anything down.

Exercise 5-1: *Calculation*
Tamiko's weight last visit (6 weeks gestation) was 125 lbs. Today she weighs 113 lbs. What percent of body weight has she lost?

Tamiko asks why she is so sick.

Exercise 5-2: *Multiple Choice Question*
The patient tells you that an elder at her church told her that is was because she was psychologically rejecting the baby. What would be the best response to the patient?
  A. "That is simply not true so never mind what was said."
  B. "In the past this was what people thought caused hyperemesis."
  C. "Tell the elder she is wrong."
  D. "How do you feel about the baby?"

Exercise 5-3: *Fill-in*
The most accepted theory of causation for hyperemesis is an excessive amount of circulating _____.

This is Tamiko's second pregnancy. The first pregnancy ended in an early complete spontaneous abortion.

The answers can be found on page 115.

Exercise 5-4: *Fill-in*

What is Tamiko's gravid and para?

G _____ P _____ T _____ A _____ L _____

Exercise 5-5: *Select All That Apply*

What are the risk factors for hyperemesis gravidarum?

❏ Elderly primips

❏ Nausea and vomiting with previous pregnancies

❏ History of not being able to tolerate oral contraceptives

❏ Singletons

❏ Multiparas

❏ Hypothyroidism

❏ GERD (Gastroesophageal reflux)

❏ Anorexia

❏ H-pylori seropositivity

Exercise 5-6: *Fill-in*

A diagnosis is made with reports of uncontrollable nausea and vomiting and _____ % weight loss.

e **eResource 5-1:**
- Go to Epocrates online [Pathway: *online.epocrates.com* → tap on the "Diseases" tab → enter "hyperemesis gravidarum" in the search field to view content about "Nausea and Vomiting in Pregnancy" → tap on "Diagnosis" and select "Approach" to learn about early intervention.]
- Open to Medscape on your mobile device. [Pathway: Medscape → select "hyperemesis gravidarum" → elect "Treatment."]

You explain to Tamiko that hyperemesis occurs in 1–2% of pregnancies and is different than regular morning sickness. You also explain that since the dehydration it produces can lead to other complications, it is serious and she should go to the hospital for admission. Tamiko feels so terrible that she doesn't object. She goes to the hospital and is admitted to the high-risk perinatal unit for treatment.

When Tamiko arrives at the perinatal unit, she is weak and has vertigo.

Exercise 5-7: *Select All That Apply*

Upon admission, the following issues must be addressed:

❏ Intimate partner abuse

❏ Living will

❏ Advanced directive

❏ Health Insurance Portability and Accountability Act (HIPAA)

The answers can be found on page 116.

❏ Weighing the patient

❏ Patient's bill of rights

The nurse draws blood, obtains a urinalysis, and starts an IV.

Exercise 5-8: *Select All That Apply*
What laboratory finding would you expect on a patient that is vomiting and dehydrated?

❏ Elevated liver enzymes—aspartate aminotransferase (AST) and alanine aminotransferase (ALT).

❏ Decrease in liver enzymes—aspartate aminotransferase (AST) and alanine aminotransferase (ALT).

❏ CBC shows elevated RBCs and Hct.

❏ CBC shows a decrease in RBCs and Hct.

❏ BUN (blood urea nitrogen) is increased.

❏ BUN is decreased.

❏ Electrolytes—sodium, potassium, and chloride are elevated.

❏ Electrolytes—sodium, potassium, and chloride are depleted.

e **eResource 5-2:**
■ To learn more about lab results likely to be obtained to confirm diagnosis hyperemesis gravidarum, use your mobile device, open MerckMedicus, and go to Harrison's Practice [Harrison's Practice → Topics → enter "hyperemesis" and select "hyperemesis gravidarum", →, select "Diagnosis" in the upper-right corner drop-down menu, select "Diagnosis" → scroll down to locate "Laboratory tests."]

■ Open Medscape on your mobile device. [Pathway: Medscape → select "hyperemesis gravidarum" → select "Workup" to view Laboratory Studies.]

■ Go to the National Guidelines Clearinghouse (NGC) to view established practice guidelines for hyperemesis gravidarum [*guideline .gov* → enter "hyperemesis gravidarum" into search field → tap to select the guideline "Nausea and Vomiting of Pregnancy."]

Tamiko provides a urine specimen that shows a specific gravity greater than 1.025 and ketones.

Exercise 5-9: *Calculation*
The IV ordered is 1,000 mL of lactated Ringers/D%W with vitamins and electrolytes at 250 mL per hour. How many hours should the IV last?

If there was no IV pump available and the gtt factor was 10, how many gtts per minute should it run?

The answers can be found on page 116.

eResource 5-3: To calculate the IV infusion rate
- Go to *MedCalc.com* and use the online calculator [Pathway: *medcalc.com* → select "Fluids/Electrolytes" → select "IV Rate" calculator.]
- On your mobile device, open Archimedes [Pathway: Archimedes → select "Main Index" → enter "IV" into the search field → select "IV Calc: Infusion rate mL/hr."]

The order is for Tamiko to receive Promethazine (Phenergan) 25 mg rectal suppository. Promethazine (Phenergan) is a category C drug but in this case the benefits outweigh the risks.

 eResource 5-4:
- On your mobile device, go to Medscape [Pathway: Medscape → enter "Phenergan" into the search field → select "Adult Dosing and Uses" and "Pregnancy and Lactation." Note: it is a good idea to check "Adverse Effects" and "Contraindications & Warnings."]
- Go to Epocrates online [Pathway: *online.epocrates.com* → tap on the "Diseases" tab → enter "hyperemesis gravidarum" in the search field to view content about "Nausea and Vomiting in Pregnancy" → tap on "Diagnosis" and select "Approach" to learn about early intervention.]

Exercise 5-10: *Ordering*
Order the steps in the intervention of administering a suppository.

_____ Lubricate the suppository with water-soluble lubricant.

_____ Explain the procedure to the patient.

_____ Provide privacy.

_____ Insert the suppository 1–1.5".

_____ Don clean cloves.

_____ Wash your hands.

_____ Drape the patient.

_____ Identify the patient with two identifiers.

_____ Remove outer wrapper from medication.

The nurse places the side rails up.

Exercise 5-11: *Fill-in*
What are some of Tomiko's fall risks?

_____

_____

_____

 eResource 5-5: For information about fall risk assessment and available tools, go to the U.S. Department of Veteran's Affairs [Pathway: *www4.va.gov* → enter "Fall Prevention" into the search field and click

The answers can be found on page 117.

on "search this site" → select "National Center for Patient Safety—Fall Prevention and Management" to access this rich resource.]

After the suppository, Tamiko sleeps for approximately 2.5 hours. When she wakes up she starts vomiting again even though she has been NPO. The nurse calls the primary care practitioner (PCP) for further orders. When the PCP answers the phone, the nurse uses SBAR to inform him or her of the situation.

Exercise 5-12: *Fill-in*

S (Situations)—The patient is _____

B (Background)—The patient has been _____

A (Assessment)—The patient is c/o, labs and diagnostic tests _____

R (Recommendation)—I think the patient would benefit from _____

Exercise 5-13: *Calculation*

Odansetran (Zofran) is ordered IV. 0.15 mg/kg now to run over 15 minutes. How much medication should you put in a 100 mL mini bag? How many gtts/min should the 100 mL mini bag be run piggyback with the drop factor still at 10gtts/mL?

 eResource 5-6: To calculate the dose and IV infusion rate (refer back to eResource 5-3):
- Go to *MedCalc.com* and use the online IV infusion rate calculator.
- On your mobile device, open Archimedes, locate and use "IV Calc: Infusion rate mL/hr" calculator.

Odansetran (Zofran) is a category B drug. The nurse hangs the medication and darkens the room to allow Tamiko to rest. Visitors are allowed in as Tamiko requests. The call bell is placed within reach and she is told she must be assisted out of bed (OOB). The following day, Tamiko's urine is less concentrated, but she is still unable to hold down any food. Total parental nutrition (TPN) is ordered in order to provide the nutrients needed to sustain a healthy pregnancy. TPN is calculated for each patient individually and mixed by the pharmacy.

 eResource 5-7: To learn more about TPN:
- Use your mobile device, open MerckMedicus and go to the Merck Manual [Merck Manual → Topics → enter "Total Parental" into the search field → select "Total parental nutrition (TPN)" → select "Total parental nutrition (TPN)" again to review content.]
- To supplement patient education for Tamiko, you may want to show her a video clip about TPN from a patient's perspective which provides a very good overview in a way that is easy to understand: *youtu.be/haWyRCPLlnU*

Exercise 5-14: *Calculation*

Normal TPN need is 25–30 Kcal/kg/day. What range of Kcals will Tamiko need in 24 hours?

The answers can be found on page 117.

Exercise 5-15: *Calculation*
If Tamiko needs 1.2 g/kg/day of protein, how much should be in her TPN?

Exercise 5-16: *Multiple Choice Question*
Prolonged TPN should contain which two amino acids?
>   A. Glutamine and choline
>   B. Arginine and proline
>   C. Glutamine and proline
>   D. Arginine and glutamine

Exercise 5-17: *Calculate*
Tamiko should receive 30 mL of fluid /kg/day to maintain hydration, so the order is for 50 mL/kg/day due to the fact that she needs replacement fluid. How much fluid should she have?

Along with her TPN fluid, a 10% fat emulsion is ordered and is prepared and sent to the unit in a 250-mL bottle. The nurse explains to Tamiko that TPN is needed for nutrition. Tamiko asks what would happen if she continues to vomit. The nurse explains that in very rare cases a gastric tube is inserted below the stomach; but most women are helped with Zofran, TPN, and bed rest.

Tamiko remains NPO in the hospital for a week. Gradually food is reintroduced. She tolerated the food and the TPN is decreased. Tamiko is discharged to go home on the 13th day.

Exercise 5-18: *Select All That Apply*
Discharge teaching includes:
>   ❑ Home care needs
>   ❑ Medication reconciliation
>   ❑ Outpatient health care appointments
>   ❑ Emergency number to call
>   ❑ The nurse's phone number
>   ❑ The hospital unit's number

The answers can be found on page 118.

Answers

Exercise 5-1: *Calculation*

Tamiko's weight last visit (6 weeks gestation) was 125 lbs. Today she weighs 113 lbs. What percent of body weight has she lost? **___9%___**

Exercise 5-2: *Multiple Choice Question*

The patient tells you that an elder at her church told her that is was because she was psychologically rejecting the baby. What would be the best response to the patient?

A. "That is simply not true, so never mind what was said."—NO, this discredits other people in a disrespectful manner.

B. **"In the past this was what people thought caused hyperemesis."—YES, this is true and explains why someone would imply that it was a psychological issue.**

C. "Tell the elder she is wrong."—NO, this would be disrespectful also.

D. "How do you feel about the baby?"—NO, this would insinuate that you also thought her adjustment was a problem.

Exercise 5-3: *Fill-in*

The most accepted theory of causation for hyperemesis is an excessive amount of circulating **human chorionic gonadotropin (hCG)**

Exercise 5-4: *Fill-in*

What is Tamiko's gravid and para?

G 2 P 0 T 0 A 1 L 0

Exercise 5-5: *Select All That Apply*

What are the risk factors for hyperemesis gravidarum?

❏ Elderly primips—NO, it is young primiparas.

☑ **Nausea and vomiting with previous pregnancies—YES.**

☑ **History of not being able to tolerate oral contraceptives—YES.**

❏ Singletons—NO, it is more common with multiples.

❏ Multiparas—NO.

❏ Hypothyroidism—NO, hyperthyroidism is a risk factor.

☑ **GERD (Gastroesophageal reflux)—YES.**

❏ Anorexia—NO, actually obesity is a risk factor.

☑ **H-pylori seropositivity—YES.**

Exercise 5-6: *Fill-in*

Diagnosis is made with reports of uncontrollable nausea and vomiting and ____5____ % weight loss.

Exercise 5-7: *Select All That Apply*

Upon admission the following issues must be addressed:

☑ **Intimate partner abuse—YES, this must be a question for every woman.**

☑ **Living will—YES, every patient should be asked if he or she has a living will.**

☑ **Advanced directive—YES, every patient should be asked.**

☑ **Health Insurance Portability and Accountability Act (HIPAA)—YES, every patient should have this information.**

☑ **Weighing the patient—YES, every patient should be weighed for medication administration.**

☑ **Patient's bill of rights—YES, every patient should be given a copy.**

Exercise 5-8: *Select All That Apply*

What laboratory finding would you expect on a patient that is vomiting and dehydrated?

☑ **Elevated liver enzymes—aspartate aminotransferase (AST) and alanine aminotransferase (ALT)—YES, these are elevated in hyperemesis.**

❏ Decrease in liver enzymes—aspartate aminotransferase (AST) and alanine aminotransferase (ALT)—NO.

☑ **CBC shows elevated RBCs and Hct—YES, these are elevated due to dehydration.**

❏ CBC shows a decrease in RBCs and Hct—NO.

☑ **BUN (Blood urea nitrogen) is increased—YES, due to dehydration.**

❏ BUN is decreased—NO.

❏ Electrolytes—sodium, potassium and chloride are elevated—NO.

☑ **Electrolytes—sodium, potassium, and chloride are depleted—YES, due to vomiting.**

Exercise 5-9: *Calculation*

The IV ordered is 1,000 mL of lactated Ringers/D%W with vitamins and electrolytes at 250 mL per hour. How many hours should the IV last?

1,000 mL divided by 250 mL = 4 hours

If there was no IV pump available and the gtt factor was 10, how many gtts per minute should it run?

250 mL × 10 gtts/ mL = 2,500 gtts divided by 60 min = 42 gtts/min

Exercise 5-10: *Ordering*

Order the steps in the intervention of administering a suppository.

_____**8**_____ Lubricate the suppository with water-soluble lubricant.

_____**3**_____ Explain the procedure to the patient.

_____**4**_____ Provide privacy.

_____**9**_____ Insert the suppository 1–1.5".

_____**6**_____ Don clean cloves.

_____**1**_____ Wash your hands.

_____**5**_____ Drape the patient.

_____**2**_____ Identify the patient with two identifiers.

_____**7**_____ Remove outer wrapper from medication.

Exercise 5-11: *Fill-in*

What are some of Tomiko's fall risks?

_____Unfamiliar surroundings_____

_____Vertigo_____

_____IV_____

Exercise 5-12: *Fill-in*

S (Situations)—The patient is _____

A G-2 P -0 10 weeks gestational age with hyperemesis gravidarum

B (Background)—**The patient has been given Phenergan 25 mg and slept for a couple of hours but woke up vomiting.**

A (Assessment)—**The patient is c/o, labs and diagnostic tests. She has an IV with electrolytes and has a high Hct, and liver enzymes.**

R (Recommendation)—I think the patient would benefit from **different medication for the vomiting.**

Exercise 5-13: *Calculation*

Odansetran (Zofran) is ordered IV. 0.15 mg/kg now to run over 15 minutes.

113 pounds divided by 2.2 = 51.4 kilograms

How much medication should you put in a 100-mL mini bag?

0.15mg/kg × 51.4 kg = 7.7 mg

How many gtts/min should the 100-mL mini bag be run piggyback with the drop factor still at 10gtts/mL?

100 mL × 10 gtts/mL = 1,000 gtts divided by 15 min = 67 gtts/min.

Exercise 5-14: *Calculation*

Normal TPN need is 25–30 Kcal/kg/day. What range of Kcals will Tamiko need in 24 hours?

25 Kcal/kg × 51.4 kg = 1,285 Kcal

30 Kcal/kg × 51.4 kg = 1,542 Kcal

So the range is between 1,285 and 1,542 Kcal/day

Exercise 5-15: *Calculation*

If Tamiko needs 1.2 g/kg/day of protein, how much should be in her TPN?

1.2 g/ kg × 51.4 kg = 65 g/day

Exercise 5-16: *Multiple Choice Questions*

Prolonged TPN should contain which two amino acids?

A. **Glutamine and choline—YES, glutamine is an abundant amino acid that protects the gut epithelia tissue lining and choline helps protect the liver from hepatic fat deposits.**

B. Arginine and proline—NO.

C. Glutamine and proline—NO.

D. Arginine and glutamine—NO.

Exercise 5-17: *Calculate*

Tamiko should receive 30 mL of fluid/kg/day to maintain hydration, so the order is for 50 mL/kg/day due to the fact that she needs replacement fluid. How much fluid should she have?

50 mL/kg × 51.4 kg = 2,570 mL/day

Exercise 5-18: *Select All That Apply*

Discharge teaching includes:

☑ **Home care needs—YES, care at home is always discussed.**

☑ **Medication reconciliation—YES, this is a Joint Commission mandate.**

☑ **Outpatient health care appointments—YES, these should be made before discharge when possible.**

☑ **Emergency number to call—YES, the patient should have a place to call if something unexpected happens.**

☐ The nurse's phone number—NO, you should not give out your private number.

☐ The hospital unit's number—NO, only if the nursing unit has a set up in place to receive outside calls and is able to triage.

6

Sexually Transmitted Infections

Case Study 6 Sonia

You are working as a graduate nurse (GN) in the outpatient women's health clinic every other Friday. It is a great opportunity to see the outpatient side of your specialty. The majority of patients who come to the clinic are for obstetrical (OB) visits or prenatal care, but there are some gynecological (GYN) patients who schedule visits. The next patient on the schedule to be seen is an 18-year-old senior-high-school student named Sonia. Sonia has been sexually active with her 19-year-old boyfriend and is here because she is having pain in her vaginal area, with redness, edema, and itching.

Exercise 6-1: *Multiple Choice Question*

What is the most common bacterial sexually transmitted disease (STD) in the United States?

    A. Gonorrhea

    B. Chlamydia

    C. Trichomoniasis

    D. Herpes

eResource 6-1:

- To obtain the latest data for STDs, go to the Center for Disease Control (CDC) Web site [Pathway: *cdc.gov* → enter "STD" into the search field → scroll down to locate and select the most recent Surveillance Report.]
- To review general guidelines regarding a general gynecologic exam, open MerckMedicus and go to the Merck Manual [Merck Manual → Topics → enter "sexually transmitted" into the search field → scroll down and select "sexually transmitted diseases" → select "general gynecologic Evaluation."]

A sexual history is obtained. Sonia has been with the same boyfriend for a year. She is on oral contraceptives. She gives a history of vaginal and oral sex. An examination is done on her and her labia are edematous with small, painful open lesions. A culture is taken of the lesions as well as a vaginal and rectal culture.

The answer can be found on page 125.

119

eResource 6-2:
- Go to the National Guidelines Clearinghouse (NGC) to view established practice guidelines for STDs. [Pathway: *guideline.gov* → enter "STD" into search field → scroll down to locate and view current treatment guidelines.]
- To learn about laboratory studies for STDs, go to Medscape from WebMD on your mobile device. [Pathway: Medscape → enter "std" into the search field → select "STD's" → tap on the "Workup" tab → select "Laboratory Studies."]
- In addition, you may want to review the following CDC Resources:
  - The latest CDC evidence-based guidelines for the treatment of STDs, go to the CDC Web site [Pathway: *www.cdc.gov/std* → scroll down and select "Download Treatment Guidelines" to view the STD Treatment Guidelines.]
  - Webinar/Podcast: Stay on the same page, scroll down and select:
    - CDC Expert Commentary: The Latest STD Treatment Guidelines Webinar or
    - Podcast featuring Dr. Kimberly Workowski, lead author of the guidelines.

Exercise 6-2: *Multiple Choice Question*

What diagnosis would you suspect?

    A. Gonorrhea

    B. Chlamydia

    C. Trichomoniasis

    D. Herpes

Sonia is prescribed a systemic and local analgesic and an antiviral valacyclovir (Valtrex) 1000 mg stat and 500 mg daily until the cultures are back to confirm the causative organism.

eResource 6-3: Go to the Epocrates online [Pathway: *online.epocrates .com* → tap on the "Drugs" tab → enter "valtrex" in the search field → tap on "valtrex" again to view information about this medication. Note: tap on "Patient Education" to review what you should be teaching Sonia.]

Exercise 6-3: *Matching*

Match the symptoms to the STD.

    _____ Thin white vaginal discharge with fishy odor.

    _____ 70–80% are asymptomatic, but many are symptomatic there is a mucopurulent discharge.

    _____ 50–90% are asymptomatic. Those with symptoms report an "abnormal vaginal discharge."

    _____ Painless ulcer (chancre).

    _____ Itching and lice or nits in pubic hair.

    _____ Intense itching with small papule lesions.

The answers can be found on page 125.

    A. Chlamydia

    B. Pediculosis pubis

    C. Bacterial vaginosis

    D. Scabies

    E. Syphilis

    F. Gonorrhea

Before Sonia leaves the clinic you provide teaching about STDs and safe sex practices.

Exercise 6-4: *Select All That Apply*

To assist young adults to decrease the spread of STDs, you should discuss:

    ❏ Leaving their partners.

    ❏ The importance of taking all the medication.

    ❏ Barriers such as condoms to decrease spread.

    ❏ Treatment of partners.

    ❏ Voluntarily telling their parents.

    ❏ Offer minimal information so they are not overwhelmed.

e

eResources 6-4:

■ To supplement patient teaching regarding STDs, open a browser and go to MerckMedicus online [Pathway: *merckmedicus.com* → select "Patient Education" tab → "Searchable Patient Handouts" → enter "STD" into the search field → scroll down to locate Women's Health Advisor handouts or any other relevant patient education handout.]

■ To locate additional material to help you understand the disease process and issues surrounding the care of patients with STDs, select the "Clinical Resources" tab in MerckMedicus and enter "STD" into the search field → browse search results to supplement your understanding.]

Exercise 6-5: *Multiple Choice Question*

The nurse understands that the patient needs more teaching when she states:

    A. "I should call if my symptoms have not decreased in 48 hours."

    B. "I should call if I think a lesion is infected."

    C. "I should call if my boyfriend doesn't believe me."

    D. "I should call if I have difficulty going to the bathroom."

In 48 hours Sonia's cultures come back to the clinic and the lesions on her labia were positive for herpes virus, but also her vaginal culture was positive for chlamydia.

Exercise 6-6: *Fill-in*

What STD is commonly found to co-exist with chlamydia? _____

The answers can be found on page 126.

eResource 6-5: To learn more about chlamydia, use your mobile device, open MerckMedicus and go to Harrison's Practice [Harrison's Practice → Topics → enter "sexually transmitted" and select "Sexually transmitted infections" → select "Chlamydia trachomatis" → scroll down to "Signs and Symptoms."]

Sonia is called back to the clinic for treatment of the chlamydia. Doxycycline is ordered.

 eResource 6-6: Go back to the Epocrates online [Pathway: *online .epocrates.com* → tap on the "Drugs" tab → enter "doxycycline" in the search field → tap on "doxycycline" again to view information about this medication. Note: tap on "Patient Education" to review what you should be teaching Sonia.]

Exercise 6-7: *Calculation*
Doxycycline 100 mg orally twice a day for 7 days.
How many mg will Sonia take in total?

Exercise 6-8: *Multiple Choice Question*
Sonia states that she is not sure her partner will go get treatment. An acceptable alternative is to:
    A. Give Sonia a double dose.
    B. Tell her to tell him that a warrant will be put out for him.
    C. Refer her to a social worker.
    D. Provide her with a prescription for him.

You explain to Sonia the importance of taking the entire dosage of medication.

Exercise 6-9: *Select All That Apply*
The complications of untreated chlamydia include:
❑ PID (pelvic inflammatory disease)
❑ Ectopic pregnancy
❑ HIV infections
❑ Abruptions
❑ Infertility

While Sonia is in the clinic you talk to her about immunizing her for human papillomavirus (HPV).

Exercise 6-10: *Multiple Choice Question*
HPV (Gardasil) immunization is available for:
    A. Women over the age of 18 years
    B. Men and women 9–26 years
    C. Women 9–26 years old
    D. Men over the age of 18 years

The answers can be found on page 127.

eResource 6-7: Go back to the Epocrates online [Pathway: *online .epocrates.com* tap on the "Drugs" tab; enter "Gardasil" in the search field → tap on "Gardasil" again to view information about this medication. Note: tap on "Patient Education" to review what you should be teaching Sonia.]

The vaccine is given in three doses, so a follow-up appointment is made for Sonia.

Exercise 6-11: *Multiple Choice Question*
The HPV vaccine should be given over what time period?
>   A. 2 months
>   B. 3 months
>   C. 6 months
>   D. 1 year

When Sonia returns for her follow-up visit and dose 2 of her HPV vaccine, she asks for more information about her herpes infection.

Exercise 6-12: *Multiple Choice Question*
The nurse understands that further teaching about genital herpes is needed when the patient states:
>   A. "I know I am cured now that I took the medication."
>   B. "I know that stress may bring it back."
>   C. "It may come back when I get my period."
>   D. "My boyfriend is susceptible."

She is counseled to take her valacyclovir (Valtrex) whenever she feels symptoms of the infection. She is scheduled for her third appointment for her immunization and a repeat cervical culture for chlamydia will be done at that time.

The answers can be found on page 127.

Answers

Exercise 6-1: *Multiple Choice Question*

What is the most common bacterial sexually transmitted disease (STD) in the United States?

A. Gonorrhea—NO.

B. Chlamydia—YES, almost 4 million new cases each year in the United States.

C. Trichomoniasis—NO.

D. Herpes—NO.

Exercise 6-2: *Multiple Choice Question*

What diagnosis would you suspect?

A. Gonorrhea—NO, this is usually a vaginal discharge.

B. Chlamydia—NO, this is usually a vaginal discharge.

C. Trichomoniasis—NO, this is usually a vaginal discharge.

D. Herpes—YES, the lesions, edema, and pain are typical of a primary outbreak.

Exercise 6-3: *Matching*

Match the symptoms to the STD.

   C   Thin white vaginal discharge with fishy odor.

   A   70–80% are asymptomatic, but many are symptomatic if there is a mucopurulent discharge.

   F   50–90% are asymptomatic. Those with symptoms report an "abnormal vaginal discharge."

   E   Painless ulcer (chancre).

   B   Itching and lice or nits in pubic hair.

   D   Intense itching with small papule lesions.

A. Chlamydia

B. Pediculosis pubis

C. Bacterial vaginosis

D. Scabies

E. Syphili

F. Gonorrhea

Exercise 6-4: *Select All That Apply*

To assist young adults to decrease the spread of STDs you should discuss:

❑ Leaving their partners—NO.

☑ **The importance of taking all the medication—YES, to make sure the STD is resolved.**

☑ **Barriers such as condoms to decrease spread—YES, barrier methods help decrease the spread.**

☑ **Treatment of partner—YES, partners should be treated whenever possible.**

❑ Voluntarily telling their parents—NO, this is against many state laws.

❑ Offer minimal information so they are not overwhelmed—NO, provide them with age-appropriate information.

Exercise 6-5: *Multiple Choice Question*

The nurse understands that the patient needs more teaching when she states:

A. "I should call if my symptoms have not decreased in 48 hours."—NO, the medication should decrease the symptoms.

B. "I should call if I think a lesion is infected."—NO, this is a good reason to call.

C. **"I should call if my boyfriend doesn't believe me."—YES, this cannot be discussed over the phone with him.**

D. "I should call if I have difficulty going to the bathroom."—NO, this is a good reason to call.

Exercise 6-6:Fill-in

What STD is commonly found to co-exist with chlamydia? **Gonorrhea.**

Exercise 6-7: *Calculation*

Doxycycline 100 mg orally twice a day for 7 days

How many mg will Sonia take in total?

200/day × 7 = 14,000 mg

Exercise 6-8: *Multiple Choice Question*

Sonia states that she is not sure her partner will go get treatment. An acceptable alternative is to:

A. Give Sonia a double dose—NO, this will not help him.

B. Tell her to tell him that a warrant will be put out for him—NO, this is never done.

C. Refer her to a social worker—NO, this is against privacy acts.

D. **Provide her with a prescription for him—YES, this is the best alternative.**

Exercise 6-9: *Select All That Apply*

The complications of untreated chlamydia include:

☑ **PID (pelvic inflammatory disease)—YES.**

☑ **Ectopic pregnancy—YES.**

❏ HIV infections—NO, promiscuous sex does present this risk, but not chlamydia.

❏ Abruptions—NO.

☑ **Infertility—YES.**

Exercise 6-10: *Multiple Choice Question*

HPV immunization is available for:

A. Women over the age of 18 years—NO.

B. **Men and women 9–26 years—YES, it is FDA approved for both.**

C. Women 9–26 years old—NO.

D. Men over the age of 18 years—NO.

Exercise 6-11: *Multiple Choice Question*

The HPV vaccine should be given over what time period?

A. 2 months—NO.

B. 3 months—NO.

C. **6 months—YES.**

D. 1 year—NO.

Exercise 6-12: *Multiple Choice Question*

The nurse understands that further teaching about genital herpes is needed when the patient states:

A. **"I know I am cured now that I took the medication."—YES, this virus is not curable.**

B. "I know that stress may bring it back."—NO, this is true.

C. "It may come back when I get my period."—NO, this is true.

D. "My boyfriend is susceptible."—NO, this is true.

7

Labor and Delivery

Case Study 7 ▰ Karen

You are assigned to work in labor and delivery today and are very excited. When you arrive at 7 a.m., the night-shift nurse gives you a hand-off. You will be taking care of Karen, a 26-year-old woman who just arrived 15 minutes ago in early labor. She is currently in the bathroom, putting on her hospital gown and leaving a urine specimen. Her background is as follows: she is at 38-week's gestation. Her antepartum course was complicated socially. Her husband was abusive and there is a protection from abuse (PFA) order on him so he cannot visit. Karen's mother is with her and is very supportive. Her uterine contractions (UCs) are mild, 30–40 seconds every 5–7 minutes. They started 5 hours ago and she called the primary care practitioner (PCP) who told her to come in to the hospital and get checked.

Karen has a birth plan that outlines what she would prefer during this experience.

Exercise 7-1: *Multiple Choice Question*
The nurse understands that a birth plan is a:
- A. Legally binding document between the patient and nurse.
- B. Contract that is voluntary between the patient and nurse.
- C. Wish list that is abided by if possible between the patient and nurse.
- D. Method of communication between patient and nurse.

Karen is in bed when you enter the room and her mother is in the chair. You introduce yourself and you can see that Karen is very anxious. She is holding tight to the side rails. You quietly put your hand on her abdomen and wait for the next UC.

Exercise 7-2: *Multiple Choice Question*
The best nursing diagnosis for Karen in the latent phase of labor is:
- A. Impaired mobility related to labor as evidenced by voluntary bed rest.
- B. Low situational self-esteem related to domestic abuse evidenced by anxiety.
- C. Anxiety related to impending delivery as evidenced by a tight grip on the handrails.
- D. Powerlessness related to labor as evidenced by a tight grip on the handrails.

The answers can be found on page 141.

Karen seems to relax with your therapeutic touch. You explain to her that you are going to do a quick assessment and then you will take her assessment history. First, you take her vital signs which are within normal limits (WNL).

Exercise 7-3: *Ordering*

Place the next assessments in priority order:

_____ Perform a sterile vaginal exam (SVE).

_____ Place her in a lithotomy position.

_____ Use litmus paper to check for rupture of membranes (ROM).

_____ Check fetal heart tones (FHT).

_____ Don sterile gloves.

_____ Drape patient.

_____ Lubricate gloves.

e **eResource 7-1:** Go to MerckManuals.com and select the Merck Manual for health care professionals [Pathway: *merckmanuals.com* → select the manual for health care professionals → enter "management of labor" into search field → select "management of normal labor" scroll down to view "beginning of labor" and "stage 1."]

Karen is placed on the external fetal monitor and is 2 cm dilated, 0 station, and 50% effaced. Her UCs are recording at 4–7 minutes' frequency lasting 30–50 seconds. Litmus paper is negative for ROM.

Exercise 7-4: *Multiple Choice Question*

What would be an appropriate nursing intervention at this stage of labor?

A. Teach patterned breathing.

B. Offer her pain medication.

C. Encourage her to get out of bed (OOB) and walk.

D. Apply sacral pressure.

You explain to Karen and her mother that you are going to take her assessment history. The night nurse had already noted the date and time that Karen arrived. Next you ask her about her obstetrical history. She has been pregnant a total of four times. One pregnancy ended in a spontaneous abortion, another in an induced abortion, and the third was preterm twins who did not survive at 22-week's gestation.

Exercise 7-5: *Fill-in*

Karen is considered a:

G _____ P _____ T _____ A _____ L _____.

You take Karen's height and weight and ask her about allergies. Karen tells you that she is allergic to penicillin and her mother confirms this. Karen relates that when she was younger she was given penicillin and broke out in uticaria all over.

The answers can be found on pages 141–142.

Exercise 7-6: *Multiple Choice Questions*

Patients that are allergic to penicillin should be given which category of antibiotics with caution?

    A. Cephalosporins

    B. Lincosamides

    C. Glycopeptides

    D. Aminoglycosides

 eResource 7-2: To learn more about penicillin and precautions, go to Epocrates online [Pathway: *online.epocrates.com* → tap on the "Drugs" tab → enter "penicillin VK" in the search field to view content → tap on "Patient Education" to view precautions.]

Next you ask Karen about the onset of labor. She states that it started approximately 5 hours ago but the UCs have become more regular in the last two. She had a small bloody show this morning and lost her mucus plug yesterday. Her prenatal records reveal that she is rubella immune and A+ blood type. Karen denies use of drugs and alcohol but admits to smoking a half pack of cigarettes each day. You perform a head-to-toe assessment on Karen. Karen rates her pain as a 3–4 with UCs.

Social history indicates that Karen lives with her mother and will collect child support from her husband. She has not seen her husband in a month but is afraid he will find out she is in the hospital and will try to come to see the baby.

Exercise 7-7: *Multiple Choice Question*

A prudent step for the nurse to take in this situation is to:

    A. Call the local police and inform them of the situation.

    B. Call the nursery and tell them the situation so they can lock the door.

    C. Let hospital security know the situation.

    D. Lock the patient's hospital door to prevent the husband from entering.

While Karen is walking around you have a chance to review her prenatal chart and find out that she is Group B streptococcus (GBS) +, so the next time she is due for her intermittent fetal monitor strip to be run on the external fetal monitor you tell her the treatment plan.

 eResource 7-3:

    ■ To view the latest guidelines from the CDC regarding perinatal group B streptococcus, go to *www.cdc.gov* [Pathway: enter "perinatal group B strep" into the search field → scroll down to locate the current guidelines]

    ■ To view Dr. Jennifer Verani, medical epidemiologist in the Respiratory Diseases Branch (RDB), National Center for Immunization and Respiratory Diseases (NCIRD), Centers for Disease Control and Prevention (CDC) expert commentary regarding Updated Guidelines for Prevention of Perinatal Group B Strep Disease go to: *www.medscape.com/viewarticle/731791* Note: you must sign up for a free medscape account if you have not already done so.

The answer can be found on page 142.

- To supplement your patient teaching, go to American Congress of Obstetrics and Gynecologists (ACOG) [Pathway: *www.acog.org* → select "ACOG Patient Page" → select "patient education pamphlets" → scroll down and select "Fetal Heart Monitoring during Labor"; Note: you can also simply enter "Fetal Heart Monitoring" into the search field]
- In addition, you may want to supplement your patient teaching with this video from The Pregnancy Show [Pathway: *thepregnancyshow.com* → select "pregnancy complications" from the menu on the left side of the screen → scroll down and click on "Pregnancy: Group B Strep"]

Exercise 7-8: *Multiple Choice Question*

Complications from untreated GBS include:

  A. Endometriosis
  B. Mastitis
  C. Neonatal neurologic syndrome
  D. Neonatal sepsis

 eResource 7-4: On your mobile device, open MerckMedicus and go to the Merck Manual [Merck Manual → Topics → enter "streptococcus" into the search field → scroll down and select "neonatal sepsis" → review content regarding etiology → tap on the drop-down menu in the upper right corner of the screen and select "Pathophysiology" and "Treatment" to learn more about the effects and treatment of GBS in the neonate.]

While you are explaining the treatment, you run a fetal monitor strip that looks like the following:

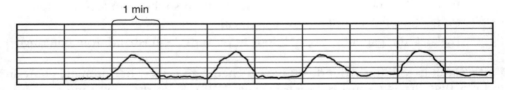

Exercise 7-9: *Fill-in*

How far apart are the UCs? _____

Exercise 7-10: *Fill-in*

What is the UC's duration? _____

 eResource 7-5: To learn more about interpreting a fetal heart rate strip,
- Go to Fetalmonitorstrips.com [Pathway: *www.fetalmonitorstrips.com* → click on "Learn more about monitor patterns and fetal distress" located at the top of the screen] or
- Go to, Monitorart.org [Pathway: *www.monitorart.org* → scroll down and select "How to interpret the fetal heart monitor tracing" from the menu on the left.]

You prepare to start an IV so that you can administer the antibiotics.

The answers can be found on pages 142–143.

Exercise 7-11: *Calculation*

The order from the PCP reads: 1,000 mL D51/2 NS at 130 mL/hr. The gtt factor is 15 gtts/mL. At how many gtts/min should you administer the IV? _____

eResource 7-6: To use an IV infusion calculator, go to:
- MedCalc.com for an online calculator [Pathway: *www.medcalc.com* → Tap on "Fluids/Electrolytes" → "IV Rate" to access the calculator.]
- Skyscape's Archimedes on your mobile device [Pathway: Archimedes → enter "IV" into the Main Index →scroll down to "IV Calc: Infusion rate mL/hr."]
- MedCalc on your mobile device [Pathway: MedCalc → tap on "I" → select "Infusion: IV Drip Rate."]

Exercise 7-12: *Multiple Choice Question*

In anticipation that a patient might need blood or blood by-products, what size angiocatheter should you use to start the IV?

    A. 24-gauge 1 inch

    B. 22-gauge 1.5 inch

    C. 20-gauge 1 inch

    D. 18-gauge 1.5 inch

Exercise 7-13: *Calculation*

The antibiotic order is Clindamycin hydrochloride (Cleocin) 300-mg IVPB (IV Piggyback) in 50 mL RL to run for 30 min. The nurse hangs the IVPB above the primary IV bag and regulates the gtts/min. At what level should the nurse set the gtts/min?

eResource 7-7: Refer back to eResource 7-7 to use an IV infusion calculator.

After the IVPB is infused you assess Karen's vital signs (VS) and fetal heart rate (FHR) and encourage her to get OOB and walk. After 30 minutes of walking in the hall you hear Karen's mother call you. Karen has spontaneously ruptured membranes and you escort her back to bed. The FHR is WNL, but the fluid discharge from Karen's vagina is moderately meconium stained. She is now 4–5 cms dilated and is getting increasingly uncomfortable. The PCP arrives and you explain to Karen and her mother that she is going to be confined to bed now that her membranes have ruptured and the fluid has meconium. The PCP puts in an intrauterine pressure catheter (IUPC) with a double lumen and an internal fetal electrode.

eResource 7-8:
- Go to MerckManuals.com and select the Merck Manual for health care professionals. [Pathway: *merckmanuals.com* → Enter "intrauterine pressure catheter" into the search field → select "Protracted labor" and scroll down, relevant text will be highlighted.]
- Go to MerckMedicus online to view related publications [Pathway: *merckmedicus.com* → enter "fetal monitoring" into search field to view "Women's Health Advisor: Internal Fetal Monitoring." Note: you can also review the information regarding external fetal monitoring.]

The answers can be found on page 143.

■ Go to MerckManuals.com and select the Merck Manual for health care professionals [Pathway: *merckmanuals.com* → enter "fetal monitoring" into search field to view recent publications related to presenting s/s, physical assessment, diagnosis, and treatment.]

Exercise 7-14: *Multiple Choice Question*

The intrauterine pressure is a device that assists with meconium stained amniotic fluid by:

A. Instilling cold fluid to coagulate the meconium.

B. Extracting the meconium with mild suction.

C. Instilling warm fluid to dilute the meconium.

D. Extracting the fluid so the meconium solidifies.

Fetal meconium is a sign of fetal distress or postdates.

Exercise 7-15: *Multiple Choice Question*

Meconium occurs because the fetus:

A. Has weak abdominal muscles.

B. Bears down in an attempt to move.

C. Releases adrenaline.

D. Does not release cortisol.

After the amniotic infusion is started Karen gets increasingly uncomfortable. The SVE reveals that she is 6 cms dilated.

Exercise 7-16: *Multiple Choice Question*

What stage and phase of labor is Karen in?

A. Stage 1: Phase 1

B. Stage 1: Phase 2

C. Stage 1: Phase 3

D. Stage 2

 eResource 7-9: On your mobile device, open Medscape [Pathway: Medscape → enter "Labor" into the search field at the top of the screen → select "Labor and Delivery, Normal Delivery . . ." → select "Technique" and scroll down to read content and view images.]

Exercise 7-17: *Multiple Choice Question*

What does the nurse expect Karen's affect to be like at this point?

A. Talkative

B. Self-absorbed

C. Irritable

D. Content

You discuss with Karen and her mother the pain relief options, which include opioids such as butorphanol (Stadol), regional anesthesia (Epidural), or breathing and relaxation techniques. Karen chooses to have an epidural so you notify the nurse anesthetist.

The answers can be found on pages 143–144.

eResource 7-10:
- Go to MerckMedicus online to view related publications [Pathway: *merckmedicus.com* → tap on "Patient Education" → enter "labor pain" and select "Women's Health Advisor Pain Relief in Labor and Delivery."]
- Go to Epocrates online [Pathway: *online.epocrates.com* → tap on the "Drugs" tab → enter "sufentanil" in the search field to view content.]
- Go to MedicalVideos to view the procedure for administering epidural anesthesia: *www.medicalvideos.us/play.php?vid=1884*

Exercise 7-18: *Ordering*
Place in order the nursing interventions to ready the patient for an epidural:
_____ Explain the procedure to the patient.

_____ Infuse a bolus dose of 500 mL of IV fluid.

_____ Have the anesthesiologist obtain consent.

_____ Position in a spinal curved position.

_____ Coach through the procedure.

_____ Reposition without disrupting the catheter.

After the epidural you reposition the patient in bed.

Exercise 7-19: *Multiple Choice Question*
The best position for the patient post epidural or spinal anesthesia is:
- A. Sitting up
- B. Lying flat
- C. Lying on side
- D. Semi-Fowler's

Exercise 7-20: *Select All That Apply*
Select all the common side effects of epidural anesthesia:
- ❑ High blood pressure
- ❑ Bladder distention
- ❑ Increased uterine contractibility
- ❑ Headaches
- ❑ Site infection

The answers can be found on page 144.

Following the epidural, Karen's fetal monitor strip looks like this:

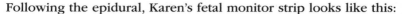
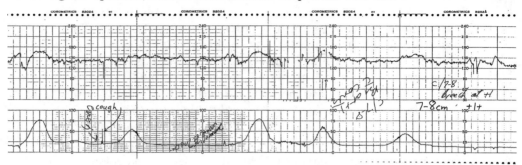

Exercise 7-21: *Fill-in*

What is the frequency of Karen's UCs? _____ minutes apart.

 eResource 7-11: To review the interpretation of a fetal heart rate strip, go back to eResource 7-5.

Since Karen's UCs have slowed down, the PCP has decided to augment labor with oxytocin (Pitocin).

Exercise 7-22: *Calculation*

The order reads to start oxytocin (Pitocin) at 2 mU/min IVPB. The Pitocin comes from the pharmacy premixed (30 U in 500 mL). For how many mL/hr should you set the pump _____

e **eResource 7-12:**
- Refer back to eResource 7-7 to use an IV infusion calculator.
- To learn more about oxytocin and precautions, go to Epocrates online [Pathway: *online.epocrates.com* → tap on the "Drugs" tab → enter "oxytocin" in the search field → select "Pitocin" to review content → tap on "Patient Education" to view precautions.]

The oxytocin (Pitocin) works and now Karen's fetal monitor strip looks different.

Exercise 7-23: *Hot Spot*

Put an X on the fetal heart deceleration.

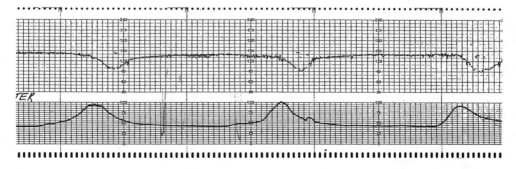

The answers can be found on pages 144–145.

Exercise 7-24: *Multiple Choice Question*
What type of deceleration is on the fetal monitor strip in Exercise 7-23?
    A. Early
    B. Late
    C. Variable
    D. Sinusoidal

Exercise 7-25: *Multiple Choice Question*
Due to the deceleration noted on the fetal monitor strip in Exercise 7-23, what should the nurse do first?
    A. Call the PCP.
    B. Stop the oxytocin (Pitocin).
    C. Turn the patient.
    D. Give the patient oxygen.

Once the deceleration is corrected, an SVE is done on Karen and she is now fully dilated and 100% effaced.

Exercise 7-26: *Select All That Apply*
What interventions should the nurse complete to get the patient who has epidural anesthesia ready to push during the second stage of labor?
    ❑ Have her pant.
    ❑ Place her in a lithotomy position.
    ❑ Check her bladder and catheterize if needed.
    ❑ Provide clean pads under her perineum.
    ❑ Encourage her to verbalize her feeling.
    ❑ Get the neonatal bed warmed and ready.
    ❑ Ask her mother to leave.

Karen does well pushing three times with each UC. She is making slight progress with each UC. The epidural drip is turned down by the nurse anesthetist so Karen can feel more of the "urge" to push. After approximately 2 hours of pushing the fetal head is beginning to crown. You call the PCP to come and you begin to prep Karen's perineum front to back and set up the delivery instruments.

Exercise 7-27: *Multiple Choice Question*
What type of precautions are used in a delivery room?
    A. Standard
    B. Isolation
    C. Droplet
    D. Blood and body fluid

The PCP holds her hand over the perineum and applies counterpressure to prevent tearing.

The answers can be found on pages 145–146.

Exercise 7-28: *Fill-in*

The maneuver is called the _____ maneuver.

After three more pushes the fetal head is delivered over an intact perineum. You stop Karen from pushing and tell her to pant so the infant's mouth and nose can be cleared and the PCP can check for a nuchal cord.

Exercise 7-29: *Multiple Choice Question*

A nuchal cord is one that:

      A. Has a true knot.

      B. Is around the fetal head.

      C. Has a false knot.

      D. Is around the fetal shoulder.

Next the PCP applies downward pressure to assist the delivery of the anterior shoulder. After the anterior shoulder the posterior shoulder slides out as does the body and legs of the infant. The PCP clamps the cord and Karen's mom cuts the cord. The baby is placed on Karen's abdomen and she immediately reaches for the infant. The infant is a boy.

Exercise 7-30: *Multiple Choice Question*

The priority for the nurse once the infant's airway is clear should be to:

      A. Promote bonding.

      B. Conduct a physical examination.

      C. Identify the infant and mother.

      D. Prevent cold stress.

Exercise 7-31: *Fill-in*

The nurse places the infant on the warmed bed and assesses him. He is acrocyanotic, his HR is 160, RR is 64, he is flexed and pulls away from the nurse's touch. She assigns him a one-minute Apgar of _____.

eResource 7-13: To calculate the APGAR

  ■ go to MedCalc.com and use the online calculator [Pathway: *medcalc .com* → select "Pediatrics" → select "APGAR" → enter data into fields.]

  ■ On your mobile device, open MedCalc [Pathway: MedCalc → tap on "A" → scroll down to select "APGAR" → enter data into search field.]

  ■ On your mobile device, open Archimedes [Pathway: Archimedes → select "Main Index" → enter "Apgar" into the search field → select "Apgar score" → enter data into fields.]

  ■ On your mobile device, open MerckMedicus [Pathway → Merck Manual → Topics → enter "neonate" into the search field → select "Neonate" → select "Apgar score in . . ." → select "Evaluation and Care of the Normal Neonate."]

The answers can be found on pages 146–147.

After you take the infant's VS, you do a quick physical assessment to make sure it is safe to keep the infant with Karen for a period of bonding. You weigh him and he is 5 pounds and 14 ounces and 19 inches long. While you are giving the infant his Vitamin K and placing his ID bands on him, the PCP is waiting for the last stage of labor to complete.

 eResource 7-14: To learn more about the evaluation and care of the neonate,
- open MerckMedicus on your mobile device [Pathway: Merck Manual → Topics → Neonate → "evaluation of . . ."]
- View video: newborn assessment *youtu.be/ijQ43e8NbZM* [no heart and lung assessment included]

Exercise 7-32: *Multiple Choice Question*
The last stage of labor (stage 3) is from:
- A. The time the infant is crowning to the time of the birth of the placenta.
- B. The time the infant is at 0 station to the time of the birth of the placenta.
- C. The time the infant's cord is cut to the time of the birth of the placenta.
- D. The time the infant is fully delivered to the time of the birth of the placenta.

Exercise 7-33: *Select All That Apply*
The four signs of placental separation are:
- ❏ The uterus becomes globular in shape.
- ❏ The uterus clamps down in the abdomen.
- ❏ The uterus rises in the abdomen.
- ❏ The umbilical cord lengthens.
- ❏ The cervix redilates.
- ❏ There is a gush of blood.

 eResource 7-15: To view videos of a spontaneous vaginal delivery, go to MedicalVideos:
- *www.medicalvideos.us/play.php?vid=146* (no audio) and
- *www.medicalvideos.us/play.php?vid=234* (with narration). Note: this video demonstrates the delivery of the placenta.

The nurse is asked to adjust the oxytocin (Pitocin) to a postpartum dose and shut off the epidural drip.

Exercise 7-34: *Calculation*
You increase the oxytocin (Pitocin) to 100 mU/min. (Remember there is 30 U in 500 mL bag.) At how many mL/hr will you set the IV pump?

 eResource 7-16: Refer back to eResource 7-7 to use an IV infusion calculator.

You check Karen's VS and fundus every 15 minutes × 4.

The answers can be found on page 147.

Exercise 7-35: *Hot Spot*

Put an X on the two spots where you should place your hands properly to check a woman's fundus postdelivery.

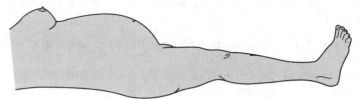

The infant is double-wrapped with a stockinet on his head and given to Karen to begin to breast-feed, which was a request from her birth plan.

 eResource 7-17: Open MerckMedicus on your mobile device and select the Merck Manual [Pathway: Merck Manual → select "Topic" → enter "Postpartum" into the search field → scroll down and select "Postpartum care" → select "Postpartum care" again and review content. Note: tap on the drop-down menu in the upper right corner and select "Initial Management."]

Exercise 7-36: *Fill-in*

At 38-week's gestation, Karen's infant is only 5 pounds and 14 ounces. Name two risk factors from Karen's history that may have contributed to a smaller infant.

1. _____
2. _____

After an hour and a half the infant's and Karen's VS are WNL. The nurse anesthetist is called to remove the epidural catheter. Karen is washed up and transferred to the postpartum unit with the infant. The nursery nurses are aware of the social situation and will only hand the infant over to a person with the correct ID band, which is Karen or her mother.

The answers can be found on page 148.

Answers

Exercise 7-1: *Multiple Choice Question*

The nurse understands that a birth plan is a:

A. Legally binding document between the patient and nurse—NO, it is not a legal document.

B. Contract that is voluntary between the patient and nurse—NO, it is not considered a contract.

C. Wish list that is abided by if possible between the patient and nurse—NO, although it is the patient's wishes, it is not just something taken that lightly.

D. **Method of communication between patient and nurse—YES, it is to open op discussion and communicate about options.**

Exercise 7-2: *Multiple Choice Question*

The best nursing diagnosis for Karen in the latent phase of labor is:

A. Impaired mobility related to labor as evidenced by voluntary bed rest—NO, she can be OOB.

B. Low situational self-esteem related to domestic abuse evidenced by anxiety—NO, she is not displaying low self-esteem.

C. **Anxiety related to impending delivery as evidenced by a tight grip on the handrails—YES, she is displaying mild to moderate anxiety.**

D. Powerlessness related to labor as evidenced by a tight grip on the handrails—NO she has not indicated that she feels powerless.

Exercise 7-3: *Ordering*

Place the next assessments in priority order:

   6   Perform a sterile vaginal exam (SVE).

   2   Place her in a lithotomy position.

   7   Use litmus paper to check for rupture of membranes (ROM).

   1   Check fetal heart tones (FHT).

   4   Don sterile gloves.

   3   Drape patient.

   5   Lubricate gloves.

Exercise 7-4: *Multiple Choice Question*

What would be an appropriate nursing intervention at this stage of labor?

A. Teach patterned breathing—NO, this will come later.

B. Offer her pain medication—NO, it is too early and can slow down labor.

C. **Encourage her to get out of bed (OOB) and walk—YES, gravity will assist decent.**

D. Apply sacral pressure—NO, this may help later.

Exercise 7-5: *Fill-in*

Karen is considered a:

G 3 P 0 T 0 A 2 L 0

Exercise 7-6: *Multiple Choice Questions*

Patients that are allergic to penicillin should be given which category of antibiotics with caution?

A. **Cephalosporins—YES, 30% of patients are also allergic to cephalosporins, so they must be used with caution.**

B. Lincosamides—NO.

C. Glycopeptides—NO.

D. Aminoglycosides—NO.

Exercise 7-7: *Multiple Choice Question*

A prudent step for the nurse to take in this situation is to:

A. Call the local police and inform them of the situation—NO, this is not necessary at this time.

B. Call the nursery and tell them the situation so they can lock the door—NO, locking the door is a fire hazard.

C. **Let hospital security know the situation—YES, the group responsible for internal security should be aware.**

D. Lock the patient's hospital door to prevent the husband from entering—NO, this is a fire hazard.

Exercise 7-8: *Multiple Choice Question*

Complications from untreated GBS include:

A. Endometriosis—NO.

B. Mastitis—NO.

C. Neonatal neurologic syndrome—NO.

D. **Neonatal sepsis—YES, this is why antibiotics are needed at least 4 hours before delivery to decrease the change of vertical transmission during birth.**

Exercise 7-9: *Fill-in*

How far apart are the UCs? **2 minutes**

Exercise 7-10: *Fill-in*

What is the UC's duration? **60 seconds**

Exercise 7-11: *Calculation*

The order form the PCP reads: 1,000 mL D51/2 NS at 130 mL/hr. The gtt factor is 15 gtts/mL. At how many gtts/min should you administer the IV?

130 mL/hr × 15 gtts/mL = 1,950 gtts/hr (60 min)

1950 divided by 60 min = **32.5 or 33 gtts/min**

Exercise 7-12: *Multiple Choice Question*

In anticipation that a patient might need blood or blood by-products, what size angio-catheter should you use to start the IV?

A. 24 gauge 1 inch—NO, too small of a lumen for blood.

B. 22 gauge 1.5 inch—NO, too small of a lumen for blood.

C. 20 gauge 1 inch—NO, the lumen may accommodate blood but the catheter is too short.

D. **18-gauge 1.5 inch—YES, this is what you should use just in case blood is needed.**

Exercise 7-13: *Calculation*

The antibiotic order is Clindamycin hydrochloride (Cleocin) 300 mg IVPB (IV Piggyback) in 50 mL RL to run for 30 min. The nurse hangs the IVPB above the primary IV bag and regulates the gtts/min. At what level should the nurse set the gtts/min?

50 mL/ 30 min × 15 gtts/ mL = 750 gtts/ 30 min = **25 gtts/min**

Exercise 7-14: *Multiple Choice Question*

The intrauterine pressure is a device that assists with meconium stained amniotic fluid by:

A. Instilling cold fluid to coagulate the meconium—NO, thick meconium is very detrimental to the infant.

B. Extracting the meconium with mild suction—NO, this is not done.

C. **Instilling warm fluid to dilute the meconium—YES, diluting the meconium makes it less detrimental to the lung alveoli.**

D. Extracting the fluid so the meconium solidifies—NO, amniotic fluid is made continuously throughout labor.

Exercise 7-15: *Multiple Choice Question*

Meconium occurs because the fetus:

A. Has weak abdominal muscles—NO, this is not the reason.

B. Bears down in an attempt to move—NO, this is not the reason.

C. **Releases adrenaline—YES, this puts the infant into a "fight or flight" mode that shunts blood away from the gut which makes it relax and they excrete meconium.**

D. Does not release cortisol—NO, the infant in distress does release cortisol.

Exercise 7-16: *Multiple Choice Question*
What stage and phase of labor is Karen in?
  A. Stage 1: Phase 1—NO, this is from 0–3 cm cervical dilatation.
  B. **Stage 1: Phase 2—YES, this is from 4–7 cm cervical dilatation.**
  C. Stage 1: Phase 3—NO, this is from 8–10 cm cervical dilatation.
  D. Stage 2—NO, this is from full dilatation of the cervix to birth of the infant.

Exercise 7-17: *Multiple Choice Question*
What does the nurse expect Karen's affect to be like at this point in time?
  A. Talkative—NO, this is in Stage 1: Phase 1.
  B. **Self-absorbed—YES, this is typical of Stage 1: Phase 2.**
  C. Irritable—NO, this is in Stage 1: Phase 3.
  D. Content—NO, this is after the birth.

Exercise 7-18: *Ordering*
Place the nursing interventions to ready the patient for an epidural in order:
  1 Explain the procedure to the patient.
  3 Infuse a bolus dose of 500 mL of IV fluid.
  2 Have the anesthesiologist obtain consent.
  4 Position in a spinal curved position.
  5 Coach through the procedure.
  6 Reposition without disrupting the catheter.

Exercise 7-19: *Multiple Choice Question*
The best position for the patient post epidural or spinal anesthesia is:
  A. Sitting up—NO, this will cause the anesthesia to only work in the lower part of the pelvis.
  B. Lying flat—NO this will cause the anesthesia to rise too high.
  C. Side lying—NO, this will cause the effect to be one sided.
  D. **Semi-Fowler's—YES, this will keep the anesthesia at the proper level.**

Exercise 7-20: *Select All That Apply*
Select all the common side effects of epidural anesthesia:
  ❏ High blood pressure—NO, it is typically a hypotensive agent.
  ☑ **Bladder distention—YES, it is difficult for the patient to feel bladder distention.**
  ❏ Increased uterine contractibility—NO, many times it slows down labor.
  ❏ Headaches—NO, this is not common but can happen.
  ❏ Site infection—NO, this can happen but is not common.

Exercise 7-21: *Fill-in*
What is the frequency of Karen's UCs? **3–4** minutes apart.

Exercise 7-22: *Calculation*

The order reads to start oxytocin (Pitocin) at 2 mU/min IVPB. The Pitocin comes from the pharmacy premixed (30 U in 500 mL). For how many mL/hr should you set the pump?

30 U = 30,000 mU

3,000 mU divided by 500 mL = 60 mU in each mL (60 mU/mL)

Desired is 2 mU/min or 120 mU/hr

On hand is 60 mU/mL

60 mU/mL divided by 120 mU/hr = **2 ml/hr**

Exercise 7-23: *Hot Spot*

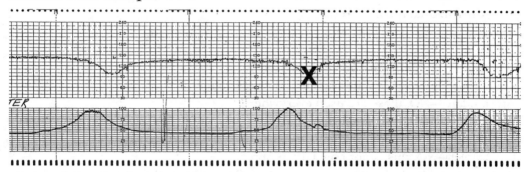

Put an X on the fetal heart deceleration.

Exercise 7-24: *Multiple Choice Question*

What type of deceleration is on the fetal monitor strip in Exercise 7-23?

A. Early—NO, it does not mirror the UC.

B. Late—NO, it is not decelerated after the UC is over.

C. **Variable—YES, it is a variable deceleration usually due to cord compression.**

D. Sinusoidal—NO, it does not have a rhythmic seesaw pattern.

Exercise 7-25: *Multiple Choice Question*

Due to the deceleration noted on the fetal monitor strip in Exercise 7-23, what should the nurse do first?

A. Call the PCP—NO, if you know the etiology you know you do not have to call unless you cannot correct it.

B. Stop the oxytocin (Pitocin)—NO, you know this may have to happen but not yet.

C. **Turn the patient—YES, you try to move the fetus off the cord.**

D. Give the patient oxygen—NO, this is not the first intervention.

Exercise 7-26: *Select All That Apply*

What interventions should the nurse complete to get the patient who has epidural anesthesia ready to push during the second stage of labor?

❑ Have her pant—NO, this is to prevent pushing.

☑ **Place her in a lithotomy position—YES, this is necessary to secure her legs, which may be numb.**

☑ **Check her bladder and catheterize if needed—YES, this is necessary every 2 hours with an epidural.**

☑ **Provide clean pads under her perineum—YES, this is necessary for infection control.**

❑ Encourage her to verbalize her feeling—NO, this is not a time to increase communication; she needs clear direction.

☑ **Get the neonatal bed warmed and ready—YES, this is the first line of defense against neonatal cold stress.**

❑ Ask her mother to leave—NO, her mom is her support system.

Exercise 7-27: *Multiple Choice Question*
What type of precautions are used in a delivery room:
A. Standard—NO, these are used everywhere.
B. Isolation—NO, this is not necessary for GBS+ moms because it is direct contact with mucus membranes.
C. Droplet—NO, this is not how GBS is spread.
D. **Blood and body fluid—YES, this is for all possible unknown bacteria, viruses and fungi that may be in someone's body fluids.**

Exercise 7-28: *Fill-in*
The maneuver is called **Ritgen's** maneuver.

Exercise 7-29: *Multiple Choice Question*
A nuchal cord is one that:
A. Has a true knot—NO.
B. **Is around the fetal head—YES, nuchal means "neck."**
C. Has a false knot—NO.
D. Is around the fetal shoulder—NO.

Exercise 7-30: *Multiple Choice Question*
The priority for the nurse once the infant's airway is clear should be to:
A. Promote bonding—NO.
B. Conduct a physical examination—NO.
C. Identify the infant and mother—NO.
D. **Prevent cold stress—YES, this is the most physiologically important step for patient safety.**

Exercise 7-31: *Fill-in*

The nurse places the infant on the warmed bed and assesses him. He is acrocyanotic, his HR is 160, RR is 64, he is flexed and pulls away from the nurse's touch. She assigns him a one-minute Apgar of <u>9</u> **(1 off for color).**

Exercise 7-32: *Multiple Choice Question*

The last stage of labor (stage 3) is from:
  A. The time the infant is crowning to the time of the birth of the placenta—NO.
  B. The time the infant is at 0 station to the time of the birth of the placenta—NO.
  C. The time the infant's cord is cut to the time of the birth of the placenta—NO.
  D. **The time the infant is fully delivered to the time of the birth of the placenta— YES, this is stage 3.**

Exercise 7-33: *Select All That Apply*

The four signs of placental separation are:

☑ **The uterus becomes globular in shape—YES, this is one of the signs.**

☐ The uterus clamps down in the abdomen—NO, the uterus rises.

☑ **The uterus rises in the abdomen—YES, this is one of the signs.**

☑ **The umbilical cord lengthens—YES, this is one of the signs.**

☐ The cervix redilates—NO, the cervix stays dilated.

☑ **There is a gush of blood—YES, this is one of the signs.**

Exercise 7-34: *Calculation*

You increase the oxytocin (Pitocin) to 100 mU/min. (Remember there is 30 U in 500 mL bag.) At how many mL/hr will you set the IV pump?

30U = 30,000 mU

30,000 mU divided by 500 mL = 60 mU/mL

Desired = 100 mU/min (60 min/hr) or 600 mU/hr

On hand = 60 mU/mL

600 mU/hr divided by 60 mU/mL = **100 mL/hr**

Exercise 7-35: *Hot Spot*

Put an X on the two spots where you should place your hands properly to check a woman's fundus postdelivery.

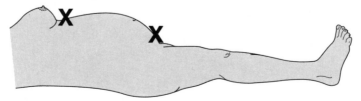

Exercise 7-36: *Fill-in*

At 38-week's gestation, Karen's infant is only 5 pounds and 14 ounces. Name two risk factors from Karen's history that may have contributed to a smaller infant.

1. **Smoking decreases infant weight.**
2. **Women who are abused have a higher incidence of low birth weight infants.**

8

First Trimester Bleeding and Previa

Case 8 ▨ Chelsea

You are the graduate nurse (GN) working in the high-risk perinatal unit on the 7 p.m. to 7 a.m. shift. The charge nurse from the emergency department (ED) calls you and gives you a report on Chelsea. Chelsea is a 28-year-old G 3, P 0, T 0, A 2, L 0 who is in 10 weeks' gestation. Chelsea started having vaginal bleeding during the night. The bleeding was slight and dark brown. She called her primary care provider (PCP) and was told to come to the ED.

Exercise 8-1: *Multiple Choice Question*
The most common cause of first trimester spontaneous abortions are:

    A. Genetic
    B. Hemorrhagic
    C. Immunosuppressant
    D. Toxemia

Chelsea is upset when you admit her to her room. You tell her all the safety precautions and ask her to call for assistance when she needs the bathroom.

Exercise 8-2: *Multiple Choice Question*
The most appropriate priority nursing diagnosis for this patient is:

    A. Sleep deprivation
    B. Risk for bleeding
    C. Anxiety
    D. Fluid volume deficit

Exercise 8-3: *Multiple Choice Question*
Chelsea asks if she should be getting up out of bed. Your best answer is:

    A. "It will not matter in the end."
    B. "It might help if you stay in bed but not that much."
    C. "Evidence says that miscarriages are not helped by bed rest."
    D. "Evidence says that getting out of bed does not alter the outcome."

The answers can be found on page 159.

Chelsea is only 10 weeks' gestation, but you use the Doppler to find the fetal heart rate. The fetal heart rate is 166 BPM. This is a good sign so you share this information with Chelsea. Chelsea sleeps during the night, but early morning at 6 a.m. she puts the call bell on because she feels as if the bleeding has picked up. You do a peri pad check, and it is still dark brown but a little heavier. You call the PCP who orders an ultrasound and an IV.

Exercise 8-4: *Calculation*
The IV order is 1,000 mL RL at 75 mL/hr. How many gtts/min is that if the drop factor on the tubing is 12 gtts/mL?

eResource 8-1:
- On your mobile device, use MedCalc to calculate the IV infusion rate: [Pathway: MedCalc → select "All Formulas" → tap on "I" → scroll down to IV Drip Rate]
- To supplement your teaching, you use your mobile device to access MedlinePlus (*nlm.nih.gov*) to provide more information regarding the ultrasound procedure [Pathway: MedlinePlus → enter "ultrasound" into the search field → scroll down and select "Fetal Development" → scroll down and select the "interactive tutorial."]

After you start the IV with an 18-gauge 1.5-inch angiocatheter you call the ultrasound technologist on call. While you are waiting for the technologist you have a discussion with Chelsea.

Exercise 8-5: *Multiple Choice Question*
The patient asks if she is going to lose her baby. The best response the nurse can give is:
- A. "No, not if it still has a heartbeat."
- B. "It is difficult to predict; 50% of these cases do not abort."
- C. "I think we should hope for the best."
- D. "Probably, because 50% of these cases go onto abort."

Exercise 8-6: *Fill-in*
What major risk factor does Chelsea have for a spontaneous abortion? _____

Exercise 8-7: *Select All That Apply*
Check the risk factors for a spontaneous abortion
- ❑ Smoking
- ❑ Intimate partner violence (IPV)
- ❑ Lupus
- ❑ Viruses
- ❑ Diabetes
- ❑ Exercise

The answers can be found on pages 159–160.

eResource 8-2:

■ To learn more about spontaneous abortion and care of the patient, use your mobile device, open MerckMedicus and go to Harrison's Practice [Harrison's Practice → Topics → enter "spontaneous" and select "spontaneous abortion" → scroll down to "Risk Factors." Tap on the drop-down menu located in the upper right corner of the screen and select "Treatment" and "Ongoing Care."]

■ Go to the National Guidelines Clearinghouse (NGC) to view established practice guidelines for Cesarean Section [*guideline.gov* → enter "miscarriage" into the search field → scroll down to select the guideline "The management of early pregnancy loss" to view the guidelines.]

■ On your mobile device go to the United Kingdom's National Health Services (NHS) Web site to view a video describing the incidence and psychosocial dimensions of miscarriage which can help you in caring for Chelsea: *www.nhs.uk* [Pathway: *www.nhs.uk* → select "Health A-Z" → on the female figure, select "abdomen" → select "pregnancy" → select "miscarriage."]

At 7 a.m. you give a walking report to the nurse coming on duty. You tell her about Chelsea's history, and Chelsea asks why you are saying she is a possible abortion case. You explain that "abortion" is the medical term for miscarriage.

Exercise 8-8: *Matching*
Match the term with its condition.

_____ Three or more spontaneous abortions.

_____ A first trimester fetal loss that does not abort.

_____ A second trimester induced abortion.

_____ A first trimester loss that was not induced.

_____ First trimester bleeding that is evidently not going to stop.

_____ A therapeutic abortion

A. A missed abortion

B. A habitual aborter

C. An inevitable abortion

D. A partial birth abortion

E. A spontaneous abortion

F. An induced abortion

The following day Chelsea's bleeding decreases, and by the time you return in the evening it has stopped completely. The patient and her family are very happy. Chelsea is voiding quantity sufficient (qs) and is tolerating a regular diet. If her condition stays stable, she is scheduled for discharge in the a.m.

Several months later Chelsea is readmitted to the high-risk perinatal unit and you admit her.

The answers can be found on page 160.

Exercise 8-9: *Multiple Choice Question*

The patient's last menstrual period (LMP) was December 17. According to Naegele's rule her expected date of delivery (EDD) is:

    A. September 10

    B. September 24

    C. October 10

    D. October 24

 eResource 8-3: To calculate Chelsea's EDD:

    ■ Go to *www.medcalc.com* to use the pregnancy date calculator.

    ■ On your mobile device, use Archimedes [Pathway: Archimedes → "Main Index" → enter "pregnancy" into the search field → select "Pregnancy calculator (1st day of LMP)."

    ■ MedCalc [Pathway: MedCalc → enter "pregnancy" in the search field → select "Pregnancy Wheel."]

Chelsea is admitted again to the perinatal high-risk unit at 32 weeks' gestation with vaginal bleeding. She is not having any pain and actually was surprised by the bleeding because she was not feeling any contractions.

Exercise 8-10: *Multiple Choice Question*

What would be the next assessment measure the nurse should anticipate?

    A. Ultrasound

    B. Sterile vaginal exam

    C. Cervical Foley catheter

    D. Amniotomy

Chelsea is placed on bed rest with an external fetal monitor. The fetal heart tones (FHT) are 136 beats per minute (BPM) and no uterine contractions (UCs) are recording.

Exercise 8-11: *Calculation*

After 1 hour of monitoring the nurse weighs the peri pad to determine the amount of blood. A dry peri pad weighs 15 gms and the patient's peri pad weighs 32 gms. How many mL of blood were lost? _____

Chelsea is diagnosed with a placenta previa.

Exercise 8-12: *Matching*

Match the condition with its description.

    _____ The placenta is at the edge of the internal os.

    _____ The os is somewhat covered by the placenta.

    _____ The placenta in the lower uterine segment.

    _____ The os is covered by the placenta.

The answers can be found on pages 161.

A. Total placenta previa
B. Partial placenta previa
C. Marginal placenta previa
D. Low-lying placenta previa

Chelsea is diagnosed with a marginal placenta previa.

Exercise 8-13: *Multiple Choice Question*
Choose the picture that shows a marginal previa.

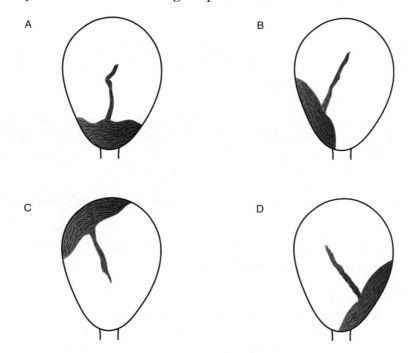

Chelsea asks many questions and is anxious. She is concerned about her baby. She asks what caused this.

eResource 8-4:
- Open a browser on your mobile device and go to: *nlm.nih.gov* to access MedlinePlus [Pathway: nlm.nih.gov → select "MedlinePlus→ enter "placenta previa" into the search field → scroll down and select topic to view.]
- Open another browser and go to the Trip Database: [Pathway: *tripdatabase.com* → enter "placenta previa" into the search field → scroll down and select topic to view (note that the content may take you to outside resources).]
- On your mobile device, open Medscape [Pathway: Medscape → Diseases and Conditions → Obstetrics and Gynecology → Obstetrical Complications → Placenta Previa.]

The answers can be found on page 162.

Exercise 8-14: *Select All That Apply*

Risk factors for a placenta previa include:

❑ Advanced maternal age (AMA)

❑ Primiparas

❑ Cocaine use

❑ Singletons

❑ Smoking

❑ Previous induced abortions

❑ Caucasian culture

 eResource 8-5: On your mobile device, open Medscape [Pathway: Medscape → Diseases and Conditions → Obstetrics and Gynecology → Obstetrical Complications → Placenta Previa → tap on the "Clinical" tab → select "Causes."]

After an hour the bleeding subsides, and Chelsea asks you what will happen next. Expectant treatment is planned. Because Chelsea has 24-hour support and transportation to the hospital, she will be discharged. Her home is 35 minutes away, but her mom is only 10 minutes away. She is discharged to her mother's house on bed rest.

At 37 weeks Chelsea is readmitted with painless vaginal bleeding. This time the first hour of observation yields 100 mL of blood loss. An IV is started.

Exercise 8-15: *Calculation*

The IV order is to start 1,000 mL of RL at 180 mL/hr with an 18-gauge 1.5-inch angiocatheter. How many gtts per min is that with a drop factor of 15 gtts/mL?

Exercise 8-16: *Hot Spot*

On the following fetal monitor strip, place an X on the late deceleration.

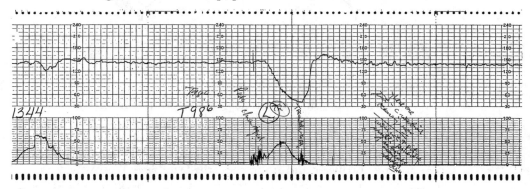

Exercise 8-17: *Ordering*

Chelsea is prepared for a Cesarean birth. Place the steps for preparation in order.

_____ Prep the abdomen.

_____ Increase the IV for the epidural anesthesia.

_____ Assist with the epidural anesthesia.

The answers can be found on pages 162–163.

_____ Place a Foley catheter.

_____ Move her to the OR.

_____ Allow her nothing by mouth (NPO).

_____ Administer Oracit (sodium citrate).

 eResource 8-6:

■ Go to the National Guidelines Clearinghouse (NGC) to view established practice guidelines for Cesarean Section [*guideline.gov* → enter "Cesarean Section" into the search field → scroll down to select the guideline.]

■ On your mobile device, open Medscape [Pathway: Medscape → Diseases and Conditions → Obstetrics and Gynecology → Labor & Delivery → Cesarean Delivery → Indications.]

Exercise 8-18: *Multiple Choice Question*

The rationale for the Oracit (sodium citrate) is:

A. To prevent nausea and vomiting

B. To neutralize the hydrochloric stomach acid

C. Bowel cleansing

D. Prevention of oral ulcers

In the OR, the fetal heart rate is down to 90 and a low-transverse Cesarean section is done.

Exercise 8-19: *Multiple Choice Question*

Pick the correct drawing showing a low-transverse uterine incision.

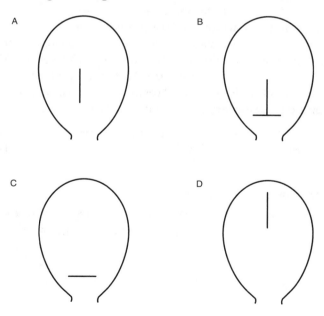

The answers can be found on pages 163–164.

eResource 8-7: Open a browser on your mobile device and go to: *nlm.nih .gov* to access MedlinePlus [Pathway: nlm.nih.gov → select "MedlinePlus → enter "fetal distress" into the search field →scroll down and select "Cesarean section" to view the video tutorial about the surgical procedure.]

Exercise 8-20: *Multiple Choice Question*

The infant was a baby girl 5 pounds and 2 ounces. At 1 minute she had a heart rate of 80, respirations were gasps, and she was limp, with some reflexes and centrally cyanotic. Identify her Apgar:

    A. 2

    B. 3

    C. 4

    D. 5

 eResource 8-8:

- On your mobile device, use Skyscape's Archimedes, to determine the infant's Apgar score. [Pathway: Archimedes → enter "APGAR" into the Main Index → select "Apgar Score."]
- On your mobile device, use MedCalGo to use an interactive online growth chart offered by MedCalc.com. [Pathway: *medcalc.com* Medcalc Home tap on "Pediatrics" "Apgar Score."]
- Learning more about the evaluation and care of the normal will help you better understand deviations from the norm. Go to MerckMedicus on your mobile device and open the Merck Manual.
- To learn more about the evaluation and care of the normal neonate. [Pathway: MerckMedicus Merck Manual → enter "neonate" into the search field → select "Neonate" → select "Apgar score" → select "Evaluation and Care of the Normal Neonate".]
- To learn more about respiratory distress in neonates, go to the Merck Manual on your mobile device. [Pathway: Go to MerckMedicus on your mobile device and open the Merck Manual enter "neonate" into the search field → select "respiratory disorders in . . ." → select "Respiratory Disorders in Neonates, Infants and Young Children."]

The infant was intubated in the delivery room; positive pressure and 100% oxygen administered. The infant responded well and no drugs were given. The infant was in first stage apnea.

Exercise 8-21: *Multiple Choice Question*

At 5 minutes the infant had a heart rate of 180, respirations were 70, and she was slightly hypotonic, with good reflexes, and acrocyanosis. What was her Apgar?

    A. 6

    B. 7

    C. 8

    D. 9

The answers can be found on page 164.

eResource 8-9:
■ Use the Apgar calculators from the previous question.
■ View a helpful video clip that will help you remember the APGAR and CHIMR screening test for newborns, go to: *youtu.be/hdAGYDzxXhw*

Chelsea's baby was taken to the neonatal intensive care unit (NICU) for observation and oxygen administration if needed.

Exercise 8-22: *Multiple Choice Question*
An infant in distress at birth is at high risk for:
    A. Hypokalemia
    B. Hypocalcaemia
    C. Hypoglycemia
    D. Hypothyroidemia

After the infant is delivered, the uterus is repaired and the fascia and skin closure done. The skin is closed with staple closure. Chelsea's total blood loss is estimated at 1,500 mL.

Exercise 8-23: *Multiple Choice Question*
What is considered normal blood loss for a delivery?
    A. Up to 250 mL
    B. Up to 500 mL
    C. Up to 750 mL
    D. Up to 1,000 mL

A stat complete blood count (CBC) is done on Chelsea and her Hct is 28%, so two units of whole blood are ordered for her. The lab calls you that the first unit is ready and you go down to pick it up. Chelsea is in the recovery room.

Exercise 8-24: *Ordering*
Place the steps for administering blood or blood products in order.
    _____ Take a 15-minute set of VS.
    _____ Administer Acetaminophen (Tylenol) if ordered.
    _____ Take VS before the unit of blood is hung.
    _____ Check the patient's blood type on the chart.
    _____ Check the IV.
    _____ Hang the blood.
    _____ ID the patient.
    _____ Have a second licensed professional ID the patient.

eResource 8-10: To learn more about spontaneous abortion use your mobile device, open MerckMedicus and go to the Merck Manual [Pathway: Merck Manual → Topics → and enter "blood" into the search field → scroll down and select "Blood transfusion" → scroll down to

The answers can be found on page 165.

"Technique" to read the proper procedure. Hit the "back button" (upper left corner) and scroll back up to "Complications of . . ." to read about complications that may occur in blood transfusions.]

After two units of blood are administered and Chelsea's patient controlled analgesic (PCA) are in place, she is transferred to the NICU to visit her infant. After the visit she is transferred to her postpartum bed.

Answers

Exercise 8-1: *Multiple Choice Question*

The most common cause of first trimester spontaneous abortions are:

A. **Genetic—YES, genetic abnormalities are estimated to count for 50% of losses.**

B. Hemorrhagic—NO, this can be a cause but is not the most common.

C. Immunosuppressant—NO, this can be a cause but is not the most common.

D. Toxemia—NO, this is a third trimester complication.

Exercise 8-2: *Multiple Choice Question*

The most appropriate priority nursing diagnosis for this patient is:

A. Sleep deprivation—NO, this is not the priority.

B. **Risk for bleeding—YES, she is at great risk for continuing to bleed.**

C. Anxiety—NO, this is not the priority.

D. Fluid volume deficit—NO, this is not the priority.

Exercise 8-3: *Multiple Choice Question*

Chelsea asks if she should be getting up out of bed. Your best answer is:

A. "It will not matter in the end."—NO, this strips all hope away.

B. "It might help if you stay in bed but not that much."—NO, this is not encouraging.

C. "Evidence says that miscarriages are not helped by bed rest."—NO, this is true but communicated poorly.

D. **"Evidence says that getting out of bed does not alter the outcome."—YES, this is the best way to communicate that bed rest may not help the situation.**

Exercise 8-4: *Calculation*

The IV order is 1,000 mL RL at 75 mL/hr. How many gtts/min is that if the drop factor on the tubing is 12 gtts/mL?

$$\frac{\text{Desired } 12 \text{ gtts/mL}}{\text{On hand } 75 \text{ mL/hr}} \times 1{,}000 \text{ mL} = \frac{12 \text{ gtts/\cancel{mL}}}{75 \text{ mL/hr}} \times 1{,}000 \text{ \cancel{mL}} = \frac{12{,}000 \text{ gtts}}{75 \text{ mL/hr}} = \frac{160 \text{ gtts}}{\text{hr or } 60 \text{ min}}$$

$= 2.7$ gtts/min or **3 gtts/min**

Exercise 8-5: *Multiple Choice Question*

The patient asks if she is going to lose her baby. The best response the nurse can give is:

A. "No, not if it still has a heartbeat."—NO, this is false reassurance.

B. **"It is difficult to predict; 50% of these cases do not abort."—YES, this is the most honest answer without taking hope away.**

C. "I think we should hope for the best."—NO, this is false reassurance.

D. "Probably because 50% of these cases go onto abort."—NO, this takes all hope away.

Exercise 8-6: *Fill-in*

What major risk factor does Chelsea have for a spontaneous abortion?

Previous spontaneous abortions

Exercise 8-7: *Select All That Apply*

Check the risk factors for a spontaneous abortion.

☑ **Smoking—YES, this is a known risk factor.**

☑ **Intimate partner violence (IPV)—YES, this is a known risk factor.**

☑ **Lupus—YES, this is a known risk factor.**

☑ **Viruses—YES, this is a known risk factor.**

☑ **Diabetes—YES, this is a known risk factor.**

☐ Exercise—NO, this is not a risk factor unless it is done in excess.

Exercise 8-8: *Matching*

Match the term with its condition.

    B   Three or more spontaneous abortions.

    A   A first trimester fetal loss that does not abort.

    D   A second trimester induced abortion.

    E   A first trimester loss that was not induced.

    C   First trimester bleeding that is evidently not going to stop.

    F   A therapeutic abortion

A. A missed abortion

B. A habitual aborter

C. An inevitable abortion

D. A partial birth abortion

E. A spontaneous abortion

F. An induced abortion

Exercise 8-9: *Multiple Choice Question*

The patient's last menstrual period (LMP) was December 17. According to Naegele's rule, her expected date of delivery (EDDD) is:

A. September 10—NO.

B. **September 24—YES, count back three months, add 7 days and sometimes a year.**

C. October 10—NO.

D. October 24—NO.

Exercise 8-10: *Multiple Choice Question*

What would be the next assessment measure the nurse should anticipate?

A. **Ultrasound—YES, virginal or abdominal may locate the placenta.**

B. Sterile vaginal exam—NO, this is dangerous and you may puncture the placenta.

C. Cervical Foley catheter—NO, dilating the cervix may increase the bleeding.

D. Amniotomy—NO, this is dangerous and you may puncture the placenta and rupturing membranes is contraindicated at 32 weeks' gestation.

Exercise 8-11: *Calculation*

After 1 hour of monitoring the nurse weighs the peri pad to determine the amount of blood. A dry peri pad weighs 15 gms and the patient's peri pad weighs 32 gms. How many mL of blood were lost?

1 gm = 1 cc or mL

32−15 = **17 mL**

Exercise 8-12: *Matching*

Match the condition with its description.

___**C**___ The placenta is at the edge of the internal os

___**B**___ The os is somewhat covered by the placenta

___**D**___ The placenta in the lower uterine segment

___**A**___ The os is covered by the placenta

A. Total placenta previa

B. Partial placenta previa

C. Marginal placenta previa

D. Low-lying placenta previa

Exercise 8-13: *Multiple Choice Question*
Choose the picture that shows a marginal previa.

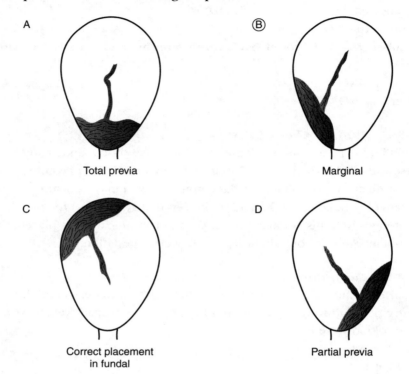

A

Total previa

Ⓑ

Marginal

C

Correct placement
in fundal

D

Partial previa

Exercise 8-14: *Select All That Apply*
Risk factors for a placenta previa include:

☑ **Advanced maternal age (AMA)—YES, this is a known risk factor.**

❑ Primiparas—NO, it is multiparas that are at risk.

☑ **Cocaine use—YES, this is a known risk factor.**

❑ Singletons—NO, carrying multiples puts a woman at risk.

☑ **Smoking—YES, this is a known risk factor.**

☑ **Previous induced abortions—YES, this is a known risk factor.**

❑ Caucasian culture—NO, minority women are at risk.

Exercise 8-15: *Calculation*

The IV order is to start 1,000 mL of RL at 180 mL/hr with an 18-gauge 1.5-inch angio-catheter. How many gtts per min is that with a drop factor of 15 gtts/mL?

$$\frac{180 \text{ mL/hr} \times 15 \text{ gtts/mL}}{60 \text{ min/hr}} = 2{,}700 \text{ gtts/hr} = \textbf{45 gtts/min}$$

Exercise 8-16: *Hot Spot*

On the flowing fetal monitor strip, place an X on the late deceleration.

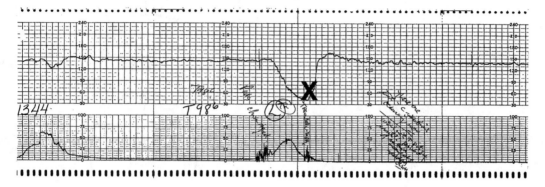

Exercise 8-17: *Ordering*

____7____ Prep the abdomen

____2____ Increase the IV for the epidural anesthesia

____5____ Assist with the epidural anesthesia

____4____ Place a Foley

____6____ Move to the OR

____1____ Keep NPO

____3____ Administer Oracit (Sodium citrate)

Exercise 8-18: *Multiple Choice Question*

The rational for the Oracit (sodium citrate) is:

A. To prevent nausea and vomiting—NO, this is not the reason.

B. **To neutralize the hydrochloric stomach acid—YES, this is the rationale.**

C. Bowel cleansing—NO, this is not the reason.

D. Prevention of oral ulcers—NO, this is not the reason.

Exercise 8-19: *Multiple Choice Question*

Pick the correct drawing showing a low-transverse uterine incision.

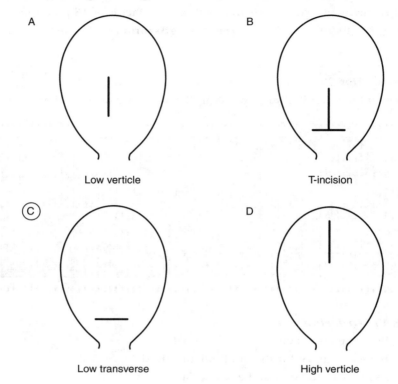

A   Low verticle

B   T-incision

C   Low transverse

D   High verticle

Exercise 8-20: *Multiple Choice Question*

The infant was a baby girl 5 pounds and 2 ounces. At 1 minute she had a heart rate of 80, respirations were gasps, and she was limp, with some reflexes and centrally cyanotic. Identify her Apgar:

A. 2—NO.

B. **3—YES, 1 off for HR, 1 off for Respirations, 2 off for muscle tone, 1 off for reflexes and 2 off for color.**

C. 4—NO.

D. 5—NO.

Exercise 8-21: *Multiple Choice Question*

At 5 minutes the infant had a heart rate of 180, respirations were 70, and she was slightly hypotonic, with good reflexes, and acrocyanosis. What was her Apgar:

A. 6—NO.

B. 7—NO.

C. **8—YES, 1 off for color and 1 off for muscle tone.**

D. 9—NO.

Exercise 8-22: *Multiple Choice Question*

An infant in distress at birth is at high risk for:

A. Hypokalemia—NO.

B. Hypocalcaemia—NO.

C. **Hypoglycemia—YES, glucose stores are used up during times of stress.**

D. Hypothyroidemia—NO.

Exercise 8-23: *Multiple Choice Question*

What is considered normal blood loss for a delivery?

A. Up to 250 mL—NO.

B. **Up to 500 mL—YES.**

C. Up to 750 mL—NO.

D. Up to 1,000 mL—NO.

Exercise 8-24: *Ordering*

Place the steps for administering blood or blood products in order.

__8__ Take a 15-minute set of VS.

__1__ Administer Acetaminophen (Tylenol) if ordered.

__3__ Take VS before the unit of blood is hung.

__2__ Check the patient's blood type on the chart.

__4__ Check the IV.

__7__ Hang the blood.

__5__ ID the patient.

__6__ Have a second licensed professional ID the patient.

9

Ectopic Pregnancy

Case Study 9 Bonita

Bonita is a 36-year-old patient who is a G-1. She had difficulty becoming pregnant due to a history of endometriosis. She arrives in the emergency department (ED) with a complaint of a right lower quadrant pain that had been increasing in severity all day. Going by her last menstrual period (LMP), Bonita is in 9 weeks' gestation. The ED primary care provider (PCP) orders:

- hCG level
- transvaginal ultrasound
- admit to the high-risk perinatal unit

You are the graduate nurse (GN) on duty in the high-risk perinatal unit. You admit Bonita to her room and take a full intake history. The ultrasound technician arrives to do a transvaginal ultrasound and an unruptured ectopic pregnancy is diagnosed by right tube mass measuring 3.5 cms, absence of gestational sac in the uterus, and low hCG levels.

Exercise 9-1: *Select All That Apply*

What are considered risk factors for ectopic pregnancies?

- [ ] Previous ectopic
- [ ] Smoking
- [ ] Previous GYN surgery
- [ ] Young age
- [ ] Sexually transmitted infections (STIs)
- [ ] Grand multiparas

e **eResource 9-1:**
- [ ] To learn more about ectopic pregnancy and patient care, open your mobile device go to MerckMedicus online: *merck.ubmed.com* and enter "ectopic" into the search field → scroll down to "Ectopic Pregnancy" → tap on "expand ectopic pregnancy" to open section content]
- [ ] Open WebMDmobile on your mobile device [Pathway: WebMDmobile → Conditions → enter "ectopic" into the search field → select "ectopic pregnancy"]

The answer can be found on page 171.

- Go to *MerckManuals.com* and select the Merck Manual for healthcare professionals [Pathway: *merckmanuals.com* → enter "management of labor" into search field → select "management of normal labor" → scroll down to view "beginning of labor" and "stage 1."]
- Go to the United Kingdom's National Health Services (NHS) Web site to view videos and materials related to ectopic pregnancy that can be used for patient teaching [Pathway: *nhs.uk* → select "Health A-Z" → on the female figure, select "abdomen" → select "pregnancy" → select "ectopic pregnancy."]

Bonita is very upset about the diagnosis and states that she does not know why "God is doing this to her."

Exercise 9-2: *Multiple Choice Question*

An appropriate nursing diagnosis for a patient in this situation is:

A. Grieving

B. Impaired religiosity

C. Ineffective coping

D. Spiritual distress

After the PCP speaks with Bonita and her family, you receive order. Bonita will be NPO (nothing by mouth) and will receive an IV to prevent dehydration during her treatment.

Exercise 9-3: *Calculation*

An IV is ordered: 1,000 mL D51/2NS at 125 mL/hr. The gtts factor is 10 gtts/mL. For how many gtts per minute do you set the IV?

eResource 9-2: To use an IV infusion calculator, go to:
- *MedCalc.com* for an online calculator [Pathway: *medcalc.com* → Tap on "Fluids/Electrolytes" → "IV Rate" to access the calculator.]
- Skyscape's Archimedes on your mobile device [Pathway: Archimedes → enter "IV" into the Main Index → scroll down to "IV Calc: Infusion rate mL/hr."]
- MedCalc on your mobile device [Pathway: MedCalc → tap on "I" → select "Infusion: IV Drip Rate."]

Exercise 9-4: *Fill-in*

You explain to Bonita that she does not need surgical removal of the fallopian tube, which is called: _____

eResource 9-3: To supplement your patient teaching, go to:
- American Congress of Obstetrics and Gynecologists (ACOG) [Pathway: *acog.org*, select "ACOG Patient Page," select "patient education pamphlets" → enter "Ectopic Pregnancy" into the search field.]

The answers can be found on page 171.

■ MedicalVideos: *www.medicalvideos.us/videos/1145/ectopic-pregnancy*

Methotrexate (Amethopterin) is ordered.

Exercise 9-5: *Multiple Choice Question*

Methotrexate (Amethopterin) is classified as what type of drug?

    A. Antineoplastic

    B. Skeletal muscle relaxant

    C. Beta-adrenergic blocking agent

    D. Antiarrhythmic

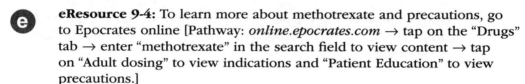 **eResource 9-4:** To learn more about methotrexate and precautions, go to Epocrates online [Pathway: *online.epocrates.com* → tap on the "Drugs" tab → enter "methotrexate" in the search field to view content → tap on "Adult dosing" to view indications and "Patient Education" to view precautions.]

Exercise 9-6: *Calculation*

Methotrexate (Amethopterin) is ordered 25 mg IM. It arrives in vials to reconstitute 20 mg per mL with NaCl. How many mL should you give? _____

After treatment Bonita is nauseous and vomits. You provide comfort care to her.

Exercise 9-7: *Multiple Choice Question*

What antidote for Methotrexate (Amethopterin) should you have on hand?

    A. Calcium gluconate

    B. Naloxone (Narcan)

    C. Calcium leucovorin

    D. Amifostine (Ethyol)

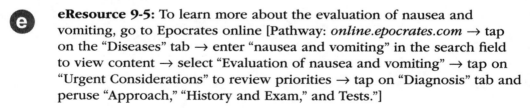 **eResource 9-5:** To learn more about the evaluation of nausea and vomiting, go to Epocrates online [Pathway: *online.epocrates.com* → tap on the "Diseases" tab → enter "nausea and vomiting" in the search field to view content → select "Evaluation of nausea and vomiting" → tap on "Urgent Considerations" to review priorities → tap on "Diagnosis" tab and peruse "Approach," "History and Exam," and Tests."]

The following morning Bonita is released after an ultrasound show that the mass in her tube has decreased by 1 cm. She is scheduled for weekly visits to her PCP in order to monitor her human Chorionic Gonadotropin (hCG) levels, which should go back to 0 before she contemplates a future pregnancy.

The answers can be found on pages 171–172.

eResource 9-6: For more information for yourself and Bonita, go to:
- WebMDmobile: [Pathway: WebMDmobile → Conditions → enter "pregnancy" into the search field → select "Ectopic pregnancy" and scroll down to "What can you expect after an ectopic pregnancy?"]
- On your mobile device, open MerckMedicus and go to:
- Harrison's Practice [Pathway → Harrison's Practice → Topics → enter "human chorionic" into the search field → select "Human chorionic gonadotropin, beta type, testing for free or total" → review information]
- Merck Manual [Pathway → Merck Manual → Topics → enter "human chorionic" into the search field → select "Human chorionic gonadotropin (hCG)" → select "in ectopic pregnancy" to review information → tap on the drop-down menu in the upper right corner to select desired sections for review. Note: be sure to review "Prognosis."]

The answer can be found on page 176.

Answers

Exercise 9-1: *Select All That Apply*

What are considered risk factors for ectopic pregnancies?

☑ **Previous ectopic—YES, this is a risk factor.**

☑ **Smoking—YES, this is a risk factor.**

☑ **Previous GYN surgery—YES, this is a risk factor.**

❏ Young age—NO, it is more likely to happen to older women.

❏ Sexually transmitted infections **(STIs)—YES, this is a risk factor.**

❏ Grand multiparas—NO, parity does not seem to be a risk.

Exercise 9-2: *Multiple Choice Question*

An appropriate nursing diagnosis for a patient in this situation is:

A. Grieving—NO, although she is grieving this is not the priority.

B. Impaired religiosity—NO, she has a belief although it is negative.

C. Ineffective coping—NO, she is demonstrating poor coping but this in not the priority.

D. **Spiritual distress—YES, she is demonstrating a typical sign of spiritual distress.**

Exercise 9-3: *Calculation*

An IV is ordered: 1,000 mL D51/2NS at 125 mL/hr. The gtts factor is 10 gtts/ mL, how many gtts per minute do you set the IV at?

125 mL / hr × 10gtts/ mL = 1,250 gtts/ hr divided by 60 min = **21 gtts/min**

Exercise 9-4: *Fill-in*

You explain to Bonita that she does not need surgical removal of the fallopian tube, which is called: __salpingostomy__

Exercise 9-5: *Multiple Choice Question*

Methotrexate (Amethopterin) is classified as what type of drug?

A. **Antineoplastic—YES, it attacks rapidly dividing cells by interfering with folic acid uptake.**

B. Skeletal muscle relaxant—NO.

C. Beta-adrenergic blocking agent—NO.

D. Antiarrhythmic—NO.

Exercise 9-6: *Calculation*

Methotrexate (Amethopterin) is ordered 25 mg IM. It arrives in vials to reconstitute 20 mg per mL with NaCl. How many mL should you give?

<u>Desired = 25 mg</u>

On hand = 20 mg/ 1mL = **1.25 mL**

Exercise 9-7: *Multiple Choice Question*

What antidote for Methotrexate (Amethopterin) should you have on hand:

A. Calcium gluconate—NO, this is the antidote for Magnesium sulfate.

B. Naloxone (Narcan)—NO, this is an antidote for narcotics.

C. **Calcium leucovorin—YES, this is an antidote for Methotrexate, but must be given within 4 hours of its administration.**

D. Amifostine (Ethyol)—NO, this decreases side effects of chemotherapy.

10

Hydatidiform Mole (Gestational Trophoblastic Disease or GTD)

Case Study 10 ▨ Lauren

Lauren is admitted to the high-risk perinatal center after being seen for the first time in the OB clinic. Lauren is a 37-year-old G 6, P 0, T 5, A 0, L 5. Her last menstrual period (LMP) was 14 weeks ago. She delayed prenatal care because she has been so busy with her children. When she came to the clinic she was worried that this time "things felt different" and that she felt like she was growing fast. She was afraid that she was carrying twins. No fetal heart tones were heard in the clinic so she was sent to the high-risk unit to verify dates or a fetal loss.

Exercise 10-1: *Fill-in*

The nurse measures the patient's abdomen and her uterus is at the level of the umbilicus. This indicates that she is _____ weeks' gestation.

Exercise 10-2: *Select All That Apply*

Other symptoms that are typical of gestational trophoblastic disease (GTD) are:

❑ Vaginal spotting

❑ Hemoconcentration

❑ Weight loss

❑ Vaginal discharge of vesicles

e **eResource 10-1:** To supplement your understanding of Hydatidiform Mole:

■ On your mobile device, go to Medscape [Pathway: Medscape → enter "hydatidiform mole" → select "Hydatidiform Mole" and read "Overview," "Clinical," and Differential Diagnosis."]

■ Open a browser on your mobile device and go to: *nlm.nih.gov* to access MedlinePlus [Pathway: nlm.nih.gov → select "MedlinePlus" → enter "Hydatidiform Mole" into the search field → scroll down and select "Hydatidiform Mole."]

The answers can be found on page 177.

Lauren is very upset that there is no heartbeat. Even though the pregnancy wasn't planned, she says she was getting used to the idea of having another baby.

An ultrasound is ordered, and vesicles are seen in the uterus which is indicative of a molar pregnancy.

Exercise 10-3: *Multiple Choice Question*
What hormonal abnormality would the nurse expect with a molar pregnancy?

    A. Elevated estriol

    B. Decreased levels of estriol

    C. Elevated hCG

    D. Decreased levels of hCG

 eResource 10-2: Remaining in Medscape on your mobile device [Pathway: Medscape → enter "hydatidiform mole" → select "Hydatidiform Mole" → select "Workup" → read "Laboratory Tests."]

Lauren asks what has caused this: "Is it because I did not come to see the doctor?"

Exercise 10-4: *Multiple Choice Question*
The best answer the nurse can give would be:

    A. "No, we do not know the pathophysiology of this condition."

    B. "No, but coming to the doctors may have helped."

    C. "No, but it may have been prevented somewhat."

    D. "No, it is actually caused by a genetic anomaly."

 eResource 10-3: To supplement your patient teaching, on your mobile device, go to:

■ MerckMedicus and open the Merck Manual [Pathway → Merck Manual → Topics → enter "hydatidiform mole" into the search field → select "Hydatidiform mole" → review overview and scroll down to "Pathology."]

■ Open a browser on your mobile device and go to: *nlm.nih.gov* to access MedlinePlus [Pathway: nlm.nih.gov → select "MedlinePlus" → enter "Hydatidiform Mole" into the search field → scroll down and select "Hydatidiform Mole" → scroll down to "Causes."]

You explain to Lauren that GTD can take different forms.

Exercise 10-5: *Matching*
Match the GTD condition with its etiology.

    _____ Malignancy from trophoblastic tissue

    _____ Triploid karyotype, 96 chromosomes (2 sperm enter one ovum)

    _____ 46 chromosomes all paternal in an ovum that has no maternal chromosomes

    A. Partial hydatidiform mole

    B. Complete hydatidiform mole

    C. Choriocarcinoma

The answers can be found on page 177.

Exercise 10-6: *Select All That Apply*

Select the risk factors for GTD:

❑ Older maternal age

❑ European descent

❑ Lack of vitamins

❑ Multiparity

Lauren complains of a headache and you dipstick her urine and it is positive (1+) for protein.

Exercise 10-7: *Multiple Choice Question*

What is the next assessment you should make for a 14-week patient with GTD who complains of a headache and is "spilling" protein in her urine?

    A. Basal body temperature

    B. Apical pulse rate

    C. CVA tenderness (costal vertebral angle)

    D. DTR (deep tendon reflexes)

 eResource 10-4: MerckMedicus and open the Merck Manual [Pathway → Merck Manual → Topics → enter "eclampsia" into the search field → select "Eclampsia" → review "preeclampsia" overview and scroll down to "Symptoms and Signs" and "Treatment."]

You also explain to Lauren and her family that the treatment will be evacuation of the molar pregnancy. Lauren's blood pressure is 160/98 so the PCP orders magnesium sulfate IV.

Exercise 10-8: *Multiple Choice Question*

Magnesium sulfate is an:

    A. Anticonvulsive

    B. Antihypertensive

    C. Antimetabolite

    D. Antipyretic

 eResource 10-5:

■ To learn more about magnesium sulfate IV and precautions, go to Epocrates online [Pathway: *online.epocrates.com* → tap on the "Drugs" tab → enter "magnesium sulfate" in the search field to view content → tap on "Adult dosing" to view indications "Safety and Monitoring," as well as "Patient Education" to view precautions.]

■ To learn more about Hydatidiform Mole, go to Epocrates online [Pathway: *online.epocrates.com* → tap on the "Diseases" tab → enter "Hydatidiform" in the search field to view content → select "Hydatidiform Mole" to view "Highlights" → scroll down and select "Treatment Options" and review "Treatment Options: Acute."]

The answers can be found on page 178.

■ Go to the National Guidelines Clearinghouse (NGC) to view established practice guidelines for Hydatidiform Mole [Pathway: *guideline.gov* → enter "hydatidiform mole" into search field → tap to select the guideline "Diagnosis and treatment of gestational trophoblastic disease" or the most current listed guideline.]

Exercise 10-9: *Calculation*

Magnesium sulfate is ordered 4 GM/hr and comes 40 GM/1,000 mL. For how many mL/hr should you set the pump? _____

 eResource: 10-6: To use an IV infusion calculator, go to:
■ *MedCalc.com* for an online calculator [Pathway: *medcalc.com* → Tap on "Fluids/Electrolytes" → "IV Rate" to access the calculator.]
■ Skyscape's Archimedes on your mobile device [Pathway: Archimedes → enter "IV" into the Main Index → scroll down to "IV Calc: Infusion rate mL/hr."]
■ MedCalc on your mobile device [Pathway: MedCalc → tap on "I" → select "Infusion: IV Drip Rate."]

Lauren is keep NPO for surgery and the evacuation is done later that evening. Vesicles are sent to the pathophysiology laboratory to determine the type of GTD. In two days Lauren's blood pressure is down to 130/82 and she is scheduled for discharge the following day.

The next morning you go over discharge teaching with Lauren and one of the most important topics is birth control. It is imperative you tell her that she should not get pregnant for at least a year.

Exercise 10-10: *Multiple Choice Question*

The nurse understands that the patient who is post-GTD needs more teaching when she states:

A. "This cannot happen twice to the same person."
B. "It is important that my hCG levels go back to 0."
C. "If my hCG levels rise, I may need chemotherapy."
D. "My blood pressure should stay down now."

 eResource 10-7: Go to *MerckManuals.com* and select the Merck Manual for Home [Pathway: *merckmanuals.com* → enter "Hydatidiform Mole" into the search field to view an overview of the follow-up and prognosis that you can use to supplement patient teaching prior to discharge.]

The answers can be found on page 178.

Answers

Exercise 10-1: *Fill-in*

The nurse measures the patient's abdomen and her uterus is at the level of the umbilicus. This indicates that she is ____**20**____ weeks' gestation.

Exercise 10-2: *Select All That Apply*

Other symptoms that are typical of gestational trophoblastic disease (GTD) are:

☑ **Vaginal spotting—YES, many times it is brown spotting.**

❑ Hemoconcentration—NO, anemia is a sign.

❑ Weight loss—NO, weight gain from edema is a sign.

☑ **Vaginal discharge of vesicles—YES, this is a symptom.**

Exercise 10-3: *Multiple Choice Question*

What hormonal abnormality would the nurse expect with a molar pregnancy?

A. Elevated estriol—NO.

B. Decreased levels of estriol—NO.

C. **Elevated hCG—YES, the vesicles secrete very large amounts of hCG and women often have exaggerated morning sickness.**

D. Decreased levels of hCG—NO.

Exercise 10-4: *Multiple Choice Question*

The best answer the nurse can give would be:

A. "No, we do not know the pathophysiology of this condition."—NO, this is not true.

B. "No, but coming to the doctors may have helped."—NO, this is not therapeutic or true.

C. "No, but it may have been prevented somewhat."—NO, this cannot be prevented, just treated earlier.

D. **"No, it is actually caused by a genetic anomaly."—YES, it is an abnormal amount of genetic material that causes it.**

Exercise 10-5: *Matching*

Match the GTD condition with its etiology.

____**C**____ Malignancy from trophoblastic tissue.

____**A**____ Triploid karyotype, 96 chromosomes (2 sperm enter one ovum).

____**B**____ 46 chromosomes all paternal in an ovum that has no maternal chromosomes.

A. Partial hydatidiform mole

B. Complete hydatidiform mole

C. Choriocarcinoma

Exercise 10-6: *Select All That Apply*

Select the risk factors for GTD

☑ **Older maternal age—YES, this is a risk factor.**

❑ European descent—NO, it is an increased risk in Asian women.

❑ Lack of vitamins—NO, it is a lack of protein.

☑ **Multiparity—YES, with prior miscarriages and prior GTD.**

Exercise 10-7: *Multiple Choice Question*

What is the next assessment you should make for a 14-week patient with GTD who complains of a headache and is "spilling" protein in her urine?

A. Basal body temperature—NO.

B. Apical pulse rate—NO.

C. CVA tenderness (costal vertebral angle)—NO.

D. **DTR (deep tendon reflexes)—YES, this is a sign to check for impending seizure from pregnancy-induced hypertension which is common and occurs early with GTD.**

Exercise 10-8: *Multiple Choice Question*

Magnesium sulfate is an:

A. **Anticonvulsive—YES, it affects neurotransmissions.**

B. Antihypertensive—NO, this is a secondary effect.

C. Antimetabolite—NO.

D. Antipyretic—NO.

Exercise 10-9: *Calculation*

Magnesium sulfate is ordered 4 GM/hr and comes 40 GM/1,000 mL. For how many mL/hr should you set the pump?

> 1,000 mL divided by 40 GMS = 1 GM in 25 mL so 25 mL × 4 = **100 mL/hr.**

Exercise 10-10: *Multiple Choice Question*

The nurse understands that the patient who is post-GTD needs more teaching when she states:

A. **"This cannot happen twice to the same person."—YES, her chances are now increased for it to reoccur.**

B. "It is important that my hCG levels go back to 0."—NO, this is true and the most important part of teaching. Should she get pregnant, the hCG of the pregnancy can mask the hCG produced by trophoblastic cancer spread.

C. "If my hCG levels rise, I may need chemotherapy."—NO, this is true.

D. "My blood pressure should stay down now."—NO, this is true.

11

Incompetent Cervix, Abruption, and DIC

Case Study 1 ▓ Lillian

Lillian is admitted to the high-risk unit for cervical cerclage. She is 29 years old and has been pregnant twice; both ended as pregnancy losses in the second trimester.

Exercise 11-1: *Fill-in*
Fill in Lillian's gravid and para:

G _____ P _____ T _____ A _____ L _____

Lillian is 18 weeks' gestation and her cervix has been measured by ultrasound to be less than 25 mm in length. Her cervix is also funneling or beaking, which means that the internal os is opening. Lillian is nervous about the procedure being done tomorrow because she knows that it has risks to herself and the fetus.

Exercise 11-2: Hot Spot
Place an X on the internal cervical os:

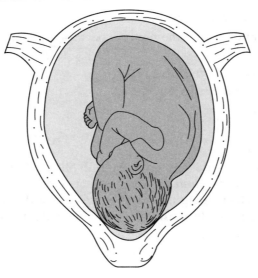

The answers can be found on page 185.

Exercise 11-3: *Select All That Apply*

Select the factors that put a woman at risk for an incompetent cervix:

❑ Diethylstilbestrol (DES) exposure is a synthetic form of estrogen, a female hormone. It was prescribed between 1938 and 1971.

❑ History of therapeutic abortions

❑ Smoking

❑ Alcohol

eResource 11-1:

■ Go to the National Guidelines Clearinghouse (NGC) to view established practice guidelines for incompetent cervix [*guideline.gov* → enter "incompetent cervix" into search field → tap to select the guideline "cervical insufficiency" to review.]

■ To learn more about cervical insufficiency and treatment, go to Epocrates online [Pathway: *online.epocrates .com* → tap on the "Disease" tab → enter "pregnancy" in the search field to view content → select on "repeated miscarriage" → review the overview and click on "urgent considerations."]

A Shirodkar procedure is done on Lillian the next morning. Purse string sutures are placed around her cervix. She is monitored for several hours and has no uterine contractions (UCs). Lillian is released to home. Lillian's prenatal course continues without incident until 36 weeks' gestation. At 36th and 37th weeks' gestation Lillian feels moderate to severe abdominal pain on her left side. She has vaginal bleeding and is taken right to the emergency department (ED) and then is transferred to the high-risk perinatal unit.

eResource 11-2: Go to Medical Videos to view a video of purse string suturing around a cervix to prevent miscarriage: *www.medicalvideos.us/ play.php?vid=887*

Exercise 11-4: *Multiple Choice Question*

What priority intervention would the nurse expect for a patient with vaginal bleeding and abdominal pain?

A. Order blood from the lab.

B. Take her blood pressure.

C. Start an IV.

D. Check her pulse.

eResource 11-3:

■ On your mobile device, go to Mobile MerckMedicus to review [Pathway: *merck.ubmed.com* → select "Pocket Guide to Diagnostic Tests" → select "Imaging Tests" → select "Abdomen-Ultrasound" and review the procedure, indications, and patient preparation.]

The answers can be found on pages 185–186.

■ To supplement patient education for Lillian, go to the American Congress of Obstetrics and Gynecologists (ACOG) [Pathway: *acog.org* select "ACOG Patient Page" select "patient education pamphlets" → enter "Repeated Miscarriage."]

Next you check the fetal heart rate (FHR) and it is 114 BPM. The ultrasonographer indicates that it is a partial abruption, and at this point the bleeding and pain are lessening. The abruption is estimated at 20% of the placenta.

Exercise 11-5: *Multiple Choice Question*
A 20% abruption is considered to be:

    A. Scant

    B. Mild

    C. Moderate

    D. Severe

Lillian is kept NPO and her IV of RL is maintained. She is also on the external fetal monitor continuously.

Exercise 11-6: *Calculation*
The order for Lillian reads 1,000 mL of RL at 180 mL/hr. The gtt factor is 12 gtts/mL. How many gtts/ min is this?

 eResource 11-4: To use an IV infusion calculator, go to:
■ *MedCalc.com* for an online calculator [Pathway: *medcalc.com* → Tap on "Fluids/Electrolytes" → "IV Rate" to access the calculator.]
■ Skyscape's Archimedes on your mobile device [Pathway: Archimedes → enter "IV" into the Main Index → scroll down to "IV Calc: Infusion rate mL/hr."]
■ MedCalc on your mobile device [Pathway: MedCalc → tap on "I" → select "Infusion: IV Drip Rate."]

Exercise 11-7: *Fill-in*
What is the fetal heart baseline on this external fetal monitor strip?

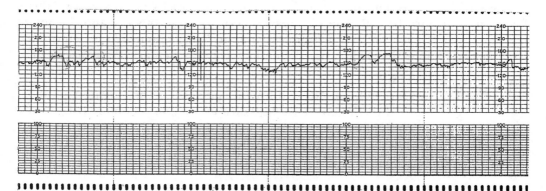

The answers can be found on page 186.

Labs are drawn on Lillian. She is typed and X-matched, a CBC is done, and a Kleihauer-Betke test is completed.

 eResource 11-5: Let's review how to interpret a fetal heart rate strip:
■ Go to *Fetalmonitorstrips.com* [Pathway: *fetalmonitorstrips.com* → click on "Learn more about monitor patterns and fetal distress" located at the top of the screen] or
■ Go to *Monitorart.org* [Pathway: *monitorart.org* → scroll down and select "How to interpret the fetal heart monitor tracing" from the menu on the left.]

Exercise 11-8: *Multiple Choice Question*
A Kleihauer-Betke test detects the degree of:
A. Hemorrhage
B. Clotting factors
C. Kidney involvement
D. Fetal-maternal hemorrhage

Exercise 11-9: *Multiple Choice Question*
A Kleihauer-Betke test is most important for a woman who is:
A. Receiving blood
B. Rh positive
C. Rh negative
D. Autoimmune compromised

 eResource 11-6: Open a browser on your mobile device and go to the National Library of Medicine to access MedlinePlus [Pathway: *nlm.nih .gov* → select "MedlinePlus" → enter "Kleihauer-Betke" into the search field → scroll down and select "Fetal-maternal erythrocyte distribution" to view information regarding Kleihauer-Betke test.]

During the night the bleeding increases again and a biophysical profile (BPP) is done on the fetus, and it is a total of 6. A choice is made to do a Cesarean section due to the cervical cerclage. Removing it at this point may just produce more unnecessary blood loss. Fibrinogen levels and a PT and a PTT are drawn on Lillian. She is moved into the OR. The Cesarean section is done quickly and the infant has a 3 Apgar at 1 minute and is intubated and an 8 at 5 minutes. It is determined from her lab results that Lillian has disseminated intravascular coagulation (DIC).

 eResource 11-7:
■ To learn more about DIC and how it is diagnosed and treated, go to the National Institute of Health [Pathway: *nih.gov* → enter "DIC" into the search field → select "Disseminated Intravascular Coagulation" and review content. Note: be sure to click on "Causes," "Who is at risk?," and "Key Points."]

The answers can be found on page 186.

■ Go to the National Guidelines Clearinghouse (NGC) to view established practice guidelines for DIC [*guideline.gov* → enter "disseminated intravascular coagulation" into the search field → tap to select the current guideline for management of DIC to review.]

Exercise 11-10: *Multiple Choice Question*
The nurse would expect the fibrinogen and platelet levels to be as follows:

    A. Fibrinogen to be decreased and platelets increased.

    B. Fibrinogen to be decreased and platelets decreased.

    C. Fibrinogen to be increased and platelets increased.

    D. Fibrinogen to be increased and platelets decreased.

 eResource 11-8: On your mobile device, go to Medscape [Pathway: Medscape → enter "DIC" → select "DIC" and review "Overview," "Clinical," and "Workup." Note: in Workup there is a diagnostic algorithm for DIC.]

It is determined that Lillian will benefit from fresh frozen plasma and platelets.

Exercise 11-11: *Fill-in*
In DIC, fibrin split products are _____ (increased or decreased).

Exercise 11-12: *Multiple Choice Question*
Normal platelet results are:

    A. 130,000–400,000mm3

    B. 200,000–500,000mm3

    C. 300,000–600,000mm3

    D. 400,000–700,000mm3

Because Lillian's platelets are low and her coagulation studies are not within normal range, after the Cesarean and the removal of the cerclage, she is transferred to the ICU for monitoring of homeostasis.

 eResource 11-9:
    ■ On your mobile device, go to Mobile MerckMedicus to review [Pathway: *merck.ubmed.com* → select "Pocket Guide to Diagnostic Tests" → select "Laboratory Tests" → select "Platelets" and review other relevant laboratory tests as well.]

    ■ Now, come out of Pocket Guide to Diagnostic Tests and enter "Coagulation Studies" in the main search field → scroll down and select "Bleeding and Thrombosis" to learn more about these important studies.]

    ■ MerckMedicus and open Harrison's Practice [Pathway: Harrison's Practice → Topics → enter "platelet" into the search field → select "Platelet count decreased" → review the basics; tap on the drop-down menu in the upper right corner to locate section content. Pay particular attention to the PEARLS.]

The answers can be found on page 187.

■ To learn more about the blood tests, go to LabTests Online: [Pathway: *labtestsonline.org* → enter "Platelets" into the search field.]

Exercise 11-13: *Multiple Choice Question*
An elevated Kleihauer-Betke result would indicate the need for:

      A. Another unit of platelets.

      B. Another unit of plasma.

      C. Extra RhoGAM.

      D. Hyperthyroid medication.

(e) **eResource 11-10:** MerckMedicus and open the Merck Manual [Pathway: Merck Manual → Topics → enter "Kleihauer" into the search field → select "Kleihauer-Betke test" → review the basics; tap on the drop-down menu in the upper right corner to locate section content. Pay particular attention to the PEARLS.]

After Lillian is treated for the Kleihauer-Betke, she will spend the night in the ICU until her blood pressure is stable and her coagulation profile is within normal limits (WNL). Her Foley output is low during the night.

Exercise 11-14: *Fill-in*
Adequate urinary output for an adult is considered to be _____ mL/hr.

In the morning, she complains of pain, which is treated. Her coagulation studies are WNL and she is moved to the postpartum floor to be with her infant.

The answers can be found on page 187.

Answers

Exercise 11-1: *Fill-in*

Fill in Lillian's gravid and para:

G _____ **3** _____ P _____ **0** _____ T _____ **0** _____ A _____ **2** _____ L _____ **0** _____

Exercise 11-2: *Hot spot*

Place an X on the internal cervical os.

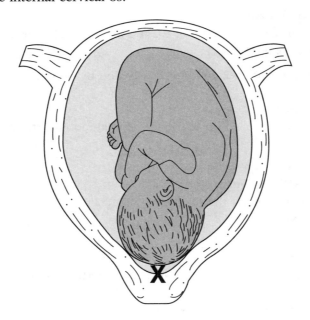

Exercise 11-3: *Select All That Apply*

Select the factors that put a woman at risk for an incompetent cervix:

☑ **Diethylstilbestrol (DES) exposure is a synthetic form of estrogen, a female hormone. It was prescribed between 1938 and 1971—YES, this is a known risk factor.**

☑ **History of therapeutic abortions—YES, this is a known risk factor.**

☐ Smoking—NO, this is not a known risk factor.

☐ Alcohol—NO, this is not a known risk factor.

Exercise 11-4: *Multiple Choice Question*

What priority intervention would the nurse expect for a patient with vaginal bleeding and abdominal pain?

A. Order blood from the lab—NO, this would not be first.

B. Take her blood pressure—NO, this would not be first.

C. **Start an IV—YES, and access is most important.**

D. Check her pulse—NO, this is important but would not be first.

Exercise 11-5: *Multiple Choice Question*

A 20% abruption is considered to be:

A. Scant—NO, this terminology is not used.

B. **Mild—YES, 0–20% is mild.**

C. Moderate—NO, this is 20–50%.

D. Severe—NO, this is over 50%.

Exercise 11-6: *Calculation*

The order for Lillian reads 1,000 mL of RL at 180 mL/hr. The gtt factor is 12 gtts/mL. How many gtts/min is this?

180 mL/hr $\times$ 12gtts/mL = 2,160 gtts/hr divided by 60 min/hr = **36 gtts/min.**

Exercise 11-7: *Fill-in*

What is the fetal heart baseline on this external fetal monitor strip?

140–150 BPM

Exercise 11-8: *Multiple Choice Question*

A Kleihauer-Betke test detects the degree of:

A. Hemorrhage—NO.

B. Clotting factors—NO.

C. Kidney involvement—NO.

D. **Fetal-maternal hemorrhage—YES, it detects maternal-fetal transfusion.**

Exercise 11-9: *Multiple Choice Question*

A Kleihauer-Betke test is most important for a woman who is:

A. Receiving blood—NO.

B. Rh positive—NO.

C. **Rh negative—YES, it detects maternal-fetal transfusion.**

D. Autoimmune compromised—NO.

Exercise 11-10: *Multiple Choice Question*

The nurse would expect the fibrinogen and platelet levels to be:

A. Fibrinogen to be decreased and platelets increased—NO.

B. **Fibrinogen to be decreased and platelets decreased—YES, they are both decreased.**

C. Fibrinogen to be increased and platelets increased—NO.

D. Fibrinogen to be increased and platelets decreased—NO.

Exercise 11-11: *Fill-in*

In DIC, fibrin split products are **increased** (increased or decreased).

Exercise 11-12: *Multiple Choice Question*

Normal platelet results are:

A. **130,000–400,000mm3—YES.**

B. 200,000–500,000mm3—NO.

C. 300,000–600,000mm3—NO.

D. 400,000–700,000mm3—NO.

Exercise 11-13: *Multiple Choice Question*

An elevated Kleihauer-Betke results would indicate the need for:

A. Another unit of platelets—NO, it does not detect coagulation issues.

B. Another unit of plasma—NO, it does not detect hypovolemia.

C. **Extra RhoGAM—YES, it detects the amount of maternal-fetal transfusion.**

D. Hyperthyroid medication—NO, it does not detect thyroid dysfunction.

Exercise 11-14: *Fill-in*

Adequate urinary output for an adult is considered to be **30** mL/hr.

12

Gestational Hypertension and HELLP

Case 12 ■ La-Neisha

La-Neisha is a 24-year-old Gravida-1. She presents to the high-risk perinatal unit after being seen in the office of her primary care provider (PCP). La-Neisha is 30 weeks' gestation and her prenatal record is sent to the hospital with her.

Exercise 12-1: *Exhibit Question*

Circle seven clinical signs of gestational hypertension.

Date	Weeks	Weight	Blood Pressure (B/P)	FHR	Urinalysis (UA)	Hct	Comments
11-11	6	122	106/62		N/N	42%	C/O sl N&V. Instructions given to eat before rising
12-10	10	124	108/70		N/N		N&V continue but able to keep some food down
1-6	14	126	110/60	164 BPM	N/N		Feeling better. Increased frequency of urination
2-4	18	128	108/72	154 BPM	N/N		No complaints
3-4	22	131	112/80	150 BPM	N/tr		No complaints— feels baby kick!

Continued

Continued

Date	Weeks	Weight	Blood Pressure (B/P)	FHR	Urinalysis (UA)	Hct	Comments
4-1	26	136	128/86	155 BPM	N/tr	41.5%	No complaints. Told to call if headache develops
4-29	30	145	140/92	152 BPM	N/1+		C/O headache and shoes being tight. To high-risk unit

When La-Neisha arrives on the unit her B/P is 142/90.

Exercise 12-2: *Fill-in*

The diagnosis of gestational hypertension is made when there are two B/Ps 140/90 at least _____ hours apart.

eResource 12-1:
- To learn more about gestational hypertension, go to Epocrates online [Pathway: *online.epocrates.com* → tap on the "Diseases" tab → enter "gestational" in the search field to view content → select "gestational hypertension" to view "Key Highlights" → scroll down and select "Treatment Options" and review "Treatment Options: Acute"; also review "Prevention."]
- To learn more about the recommended guidelines for care go to the National Guidelines Clearinghouse (NGC) to view established practice guidelines for gestational hypertension [Pathway: *guideline.gov* → enter "gestational hypertension" into search field → tap to select the guideline "Treatment of the hypertensive disorders of pregnancy . . ." or the most current listed guideline.]
- Open a browser on your mobile device and go to: *nlm.nih.gov* to access MedlinePlus [Pathway: nlm.nih.gov → select "MedlinePlus" → enter "gestational hypertension" into the search field → scroll down and select "gestational hypertension."]

Exercise 12-3: *Fill-in*

The nurse understands that the patient is not a chronic hypertensive because if she were, her B/P would have been elevated before the _____ week of gestation.

The answers can be found on page 200.

La-Neisha's mother is with her and asks you if this is "toxemia," which she had when she was pregnant with La-Neisha.

Exercise 12-4: *Multiple Choice Question*

The best response the nurse can give to the patient's mother is:

    A. "We have not called it that in years."

    B. "I am not sure if it is the same condition."

    C. "I would ask the doctor."

    D. "Yes, it is now called gestational hypertension."

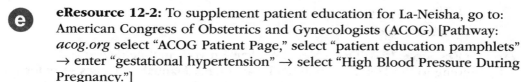 **eResource 12-2:** To supplement patient education for La-Neisha, go to: American Congress of Obstetrics and Gynecologists (ACOG) [Pathway: *acog.org* select "ACOG Patient Page," select "patient education pamphlets" → enter "gestational hypertension" → select "High Blood Pressure During Pregnancy."]

Exercise 12-5: *Matching*

Match the currently used term to the condition.

    _____ Characterized by seizures

    _____ Characterized by B/Ps 160/100

    _____ Characterized by B/Ps 140/90

    A. Severe preeclampsia

    B. Mild preeclampsia

    C. Eclampsia

Besides elevated B/Ps the second symptoms to look at for a diagnosis of gestational hypertension is protein in the urine. La-Neisha is ordered to bed rest with bathroom privileges and she is collecting a 24-hour urine sample for total protein.

 eResource 12-3: Additional educational information for La-Neisha can be obtained by:

    ■ Viewing a March of Dimes video on gestational hypertension: *youtu.be/CCxwP2Zpb3I*

    ■ Reading the supplemental materials: "Preeclampsia: High blood pressure and preeclampsia" provided on the same March of Dimes Web site. [*marchofdimes.com* → enter "preeclampsia" into the search field → scroll down and select "Preeclampsia"]

Exercise 12-6: *Fill-in*

    A. For mild preeclampsia, the diagnosis is made if there is more than _____ mg protein in a 24-hour urine.

    B. For severe preeclampsia, the diagnosis is made if there is more than _____ mg protein in a 24-hour urine.

Unfortunately La-Neisha has many of the risk factors for gestational hypertension.

The answers can be found on page 200.

Exercise 12-7: *Select All That Apply*

Select the risk factors for gestational hypertension:

❑ Primiparous

❑ Singletons

❑ Family history

❑ Lower socioeconomic status

❑ Coexisting conditions: diabetes, kidney disease, etc.

❑ Caucasian women

❑ Obese women

❑ Age extremes

e **eResource 12-4:** Open MerckMedicus on your mobile device and going to the Merck Manual [Pathway: Merck Manual → Topics → enter "pregnancy" into the search field → select "hypertension during . . ." → select "Risk factors."]

Exercise 12-8: *Multiple Choice Question*

Because women with gestational hypertension experience vasospasms and hypoperfusion, the best position to maintain them while on bed rest is:

A. Fowlers

B. Sims

C. Prone

D. Supine

Exercise 12-9: *Multiple Choice Question*

La-Neisha complains of right upper quadrant discomfort, the nurse would expect the following to be ordered:

A. Gastric acid essay

B. Pulmonary function tests

C. Cardiac enzyme tests

D. Liver function tests

Exercise 12-10: *Multiple Choice Question*

Cerebral signs that women with gestational hypertension may experience are:

A. Tinnitus

B. Blurred vision

C. Somnolence

D. Forgetfulness

e **eResource 12-5:** To supplement your understanding, return to Epocrates online [Pathway: *online.epocrates.com* → tap on the "Diseases" tab → enter "gestational" in the search field to view content → select "gestational hypertension" to review material.]

The answers can be found on pages 200–201.

Exercise 12-11: *Multiple Choice Question*

The nurse finds that La-Neisha's deep tendon reflexes (DTR) are slightly hyperreflexic. The nurse would record this as:

    A. 1+ DTR

    B. 2+ DTR

    C. 3+ DTR

    D. 4+ DRT

 eResource 12-6: To review the steps involved in doing a deep tendon reflex assessment, go to:

    ■ The Precise Neurological Exam (Russell & Triola, 1995–2006): *cloud.med.nyu.edu/modules/pub/neurosurgery/index.html* → scroll down and select "Module VI: Reflexes, including deep tendon reflexes . . ." to view content.

    ■ To view a video demonstration of deep tendon reflexes assessment, go to *www.utoronto.ca/neuronotes/NeuroExam/motor_6.htm*

La-Neisha is attached to the external fetal monitor in order to allow for continuous fetal evaluation. You receive an order to place a Foley catheter to collect continuous urine drainage in order to maintain an accurate output.

 eResource 12-7: This video can provide a good review of fetal heart monitoring: *youtu.be/DvcDXvlCXAE*

Exercise 12-12: *Multiple Choice Question*

You understand that the decreased perfusion to the kidneys will result in increased excretion of:

    A. Urea

    B. Nitrogen

    C. Sodium

    D. Albumin

You assess La-Neisha's feet and hands and they are edematous but when indented return to the surface within 15 seconds.

Exercise 12-13: *Multiple Choice Question*

The proper way to document La-Neisha's edema is:

    A. 1+

    B. 2+

    C. 3+

    D. 4+

Exercise 12-14: *Multiple Choice Question*

Later that evening La-Neisha is diagnosed with clonus. The nurse understands that this is:

    A. Fasciculations after dorsiflexion

    B. Spots in front of her eyes

    C. Sacral edema

    D. Decrease response to stimuli

The answers can be found on pages 201–202.

La-Neisha is started on magnesium sulfate ($MgSO_4$).

Exercise 12-15: *Calculation*

The $MgSO_4$ is ordered: Give a 4-gm bolus in 20 minutes and then 4 gms/hour. The dose comes premixed by the pharmacy as 40 gms/500 mL.

    A. At what mL/hr level should the nurse set the pump for the first 20 minutes?

    B. At what level should the nurse set the pump for the remainder of the time?

 eResource 12-8: Remember, you can use an IV infusion calculator:

- *MedCalc.com* for an online calculator [Pathway: *medcalc.com* → Tap on "Fluids/Electrolytes" → "IV Rate" to access the calculator.]
- Skyscape's Archimedes on your mobile device [Pathway: Archimedes → enter "IV" into the Main Index → scroll down to "IV Calc: Infusion rate mL/hr."]
- MedCalc on your mobile device [Pathway: MedCalc → tap on "I" → select "Infusion: IV Drip Rate."]

Exercise 12-16 *Select All That Apply*

Some of the appropriate nursing interventions for La-Neisha are to:

    ❏ Provide a quiet, dark environment.

    ❏ Allow as many visitors as she would like.

    ❏ Keep NPO.

    ❏ Assist OOB (out of bed) to the chair.

    ❏ Keep Naloxone (Narcan) close at hand.

Exercise 12-17: *Multiple Choice Questions*

The nurse understands that the first sign of $MgSO_4$ toxicity is:

    A. Decrease respirations.

    B. Decreased affect.

    C. Decreased DTR.

    D. Decreased B/P.

La-Neisha's mother stays at the hospital with her. During the night La-Neisha's mother calls the rapid response team (RRT). She uses the code numbers on the phone because, she says, "La-Neisha is staring into space and not answering." La-Neisha has had a seizure.

Exercise 12-18: *Multiple Choice Question*

The priority during the seizure is to:

    A. Provide oxygen.

    B. Call a full-blown cardiac code.

    C. Pad the bed rails.

    D. Turn to the left side.

After the seizure La-Neisha is in a postictal state, and oxygen is provided at 10 L via mask. Hydrazaline (Apresoline) is given stat.

The answers can be found on pages 202–203.

eResource 12-9: To review drug information about Apresoline, go to Medscape on your mobile device [Pathway: Medscape → enter "Apresoline" in the search field → tap on "Apresoline" to view dosage, drug interactions and contraindications and warnings]

Exercise 12-19: *Fill-in*

The fetal monitor strip below shows the fetal heart rate (FHR) during the seizure.

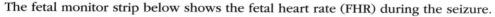

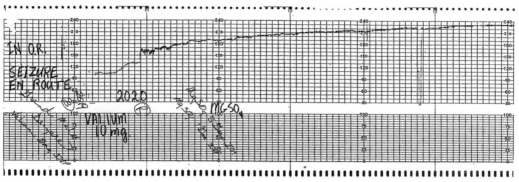

The fetal heart rate is _____

After the seizure, the fetal heart rates are within normal limits (WNL). So the decision is made to prepare La-Neisha for a Cesarean birth in the morning. The NICU staff is notified because she is only 30-1/7 weeks' gestation.

Exercise 12-20: *Multiple Choice Question*

During the next assessment, La-Neisha's respiration rate is 14, the nurse should:

      A. Continue the $MgSO_4$ infusion.

      B. Decrease the $MgSO_4$ infusion.

      C. Increase the $MgSO_4$ infusion.

      D. Stop the $MgSO_4$ infusion.

 eResource 12-10: To review drug information about magnesium sulfate IV, go to Epocrates online [Pathway: *online.epocrates.com* → tap on the "Drugs" tab → enter "magnesium sulfate" in the search field to view content → tap on "Adult dosing" to view indications "Safety and Monitoring," as well as "Patient Education" to view precautions.]

Labs results are obtained for La-Neisha. The results reveal she has HELLP syndrome.

Exercise 12-21: *Fill-in*

Fill in the conditions that the acronym HELLP stands for:

      A. H _____

      B. E _____

      C. L _____

      D. L _____

      E. P _____

The answers can be found on page 203.

eResource 12-11: To learn more about the HELLP syndrome, open a browser on your mobile device and go to the National Library of Medicine to access MedlinePlus [Pathway: *www.nlm.nih.gov* → select "MedlinePlus" → enter "HELLP syndrome" into the search field → scroll down and select "HELLP syndrome and your Pregnancy" and "HELLP syndrome."]

Exercise 12-22: *Multiple Choice Question*

La-Neisha's lactic acid dehydrogenase (LDH), aspartate transaminase (AST)—also called serum glutamic oxaloacetic transaminase (SGOT)—and alanine transaminase (ALT)—also called serum glutamic pyruvic transaminase (SGPT)—are elevated.

 eResource 12-12: Look these blood tests and normal values on your mobile device, go to Mobile MerckMedicus to review [Pathway: MerckMedicus → select "Pocket Guide to Diagnostic Tests" → select "Laboratory Tests" → select and review laboratory tests.]

What clinical symptom does the nurse expect to increase in severity?

    A. Headache

    B. RUQ pain

    C. CVA tenderness

    D. Muscle irritability

 eResource 12-13: To learn more about the management of HELLP syndrome,

    ■ Go to Epocrates online [Pathway: *online.epocrates.com* → tap on the "Diseases" tab → enter "HELLP" in the search field to view content → select "HELLP syndrome in pregnancy" → review "Key Highlights," "Treatment," and other relevant sections] or

    ■ On your mobile device, open MerckMedicus and go to:

        ■ Harrison's Practice [Pathway → Harrison's Practice → Topics → enter "HELLP" into the search field → select "HELLP" → review information—focusing on S/S and Treatment (be sure to look at PEARLS)]

        ■ Merck Manual [Pathway: Merck Manual → Topics → enter "HELLP" into the search field → select "HELLP syndrome" → review content.]

The decision is to move the Cesarean birth up and La-Neisha is moved to the OR. The nurse calls the blood bank for the products ordered.

Exercise 12-23: *Multiple Choice Question*

The blood products the nurse would expect to transfuse for a patient with HELLP syndrome are:

    A. Whole blood and platelets

    B. RhoGAM and whole blood

    C. Whole blood and plasma

    D. Plasma and platelets

The answers can be found on pages 203–204.

eResource 12-14: To learn more about this surgical procedure, go to
■ MerckMedicus on your mobile device and go Merck Manual [Pathway: Merck Manual → Topics → enter "cesarean" into the search field → select "Cesarean section → review content.]
■ Go to MedicalVideos to view a video of a Cesarean section: *www.medicalvideos.us/videos/99/cesarean-section.*

La-Neisha does well during the Cesarean. The infant is taken to the NICU because of his premature status. Postoperative La-Neisha is monitored in the high-risk unit.

Exercise 12-24: *Fill-in*
The nurse understands that eclamptic patients have a high risk of seizures for the first _____ hours postpartum.

 eResource 12-15: Harrison's Practice [Pathway: Harrison's Practice → Topics → enter "eclampsia" into the search field → select "Eclampsia" → review information in "Basics" section—focus on "Ongoing Care."]

The answers can be found on page 204.

Answers

Exercise 12-1: *Exhibit Question*

Circle seven clinical signs of gestational hypertension.

Date	Weeks	Weight	Blood Pressure B/P	FHR	Urinalysis (UA)	Hct	Comments
11-11	6	122	106/62		N/N	42%	C/O sl N&V. Instructions given to eat before rising
12-10	10	124	108/70		N/N		N&V continue but able to keep some food down.
1-6	14	126	110/60	164 BPM	N/N		Feeling better. Increased frequency of urination.
2-4	18	128	108/72	154 BPM	N/N		No complaints.
3-4	22	131	112/80	150 BPM	(N/tr)		No complaints— feels baby kick!
4-1	26	136	(128/86)	155 BPM	(N/tr)	41.5%	No complaints. Told to call if headache develops
4-29	30	(145)	(140/92)	152 BPM	(N/1+)		(C/O headache and shoes being tight.) To high-risk unit.

Exercise 12-2: *Fill-in*

The diagnosis of gestational hypertension is made when there are at two B/Ps 140/90 at least **6** hours apart.

Exercise 12-3: *Fill-in*

The nurse understands that the patient is not a chronic hypertensive because if she were, her B/P would have been elevated before the ___**20**___ weeks of gestation.

Exercise 12-4: *Multiple Choice Question*

The best response the nurse can give to the patient's mother is:
A. "We have not called it that in years."—NO, this is condescending.
B. "I am not sure if it is the same condition."—NO, this provides no information.
C. "I would ask the doctor."—NO, this provides no information.
D. **"Yes, it is now called gestational hypertension."—YES, this is appropriate, not condescending and provides information.**

Exercise 12-5: *Matching*

Match the currently used term to the condition.
___**C**___ Characterized by seizures
___**A**___ Characterized by B/Ps 160/100
___**B**___ Characterized by B/Ps 140/90
A. Severe pre-eclampsia
B. Mild pre-eclampsia
C. Eclampsia

Exercise 12-6: *Fill-in*

A. For mild preeclampsia the diagnosis is made if there is more than ___**300**___ mg protein in a 24-hour urine.
B. For severe preeclampsia the diagnosis is made if there is more than ___**500**___ mg protein in a 24-hour urine.

Exercise 12-7: *Select All That Apply*

Select the risk factors for gestational hypertension:
☑ **Primiparous—YES, this is a risk factor.**
☐ Singletons—NO, multiples increases the risk.
☑ **Family history—YES, this is a risk factor.**
☑ **Lower socioeconomic status—YES, this is a risk factor.**
☑ **Coexisting conditions: diabetes, kidney disease, etc.—YES, this is a risk factor.**
☐ Caucasian women—NO, African-American and Black women have increased risk.
☑ **Obese women—YES, this is a risk factor.**
☑ **Age extremes—YES, this is a risk factor.**

Exercise 12-8: *Multiple Choice Question*

Because women with gestational hypertension experience vasospasms and hypoperfusion the best position to maintain them in while on bed rest is:

A. Fowlers—NO.

B. **Sims—YES, side lying, increases blood flow to the placenta.**

C. Prone—NO.

D. Supine—NO, this compresses the vena cava and decreases placental blood flow.

Exercise 12-9: *Multiple Choice Question*

La-Neisha complains of right upper quadrant discomfort, the nurse would expect the following to be ordered:

A. Gastric acid essay—NO, this is not a Gastrointestinal (GI) problem.

B. Pulmonary function tests—NO, this is not a pulmonary condition, although gestational hypertension can lead to pulmonary edema in its later stages.

C. Cardiac enzyme tests—NO, this is not a cardiac issues

D. **Liver function tests—YES, the liver capsule is edematous from vasospasms.**

Exercise 12-10: *Multiple Choice Question*

Cerebral signs that women with gestational hypertension may experience are:

A. Tinnitus—NO, this is not a typical symptom.

B. **Blurred vision—YES, this is caused by decreased cerebral perfusion.**

C. Somnolence—NO, this is not a typical symptom but may occur with $MgSO_4$ infusion.

D. Forgetfulness—NO, this is not a typical symptom.

Exercise 12-11: *Multiple Choice Question*

The nurse finds that La-Neisha's deep tendon reflexes (DTR) are slightly hyperreflexic. The nurse would record this as:

A. 1+ DTR—NO, this is hyporeflexic.

B. 2+ DTR—NO, this is normal reflex response.

C. **3+ DTR—YES, this is slightly hyperreflexic.**

D. 4+ DRT—NO, this is severe hyperreflexia.

Exercise 12-12: *Multiple Choice Question*

You understand that the decreased perfusion to the kidneys will result in increased excretion of:

A. Urea—NO, this is retained and elevated in the central circulation.

B. Nitrogen—NO, this is retained and elevated in the central circulation.

C. Sodium—NO, this is retained and elevated in the central circulation.

D. **Albumin—YES, this is excreted at increased amounts.**

Exercise 12-13: *Multiple Choice Question*

The proper way to document La-Neisha's edema is:

A. **1+—YES, if the pitting lasts 0–15 sec.**

B. 2+—NO, if the pitting lasts 16–30 sec.

C. 3+—NO, if the pitting lasts 31–60 sec.

D. 4+—NO, is if the pitting lasts >60 sec.

Exercise 12-14: *Multiple Choice Question*

Later that evening La-Neisha is diagnosed with clonus. The nurse understands that this is:

A. **Fasciculations after dorsiflexion—YES, there are extra beats due to muscle irritation.**

B. Spots in front of her eyes—NO, this is a cerebral symptoms.

C. Sacral edema—NO, this is a vascular symptom.

D. Decrease response to stimuli—No, this is neurological.

Exercise 12-15: *Calculation*

$MgSO_4$ is ordered: Give a 4-gm bolus in 20 minutes and then 4 gms/hour. The dose comes premixed by the pharmacy as 40 gms/500 mL.

A. At what mL/hr level should the nurse set the pump for the first 20 minutes?
500 mL divided by 40 gms = 1 gm /12.5 mL × 4 = 50 mL in 20 min. or 0.3 hours
50 mL × .03 = **150 mL/hr for the first 20 minutes**

B. At what level should the nurse set the pump at for the remainder of the time?
50 mL/hr

Exercise 12-16: *Select All That Apply*

Some of the appropriate nursing interventions for La-Neisha are to:

☑ **Provide a quiet, dark environment—YES, decrease neurological stimulation.**

☐ Allow as many visitors as she would like—NO, this is one condition in which excessive stimulation should be avoided.

☑ **Keep NPO—YES, in case of a seizure to decrease aspiration.**

☐ Assist OOB (out of bed) to the chair—NO, this is not recommended if she is on $MgSO_4$.

☐ Keep Naloxone (Narcan) close at hand—NO, keep calcium gluconate on hand as the $MgSO_4$ antidote.

Exercise 12-17: *Multiple Choice Questions*

The nurse understands that the first sign of $MgSO_4$ toxicity is:

A. Decrease respirations—NO.

B. Decreased affect—NO.

C. **Decreased DTRs—Yes, this is typically the first sign so DTRs need to be assessed often.**

D. Decreased B/P—NO.

Exercise 12-18: *Multiple Choice Question*

The priority during the seizure is to:

A. Provide oxygen—NO, this could be traumatic getting it on during a seizure.

B. Call a full blown cardiac code—NO, she does not need CPR.

C. Pad the bed rails—NO, it is too late for this.

D. **Turn to the left side—YES, this will help oxygenate the fetus and keep La-Neisha's airway patent.**

Exercise 12-19: *Fill-in*

The fetal heart rate is **tachycardic** indicating a period of fetal distress.

Exercise 12-20: *Multiple Choice Question*

During the next assessment, La-Neisha's respiration rate is 14, the nurse should:

A. **Continue the $MgSO_4$ infusion.—YES, you would stop it if RR fell below 12 per minute.**

B. Decrease the $MgSO_4$ infusion.—NO.

C. Increase the $MgSO_4$ infusion.—NO.

D. Stop the $MgSO_4$ infusion.—NO.

Exercise 12-21: *Fill-in*

Fill in the conditions that the acronym HELLP stands for:

A. H **Hemolysis**

B. E **Elevated**

C. L **Liver Enzymes**

D. L **Low**

E. P **Platelets**

Exercise 12-22: *Multiple Choice Question*

La-Neisha's lactic acid dehydrogenase (LDH), aspartate transaminase (AST)—also called serum glutamic oxaloacetic transaminase (SGOT)—and alanine transaminase (ALT)—also called serum glutamic pyruvic transaminase (SGPT)—are elevated. What clinical symptom does the nurse expect to increase in severity?

A. Headache—NO, these do not indicate a cerebral condition.

B. **RUQ pain—YES, liver enlargement due to vasospasms.**

C. CVA tenderness—NO, these are not kidney function tests.

D. Muscle irritability—NO, these are not indicative of muscle function.

Exercise 12-23: *Multiple Choice Question*

The blood products the nurse would expect to transfuse for a patient with HELLP syndrome are:

A. Whole blood and platelets—NO, whole blood increases volume too rapidly.

B. RhoGAM and whole blood—NO, RhoGAM is used postpartally for Rh-patients.

C. Whole blood and packed RBCs—NO.

D. **Packed RBCs and platelets—YES, platelets are needed for clotting and packed RBCs are needed to counteract the hemolysis.**

Exercise 12-24: *Fill-in*

The nurse understands that eclamptic patients have a high risk of seizures for the first ___**24**___ hours postpartum.

Reference

Russell, S., & Triola, M. (1995–2006). *The Precise Neurological Exam,* New York University School of Medicine. Available: *http://cloud.med.nyu.edu/modules/pub/neurosurgery/index.html.*

13

Gestational Diabetes (GD)

Case Study 13 ▨ Margaret

Margaret is admitted to the high-risk perinatal unit for adjustment of her insulin. She is a gestational diabetic for the first time. Her obstetrical history includes two previous infants both over 9 pounds. She is 36 years old and is 32 weeks' pregnant. She was placed on insulin therapy at 26 weeks' gestation.

eResource 13-1:
- ■ To read the recommended guidelines for screening and care go to the National Guidelines Clearinghouse (NGC) [Pathway: *guideline.gov* → enter "gestational diabetes" into search field.]
  - ■ For screening guidelines, → tap to select the guideline "Screening for Gestational diabetes. . . ." or the most current listed screening guideline.]
  - ■ For care guidelines: → tap to select the guideline "Gestational diabetes mellitus (GDM). Evidence-based nutrition practice guideline" or the most current listed guideline.
- ■ Open a browser on your mobile device and go to: *nlm.nih.gov* to access MedlinePlus [Pathway: nlm.nih.gov → select "MedlinePlus" → enter "gestational hypertension" into the search field → scroll down and select "gestational hypertension."]

Exercise 13-1: *Multiple Choice Question*
Gestational diabetes was diagnosed at 24 weeks after a routine screening 1-hour glucose tolerance test (GTT) revealed a blood glucose level above:

    A. 130 mg/dL

    B. 135 mg/dL

    C. 140 mg/dL

    D. 150 mg/dL

eResource 13-2: To learn more about the GTT, go to MerckMedicus on your mobile device and open the Pocket Guide to Diagnostic Tests [Pathway: Pocket Guide → enter "GTT" into the search field → select "GTT" to review information. Note: be sure to look at "Comments."]

The answer can be found on page 213.   **205**

Exercise 13-2: *Matching*

Match the terms to the condition.

_____ Absolute insulin deficiency that usually appears before age 30.

_____ Glucose intolerance during pregnancy.

_____ Hyperglycemia at levels lower than what qualifies for gestational diabetes (GD).

_____ Insulin resistance or deficiency usually diagnosed after age 30.

A. Type I diabetes

B. Type II diabetes

C. Impaired glucose tolerance

D. Gestational diabetes mellitus

Exercise 13-3: *Multiple Choice Question*

Margaret's diabetes was not noticed in her first trimester because:

A. Her glucose was not routinely checked.

B. She fasted before she came for her office visit.

C. There was physiologically less insulin resistance.

D. She consumed less glucose.

Exercise 13-4: *Multiple Choice Question*

The placental hormones in pregnancy that cause insulin resistance are:

A. Human placental lactogen (hPL) and estriol.

B. Progesterone and estriol.

C. Progesterone and somatotropin.

D. Human placental lactogen and somatotropin.

Exercise 13-5: *Fill-in*

Glucose intolerance in pregnancy is most likely to occur after the _____ week of gestation.

Exercise 13-6: *Multiple Choice Question*

 eResource 13-3: To supplement patient teaching,

■ You can provide Margaret a pamphlet from American Congress of Obstetrics and Gynecologists (ACOG) [Pathway: www.acog.org select "ACOG Patient Page" select "patient education pamphlets" → enter "Diabetes and Pregnancy" → select "Diabetes and Pregnancy."]

■ In addition, you may opt to show Margaret the March of Dimes video about gestational diabetes: *bcove.me/xhnth2js*

The answers can be found on pages 213–214.

The nurse understands which of the following blood glucose levels indicates an abnormal value for a 3-hour glucose tolerance test (GTT)?

    A. Fasting glucose of 104

    B. A 1-hour glucose of 188

    C. A 2-hour glucose of 163

    D. A 3-hour glucose of 148

Margaret knows that regulating her insulin is of utmost importance because of the risks to herself and the fetus.

Exercise 13-7: *Select All That Apply*

Known maternal and fetal risks exposed to glucose intolerance are:

- ❑ Hydramnios
- ❑ Small for gestation age (SGA)
- ❑ Postdate deliveries
- ❑ Hypertension
- ❑ Fetal death
- ❑ Cord prolapsed
- ❑ Urinary tract infections (UTIs)
- ❑ Vomiting
- ❑ Vaginal yeast infections
- ❑ Precipitous labors
- ❑ Neonatal respiratory distress syndrome
- ❑ Neonatal hyperglycemia
- ❑ Neonatal polycythemia

Margaret's glycosylated hemoglobin (HbA1C) level was 15% and therefore her glucose controls need to be readjusted.

Exercise 13-8: *Fill-in*

HbA1C is an average measurement of glucose over the past _____ days.

    e   **eResource 13-4:** To learn more about the HbA1C,

        ■ Go to MerckMedicus on your mobile device and open the Pocket Guide to Diagnostic Tests [Pathway: Pocket Guide → enter "HbA1C" into the search field → select "HbA1C" to review information → tap on the drop-down menu in the upper right corner to view content sections. Note: be sure to look at "Comments."]

        ■ Go to LabsOnline [Pathway: *labtestsonline.org* → enter "HbA1C" into the search field → select "A1c and eAG: At a Glance" to review material.]

Most women such as Margaret are not candidates for oral hypoglycemics since many have teratogen effects. Insulin is usually used to maintain GD. Glyburide

The answers can be found on page 214.

(Diabeta) is an antidiabetic oral medication that is sometimes used because it is a category B drug while most of the others are category C drugs. Glyburide does not cross the placenta. Not only does Margaret's glucose need to be better controlled but a fetal surveillance schedule is set up to maintain the health of her fetus.

 eResource 13-5: To learn more about Diabeta,
- go to Epocrates online [Pathway: *online.epocrates.com* → tap on the "Drugs" tab → [Pathway: Epocrates → enter "Diabeta" into the search field → tap on "Diabeta" to view content → scroll down to view "Adverse Reactions" and to view indications "Safety and Monitoring" as well as "Patient Education" to view precautions] or
- open Epocrates on your mobile device [Pathway: Epocrates → enter "Diabeta" into the search field → tap on "Diabeta" to view content → scroll down to view "Adverse Reactions" and to view indications "Safety and Monitoring."]

Exercise 13-9: *Fill-in*

Daily fetal movement counts are to be done now every day. Margaret should feel _____ fetal movements in 2 hours.

Weekly nonstress tests (NSTs) are also scheduled to make sure there is no fetal hypoxia.

 eResource 13-6: Prior to setting Margaret up with the NST, you decide to provide some patient education by showing a brief video tutorial regarding NST: *youtu.be/DvcDXvlCXAE*

Exercise 13-10: *Exhibit Question*

The current NST done on Margaret is below. How many fetal heart accelerations are there?

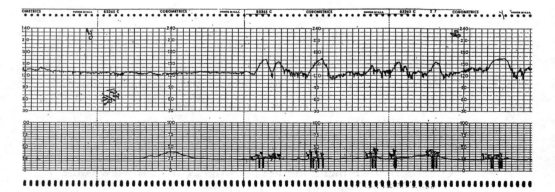

 eResource 13-7: Let's review how to interpret a fetal heart rate strip,
- Go to *Fetalmonitorstrips.com* [Pathway: *fetalmonitorstrips.com* → click on "Learn more about monitor patterns and fetal distress" located at the top of the screen] or

The answers can be found on pages 214–215.

- Go to Monitorart.org [Pathway: *monitorart.org* → scroll down and select "How to interpret the fetal heart monitor tracing" from the menu on the left.]

At home, blood glucose monitoring is reviewed with Margaret.

Exercise 13-11: *Multiple Choice Question*
The nurse understands that further teaching is needed when the patient states:
    A. "I should wash my hands before I handle the strips."
    B. "I should check my glucose before I eat if I feel weak."
    C. "I should keep concentrated glucose in my purse."
    D. "I should wear my alert band all the time."

Margaret takes Humalog and Lantus in the morning and Humulin N at night. She rotates her injection sites and is fine with giving herself insulin. The next day before discharge the registered dietician visits Margaret and explains about carbohydrate counting. She tells Margaret to take in two to four carbohydrates per meal.

eResource 13-8:
- To learn more about these medications, go to Epocrates online [Pathway: *online.epocrates.com* → tap on the "Drugs" tab → enter "Humalog", and "Lantus" and "Humulin N" in the search field one at a time to view content → tap on "Adult dosing" to view indications "Safety and Monitoring", as well as "Patient Education" to view precautions.]

Exercise 13-12: *Multiple Choice Question*
Two to four carbohydrates per meal are how many grams of carbohydrate?
    A. 15–30 g
    B. 25–50 g
    C. 30–60 g
    D. 45–90 g

Because Margaret's fetus needs glucose 24/7, she needs to consume two snacks a day that are one to two carbohydrate choices. One of the most difficult times to regulate glucose is after breakfast, so Margaret is told to monitor her glucose one hour after breakfast. If it is high she should decrease her intake by one carb and increase protein. Margaret is given a diet history tool so she can record her intake and glucose levels. Margaret is discharged with a return prenatal appointment in a week.

eResource 13-9: To locate more dietary teaching information for Margaret,
- go to the CDC [Pathway: *cdc.gov* → enter "Gestational Nutrition Guidelines" into the search field → and tap on the link to view guidelines] or
- University of Wisconsin Department of Medicine [Pathway: *www2 .medicine.wisc.edu* → enter "Diabetes Management Assist" into the search field → tap on "Diabetes Management Assist" to view content.]

The answers can be found on page 215.

Exercise 13-13: *Exhibit Question*

In 1 week, the patient's diet history looks like the following. Circle the meal that requires modification.

Date/Time	Food	Time	Glucose	Insulin
12-1 0630				4 U Humalog and 6 Lantus
0700	Banana, cereal, milk, and OJ	0800	156	
1000	Apple	—	—	—
1100			94	
1200	Wheat bread low-fat turkey lettuce and tomato sandwich, diet soda			
		1300	102	
1500	5 crackers			
1800	Chicken breast, rice, corn, and pudding			
		1900	118	
2200	100-calorie pretzel snack			

The primary care practitioner (PCP) keeps a close watch on Margaret's glucose and provides her with fetal surveillance. At 37 weeks the estimated fetal weight is approaching 10 pounds. A Cesarean birth is scheduled pending an amniocentesis for fetal lung maturity.

eResource 13-10: This short video presents an overview of the process of performing and amniocentesis using ultrasound guidance: *youtu.be/ fvqJ4lX5I8o*

Exercise 13-14: *Multiple Choice Question*

The Lecithin-sphingomyelin ratio, which indicates fetal lung maturity, is:

    A. 1:1

    B. 1:2

    C. 2:1

    D. 2:3

eResource 13-11: Go to MerckMedicus on your mobile device and open the Pocket Guide to Diagnostic Tests [Pathway: Pocket Guide → enter "Lecithin" into the search field → select "Lecithin-sphingomyelin ratio" to review information → tap on the drop-down menu in the upper right corner to view content sections. Note: be sure to look at "Comments."]

The answers can be found on pages 215–216.

Exercise 13-15: *True/False*

Phosphatidylglycerol (PG) presence in amniotic fluid indicates fetal lung maturity.

True/False

The fetal tests indicate that Margaret's infant is mature and a Cesarean is done. The infant is 9 pounds and 13 ounces and is taken to the newborn nursery for assessment. Margaret does well postoperatively and is taken to the postpartum unit. Her glucose levels are checked for the first two days and are within normal range. No further insulin or glucose monitoring is ordered.

Exercise 13-16: *Multiple Choice Question*

The patient asks the nurse if her diabetes will return. The best answer is:

    A. "You are at high risk for insulin-dependent diabetes."

    B. "Probably not, since you are not having more kids."

    C. "Yes, in a year or so it is likely."

    D. "You are high risk for latent diabetes."

eResource 13-12: To supplement patient teaching regarding prognosis, go to Epocrates online [Pathway: *online.epocrates.com* → tap on the "Diseases" tab → enter "gestational" in the search field to view content → select "gestational diabetes" → tap on "Followup" to view prognosis.]

The answers can be found on page 216.

Answers

Exercise 13-1: *Multiple Choice Question*

Gestational diabetes was diagnosed at 24 weeks after a routine screening 1-hour glucose tolerance test (GTT) revealed a blood glucose level above:

A. 130 mg/dL—NO.

B. 135 mg/dL—NO.

C. **140 mg/dL—YES, this is the most common cutoff point although some PCPs are now using 135 mg/dL.**

D. 150 mg/dL—NO.

Exercise 13-2: *Matching*

Match the terms to the condition.

____**A**____ Absolute insulin deficiency that usually appears before age 30.

____**D**____ Glucose intolerance during pregnancy.

____**C**____ Hyperglycemia at levels lower than what qualifies for gestational diabetes (GD).

____**B**____ Insulin resistance or deficiency usually diagnosed after age 30.

A. Type I diabetes

B. Type II diabetes

C. Impaired glucose tolerance

D. Gestational diabetes mellitus

Exercise 13-3: *Multiple Choice Question*

Margaret's diabetes was not noticed in her first trimester because:

A. Her glucose was not routinely checked—NO.

B. She fasted before she came for her office visit—NO.

C. **There was physiologically less insulin resistance—YES, there is less resistance in the first trimester so many women are actually hypoglycemic.**

D. She consumed less glucose—NO.

Exercise 13-4: *Multiple Choice Question*

The placental hormones in pregnancy that cause insulin resistance are:

A. Human placental lactogen (hPL) and estriol—NO.

B. Progesterone and estriol—NO.

C. Progesterone and somatotropin—NO.

D. **Human placental lactogen and somatotropin—YES.**

Exercise 13-5: *Fill-in*

Glucose intolerance in pregnancy is most likely to occur after the __28th__ week of gestation.

Exercise 13-6: *Multiple Choice Question*

The nurse understands which of the following blood glucose levels indicates an abnormal value for a 3-hour glucose tolerance test (GTT)?

 A. Fasting glucose of 104—NO, less than 105 is OK.

 B. A 1-hour glucose of 188—NO, less than 190 is OK.

 C. A 2-hour glucose of 163—NO, less than 165 is OK.

 D. **A 3-hour glucose of 148—YES, it should be less than 145 mg/dL.**

Exercise 13-7: *Select All That Apply*

Known maternal and fetal risks exposed to glucose intolerance are:

☑ **Hydramnios—YES.**

❑ Small for gestation age (SGA)—NO, it the infant is usually LGA (Large for gestational age) but in cases with advanced vascular involvement the infant could be SGA.

❑ Postdate deliveries—NO, usually the large volume increases preterm delivery.

☑ **Hypertension—YES.**

☑ **Fetal death—YES.**

☑ **Cord prolapsed—YES, as a result of the hydramnios.**

☑ **Urinary tract infections (UTIs)—YES, due to increased glucose the urine is a better medium for infection.**

❑ Vomiting—NO.

☑ **Vaginal yeast infections—YES, due to increased glucose the vaginal flora is a better medium for infection.**

❑ Precipitous labors—NO, usually labors are more difficult due to infants that are LGA.

☑ **Neonatal respiratory distress syndrome—YES, increased glucose decreases surfactant production.**

❑ Neonatal hyperglycemia—NO, hypoglycemia.

☑ **Neonatal polycythemia—YES, due to increased production of RBCs to oxygenate the fetus that is LGA.**

Exercise 13-8: *Fill-in*

HbA1C is an average measurement of glucose over the past __120__ days.

Exercise 13-9: *Fill-in*

Daily fetal movement counts are to be done now every day. Margaret should feel __10__ fetal movements in 2 hours.

Exercise 13-10: *Exhibit Question*

The current NST done on Margaret is below. How many fetal heart accelerations are there? ____7____

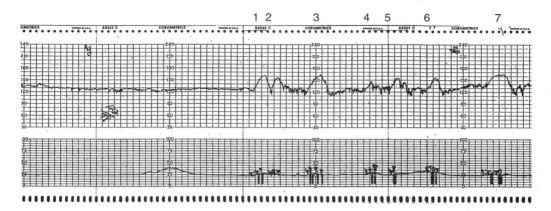

Exercise 13-11: *Multiple Choice Question*

The nurse understands that further teaching is needed when the patient states:
  A. "I should wash my hands before I handle the strips."—NO, this is correct.
  B. **"I should check my glucose before I eat if I feel weak."—YES, she should eat first.**
  C. "I should keep concentrated glucose in my purse."—NO, this is correct.
  D. "I should wear my alert band all the time."—NO, this is correct.

Exercise 13-12: *Multiple Choice Question*

Two to four carbohydrates per meal are how many grams of carbohydrate?
  A. 15–30 g—NO.
  B. 25–50 g—NO.
  C. **30–60 g—YES, each carbohydrate count is approximately 12–15 g.**
  D. 45–90 g—NO.

Exercise 13-13: *Exhibit Question*

In 1 week, the patient's diet history looks like the following. Circle the meal that requires modification.

Date/Time	Food	Time	Glucose	Insulin
12-1 0630				4 U Humalog and 6 Lantus
0700	Banana, cereal, milk, and OJ	0800	156	
1000	Apple	—	—	—
1100			94	

Date/Time	Food	Time	Glucose	Insulin
1200	Wheat bread low-fat turkey lettuce, and tomato sandwich, diet soda			
		1300	102	
1500	5 crackers			
1800	Chicken breast, rice, corn, and pudding			
		1900	118	
2200	100-calorie pretzel snack			

Exercise 13-14: *Multiple Choice Question*

The lecithin-sphingomyelin ratio, which indicates fetal lung maturity, is:

A. 1:1—NO.

B. **1:2—YES, this indicates the lungs have the correct glycoproteins to produce surfactant.**

C. 2:1—NO.

D. 2:3—NO.

Exercise 13-15: *True/False*

Phosphatidylglycerol (PG) presence in amniotic fluid indicates fetal lung maturity.

True/False—PG is a **glycerophospholipid** found in **pulmonary surfactant** and indicates fetal lung maturity.

Exercise 13-16: *Multiple Choice Question*

The patient asks the nurse if her diabetes will return. The best answer is:

A. "You are at high risk for insulin-dependent diabetes."—NO, she may not be insulin dependent.

B. "Probably not, since you are not having more kids."—NO, she may become diabetic or insulin resistant even if she does not have more children.

C. "Yes, in a year or so it is likely."—NO, many times it does not manifest for several years or decades.

D. **"You are high risk for latent diabetes."—YES, this is true.**

14

ABO Incompatibility

Case Study 14 Regina

Regina has just delivered a baby girl who is 7 pounds and 11 ounces. Regina's blood type is O negative so she received RhoGAM at 28 weeks' gestation. The cord blood is sent to the lab for typing and the results reveal that it is B+.

eResource 14-1: To learn more about screening recommendations,
- go to the U.S. Preventative Services Task Force (USPSTF) [Pathway: *www.uspreventiveservicestaskforce.org* → enter "screening Rh" → tap on "Screening: Rh(D) Incompatibility"] or . . .
- On your mobile device, open a browser and enter: *www.ahrq.gov/ clinic/pocketgd1011* → scroll down to locate Rh(D) Incompatibility (located under Obstetric and Gynecological Conditions).

Exercise 14-1: *Multiple Choice Question*
A patient is considered Rh negative when:
- A. They do not have Rh surface antigens on erythrocytes.
- B. They do have Rh surface antigens on erthyrocytes.
- C. They have Rh positive antibodies in their circulation.
- D. They have Rh negative antibodies in the circulation.

Regina as well as 15% of the U.S. population is Rh negative.

Exercise 14-2: *Multiple Choice Question*
The reason that the patient would not need a postpartum dose of RhoGAM is if:
- A. The infant was Rh positive.
- B. Her partner was Rh positive.
- C. The infant was Rh negative.
- D. Her partner was Rh negative.

The answers can be found on page 223.

eResource 14-2: To learn more about Rh incompatibility, go to:
- Open MerckMedicus and go to the Merck Manual [Merck Manual → Topics → enter "Rh" into the search field → scroll down and select "Rh blood type" → select "Erythroblastosis Fetalis" → tap on the drop-down menu in the upper right corner to navigate section content] or . . .
- Open a browser on your mobile device and go to: *nlm.nih.gov* to access MedlinePlus [Pathway: nlm.nih.gov → select "MedlinePlus → enter "Rh incompatibility" into the search field → in addition to reviewing the text, be sure to scroll down and select images].

The cord blood reveals that there is a positive direct Coombs test.

Exercise 14-3: *Multiple Choice Question*
A positive direct Coombs test noted on the cord blood indicates:
- A. Fetal blood hemolysis.
- B. Maternal blood hemolysis.
- C. The infant was Rh negative.
- D. Her mother was Rh negative.

eResource 14-3: Staying in MedlinePlus [Pathway: *nlm.nih.gov* → select MedlinePlus → enter "Rh incompatibility" into the search field → scroll down and tap on "direct COOMBS" to learn more about this test.]

Regina is given RhoGAM within 72 hours of her daughter's birth.

Exercise 14-4: *Multiple Choice Question*
The nurse would expect the RhoGAM to:
- A. Decrease the positive Coombs test.
- B. Decrease maternal sensitization.
- C. Decrease the effects of the ABO incompatibility.
- D. Decrease the number of fetal cells in the maternal circulation.

eResource 14-4: To learn more about gestational hypertension, go to Epocrates online [Pathway: *online.epocrates.com* → tap on the "Drugs" tab → enter "RhoGAM" in the search field to view content → select "RhoGAM" to view content → be sure to look at patient teaching information].

Regina is told of the infant's positive Coombs test and is told what to expect. Regina is attentive and asks multiple questions.

eResource 14-5: To supplement patient education for Regina, go to:
- KidsHealth [Pathway: *kidshealth.org* → select "Parents" → enter "Rh factor" into the search field → select "Rh incompatibility" to view content. Note: be sure to read the section on "Preventing and Treating Rh Disease of the Newborn."]

The answers can be found on page 223.

■ American Congress of Obstetrics and Gynecologists (ACOG) [Pathway: *acog.org* select "ACOG Patient Page," select "patient education pamphlets" → enter "Rh Factor" → select "The Rh FactorHigh Blood Pressure During Pregnancy."]

■ To learn more about Rh incompatibility and the Coombs test, on your mobile device, go to:

■ Pocket Guide to Diagnostic Tests on your mobile device [Pathway: Pocket Guide → enter "Coombs" into the search field → scroll down and select "Coombs, Indirect."].

■ Medscape [Pathway: Medscape → enter "Rh" into the search field → select "Rh incompatibility"].

Exercise 14-5: *Multiple Choice Question*

The priority nursing diagnosis for this patient is:

A. Risk for powerlessness

B. Ineffective parenting

C. Mild anxiety

D. Complicated grieving

Exercise 14-6: *Multiple Choice Question*

The nurse would assess an infant with positive Coomb frequently for:

A. Hypoglycemia

B. Jaundice

C. Hypocalcemia

D. Anemia

Exercise 14-7: *Exhibit*

On the following chart plot the results of the 18-hour old infant's bilirubin test, which is 7.4 mg/dL:

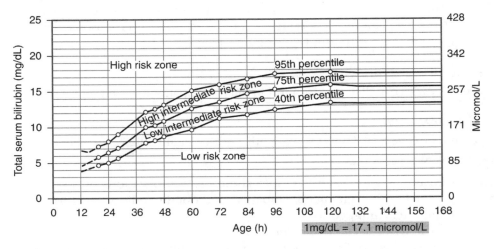

You call the PCP with the results and inform her of the bilirubin results.

The answers can be found on page 224.

Exercise 14-8: *Multiple Choice Question*

An appropriate order to expect is:

        A. Do nothing, continue to assess.

        B. Repeat the bilirubin in 1 hour.

        C. Repeat the bilirubin in 8 hours.

        D. Place under triple phototherapy.

Exercise 14-9: *Multiple Choice Question*

The best nursing intervention to prevent increasing bilirubin levels is:

        A. Do nothing, continue to assess.

        B. Place the infant by the window.

        C. Increase feedings.

        D. Keep in the newborn nursery.

The bilirubin level continues to rise and the infant is placed under phototherapy.

 eResource 14-6: On your mobile device, open WebMD [Pathway: WebMD → enter "jaundice" into the search field → select "Newborn jaundice"→ review content; be sure to scroll down and click on "Phototherapy" to view image].

Exercise 14-10: *Multiple Choice Question*

The patient asks if the infant's jaundice is because she is breast-feeding. The best answer the nurse can provide is:

        A. "No, it is not your fault, it is due to your husband's blood type."

        B. "Yes, jaundice from breast-feeding is a condition that happens."

        C. "No, it is due to the Rh factor."

        D. "No, breast-fed jaundice is a condition that can happen later."

 eResource 14-7: Remain in WebMD in the topic of Newborn Jaundice [Pathway: WebMD → enter "jaundice" into the search field → select "Newborn jaundice" → review content; be sure to scroll down and click on "Are there different types of jaundice?"]

Exercise 14-11: *Fill-in*

A severe form of jaundice that is bilirubin encephalopathy is called _____.

Exercise 14-12: *Fill-in*

Before the discovery of RhoGAM many Rh positive infants died in utero of hemolytic disease called _____.

 eResource 14-8: To learn more about the complications of severe jaundice (bilirubin encephalopathy) and obtain additional information for patient teaching, go to:

    ■ The CDC, *www.cdc.gov/jaundice*

    ■ View this brief video regarding "recognizing and treating jaundice" from the Health Science Channel, go to: *youtu.be/yjRcSSpg53Q*

The answers can be found on page 225.

The infant under phototherapy lights benefits because the lights convert unconjugated bilirubin to conjugated, which can be excreted.

Exercise 14-13: *Multiple Choice Question*

Bilirubin is excreted in the:

     A. Urine.

     B. Sweat.

     C. Stool.

     D. Saliva.

Exercise 14-14: *Multiple Choice Question*

If phototherapy fails to bring down bilirubin levels sufficiently, the next therapy that would be considered is:

     A. Exchange transfusion.

     B. Saline IV.

     C. Enemas.

     D. Diuretics.

 eResource 14-9: Return to the CDC Jaundice/Kernicterus Web site (*www.cdc.gov/jaundice*), on the menu on the right side of the screen, select "Treatment" to learn about additional treatment options.

The infant does well under phototherapy, and the nurse is careful to keep the eyes and genitals covered in order to protect the sensitive genital area and the retina from the lights. In 72 hours the bilirubin level is down significantly and the phototherapy is discontinued. Regina is provided with discharge instructions.

Exercise 14-15: *Multiple Choice Question*

The nurse understands that more teaching is needed when the patient states:

     A. "I should check the baby's abdomen to see if it is yellow."

     B. "I should continue to feed the baby every 2–4 hours."

     C. "I should keep the baby near the sunny window."

     D. "I should check the baby's feet to see if they are yellow."

 eResource 14-10: Discharge Planning

    ■ Prior to discharge, have Regina view the CDC's video "Jaundice and Your Newborn Jaundice" as a means to provide a good overview of the importance of follow-through with the prescribed regimen. *www.cdc.gov/ncbddd/jaundice/videos/index.html*

    ■ To learn more about follow-up on newborn jaundice, go to Epocrates online [Pathway: *online.epocrates.com* → tap on the "Diseases" tab → enter "jaundice" in the search field to view content → select "neonatal jaundice" → select "Follow up."]

    ■ To supplement discharge teaching, go to WebMd on your mobile device [Pathway: WebMD → enter "jaundice" into the search field → select "Newborn jaundice" → review content; be sure to scroll down and click on "How can I care for my newborn at home?" and "Jaundice in Newborns (Hyperbilirubinemia)-Home Treatment."]

The answers can be found on pages 225–226.

Answers

Exercise 14-1: *Multiple Choice Question*

A patient is considered Rh negative when:

A. **They do not have Rh surface antigens on erythrocytes—YES, this is why they build up antibodies to the Rh factor.**

B. They do have Rh surface antigens on erthyrocytes—NO, they do not.

C. They have Rh positive antibodies in their circulation—NO, they should not have circulating antibodies if treated appropriately.

D. They have Rh negative antibodies in the circulation—NO, there are no antigens to trigger antibody production.

Exercise 14-2: *Multiple Choice Question*

The reason that the patient would not need a postpartum dose of RhoGAM is if:

A. The infant was Rh positive—NO, she would need RhoGAM.

B. Her partner was Rh positive—NO, the infant's type is the determining factor since paternity is not a sure thing in all cases of pregnancy.

C. **The infant was Rh negative—YES, she would not need RhoGAM.**

D. Her partner was Rh negative—NO, the infant's type is the determining factor since paternity is not a sure thing in all cases of pregnancy.

Exercise 14-3: *Multiple Choice Question*

A positive direct Coombs test noted on the cord blood indicates:

A. **Fetal blood hemolysis—YES, this is a test of direct antiglobulins, IgG, that attach to the RBCs of the fetus and cause hemolysis.**

B. Maternal blood hemolysis—NO, the anti-A or anti-B IgG is passed from the mom through the placenta.

C. The infant was Rh negative—NO, it has nothing to do with the Rh factor.

D. Her mother was Rh negative—NO, it has nothing to do with the Rh factor.

Exercise 14-4: *Multiple Choice Question*

The nurse would expect the RhoGAM to:

A. Decrease the positive Coombs test—NO, this is for ABO incompatibility and RhoGAM does not effect it.

B. **Decrease maternal sensitization—YES, so the second Rh + fetus, if that should occur, is not effected by antibodies built up during the postpartum period.**

C. Decrease the effects of the ABO incompatibility—NO.

D. Decrease the number of fetal cells in the maternal circulation—NO.

Exercise 14-5: *Multiple Choice Question*

The priority nursing diagnosis for this patient is:

A. Risk for powerlessness—NO, asking questions is not a sign of powerlessness.

B. Ineffective parenting—NO, there is not enough evidence to implicate that the patient has ineffective parenting.

C. **Mild anxiety—YES, this is a sign of mild anxiety.**

D. Complicated grieving—NO, there is no indication that she is having a grief reaction.

Exercise 14-6: *Multiple Choice Question*

The nurse would assess an infant with positive Coomb frequently for:

A. Hypoglycemia—NO, antibodies do not affect the glucose level.

B. **Jaundice—YES, the hemolysis of the infant's RBC will increase the unconjugated bilirubin level.**

C. Hypocalcemia—NO, antibodies do not affect the calcium level.

D. Anemia—NO, it should not destroy RBCs to this extent.

Exercise 14-7: *Exhibit*

On the following chart plot the results of the 18-hour old infant's bilirubin test which is 7.4 mg/dL:

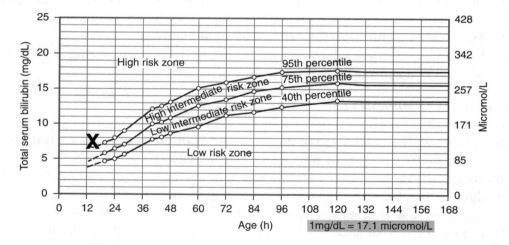

Exercise 14-8: *Multiple Choice Question*

An appropriate order to expect is:

A. Do nothing, continue to assess—NO, this level indicates that something else should be done.

B. Repeat the bilirubin in 1 hour—NO, this is too soon to evaluate a change.

C. Repeat the bilirubin in 8 hours—NO, this level indicates that something else should be done.

D. **Place under triple phototherapy—YES, treatment is indicated.**

Exercise 14-9: *Multiple Choice Question*

The best nursing intervention to prevent increasing bilirubin levels is:

A. Do nothing, continue to assess—NO.

B. Place the infant by the window—NO, this may help but evidence indicates that it is an ineffective way to decrease bilirubin.

C. **Increase feedings—YES, this increases the bilirubin excretion.**

D. Keep in the newborn nursery—NO, many phototherapies can be done in the parent's postpartum room.

Exercise 14-10: *Multiple Choice Question*

The patient asks if the infant's jaundice is because she is breast-feeding, the best answer the nurse can provide is:

A. "No, it is not your fault, it is due to your husband's blood type."—NO, blaming is never helpful.

B. "Yes, jaundice from breast-feeding is a condition that happens."—NO, breast-fed jaundice occurs at a later age, 6 days to 2 weeks and is a rare condition.

C. "No, it is due to the Rh factor."—NO, it is due to an ABO incompatibility.

D. **"No, breast-fed jaundice is a condition that can happen later."—YES, this is the best answer.**

Exercise 14-11: *Fill-in*

A severe form of jaundice that is bilirubin encephalopathy is called **Kernicterus.**

Exercise 14-12: *Fill-in*

Before the discovery of RhoGAM many Rh positive infants died in utero of hemolytic disease called **hydrops fetalis.**

Exercise 14-13: *Multiple Choice Question*

Bilirubin is excreted in the:

A. Urine—NO.

B. Sweat—NO.

C. **Stool—YES, it is conjugated in the liver and excreted in the bile to the small intestines.**

D. Saliva—NO.

Exercise 14-14: *Multiple Choice Question*

If phototherapy fails to bring down bilirubin levels sufficiently, the next therapy that would be considered would be:

A. **Exchange transfusion—YES, this is done in cases of severe jaundice to prevent kernicterus.**

B. Saline IV—NO.

C. Enemas—NO.

D. Diuretics—NO.

Exercise 14-15: *Multiple Choice Question*

The nurse understands that more teaching is needed when the patient states:

A. "I should check the baby's abdomen to see if it is yellow."—NO, this is a good place to blanch the skin and see if the underlying color is yellow.

B. "I should continue to feed the baby every 2–4 hours."—NO, this should be continued.

C. "I should keep the baby near the sunny window"—NO, this will not do any harm.

D. **"I should check the baby's feet to see if they are yellow."—YES, bilirubin collects under the skin from cephalo to caudal so waiting for the feet to turn yellow would be an advanced case.**

15

Rupture of the Membranes (ROM)

Case 15 ■ Savannah

Savannah is a 17-year-old G-1 who is 29 3/7 gestation. She comes to the high-risk perinatal unit because of possible ROM (rupture of membranes). Savannah was sleeping when she woke up with wet night clothes. Her mother drove her to the hospital where the emergency department (ED) physician sent her to the high-risk unit to be assessed by a perinatologist.

Exercise 15-1: *Matching*
Match the term with its definition.

_____ Rupture of membranes before the onset of true labor.

_____ Rupture of membranes before 37 weeks' gestation and before the true onset of labor.

_____ Rupture of membranes for more than 24 hours.

A. Preterm premature rupture of membranes (PPROM)

B. Preterm rupture of membranes (PROM)

C. Prolonged rupture of membranes

Ten percent of pregnancies experience premature rupture of membranes, and the earlier it occurs, the higher the risk to the fetus. You check the fetal heart rate (FHR) and it is 156 BPM.

Exercise 15-2: *Multiple Choice Question*
The nurse understands that an elevation in FHR is an indication of:

A. Fetal distress.

B. Possible maternal infection.

C. Lack of amniotic fluid.

D. Onset of true labor.

The answers can be found on page 235.

Exercise 15-3: *Select All That Apply*

The known risk factors for preterm rupture of membranes are:

❑ Oligohydramnios.

❑ Multiple gestation.

❑ SGA (small for gestational age).

❑ Uterine anomalies.

❑ Fetal anomalies.

❑ Incompetent cervix.

❑ Smoking.

❑ STIs (sexually transmitted infections).

 eResource 15-1: Go to the National Guidelines Clearinghouse (NGC) to view established practice guidelines for premature rupture of membranes [Pathway: *guideline.gov* → enter "premature rupture of membranes" into search field → tap to select the guideline "premature rupture of membranes" or the most current listed guideline.]

Savannah is placed on observation and a sterile speculum exam is done to determine if her membranes are ruptured.

Exercise 15-4: *Multiple Choice Question*

The nurse would expect the nitrazine paper to be what color if positive for amniotic fluid?

A. Yellow

B. Orange

C. Blue

D. Brown

 eResource 15-2: To learn more about premature rupture of membranes, go to:

■ Open MerckMedicus and go to the Merck Manual [Merck Manual → Topics → enter "premature" into the search field → scroll down and select "premature rupture of membranes" → select "Premature Rupture of Membranes (PROM)" → tap on the drop-down menu in the upper right corner to navigate section content, focusing on "Diagnosis."]

Another test for ROM is done. The vaginal fluid is placed on a microscope slide.

Exercise 15-5: *Multiple Choice Question*

Which picture indicates positive ROM?

The answers can be found on pages 235–236.

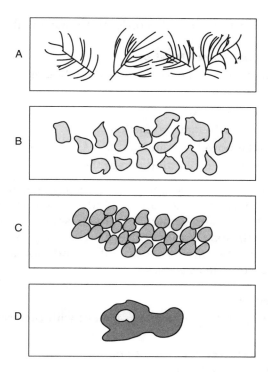

Exercise 15-6: *Multiple Choice Question*

ROM is confirmed by a transvaginal ultrasound that reveals:

    A. Oligohydramnios

    B. Hydramnious

    C. Polyhydramnios

    D. Multidramnios

Continuous external fetal monitoring is begun as well as an IV to hydrate Savannah.

Exercise 15-7: *Calculation*

The intravenous ordering is 1,000 mL Ringers Lactate at 100 mL/hr and the gtt factor is 12 gtts/mL. How many gtts/min should the nurse deliver?

 eResource 15-3: Remember, to use an IV infusion calculation, you can go to:

    ■ MedCalc.com for an online calculation [Pathway: *medcalc.com* → Tap on "Fluids/Electrolytes" → "IV Rate" to access the calculation]

    ■ Skyscape's Archimedes on your mobile device [Pathway: Archimedes → enter "IV" into the Main Index → scroll down to "IV Calc: Infusion rate mL/hr"]

    ■ MedCalc on your mobile device [Pathway: MedCalc → tap on "I" → select "Infusion: IV Drip Rate."]

The answers can be found on page 236.

Betamethasone (Corticosteroid) is also ordered for Savannah.

Exercise 15-8: *Multiple Choice Question*

The nurse knows that the indication for administering Betamethasone to a patient who may deliver preterm is to:

     A. Decrease fetal infection.

     B. Increase fetal surfactant production.

     C. Decrease fetal bowel ischemia.

     D. Increase glomerular filtration rate in the fetus.

 eResource 15-4: To learn more about Betamethasone and associated precautions, go to Epocrates online [Pathway: *online.epocrates.com* → tap on the "Drugs" tab → enter "Betamethasone" in the search field → select "betamethasone sodium phosphate." → Tap on "Adult dosing" to view indications, be sure to check "Safety and Monitoring," as well as "Adverse Reactions."]

Exercise 15-9: *Ordering*

Put in order the nursing interventions for a patient with preterm, premature rupture of membranes.

     _____ Check bladder every 2 hours.

     _____ Keep on bed rest.

     _____ Temperature every 2 hours.

     _____ Monitor vaginal discharge.

     _____ Provide dimensional activity.

Savannah's mother asks the nurse if the doctor can give Savannah antibiotics to prevent infection.

Exercise 15-10: *Multiple Choice Question*

The best answer the nurse can provide as a response to the question about antibiotics is:

     A. "Some PCPs do order antibiotics in this situation."

     B. "Antibiotic reactions can kill the fetus."

     C. "Antibiotics can mask an infection."

     D. "Antibiotics can destroy the fetal immune system."

Several hours later Savannah puts on her call bell because she is feeling "cramping." You check her fetal monitor strip.

Exercise 15-11: *Exhibit Question*

According to the following external fetal monitor strip, how far apart are the uterine contractions?

     A. Every 1–2 minutes

     B. Every 2–3 minutes

     C. Every 3–4 minutes

     D. Every 4–5 minutes

The answers can be found on page 237.

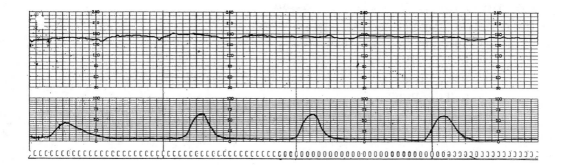

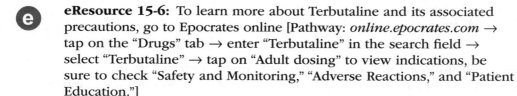

e **eResource 15-5:** Let's review again how to interpret a fetal heart rate strip.
- Go to Fetalmonitorstrips.com [Pathway: *fetalmonitorstrips.com* → click on "Learn more about monitor patterns and fetal distress" located at the top of the screen] or
- Go to Monitorart.org [Pathway: *monitorart.org* → scroll down and select "How to interpret the fetal heart monitor tracing" from the menu on the left.]

A tocolytic medication is ordered to "hold off" the delivery until the second Betamethasone injection can be administered 12 hours after the first. Terbutaline (Brethine) is given subq. × 3 and Savannah's contractions decrease. Two hours later the second dose of Betamethasone is administered, after which Savannah sleeps through most of the night. At 4 a.m. the baseline fetal heart rate is checked.

e **eResource 15-6:** To learn more about Terbutaline and its associated precautions, go to Epocrates online [Pathway: *online.epocrates.com* → tap on the "Drugs" tab → enter "Terbutaline" in the search field → select "Terbutaline" → tap on "Adult dosing" to view indications, be sure to check "Safety and Monitoring," "Adverse Reactions," and "Patient Education."]

Exercise 15-12: *Exhibit Question*
The fetal heart baseline in the strip in Exercise 15-11 would be classified as:
- A. Reassuring
- B. Bradycardic
- C. Sinusoidal
- D. Tachycardic

e **eResource 15-7:** Go back to eResource 15-5 to interpret a fetal heart rate strip.

The answers can be found on page 238.

Exercise 15-13: *Multiple Choice Question*

The priority intervention for this fetal heart rate is to:

    A. Turn the patient to the left side.

    B. Increase IV fluids.

    C. Place oxygen on the mother at 10L via mask.

    D. Call the PCP.

It is decided to do a Cesarean birth on Savannah. The NICU is called.

Exercise 15-14: *Select All That Apply*

What equipment should be ready for a preterm infant in the delivery room?

    ❑ Warmed transport incubator

    ❑ Phototherapy

    ❑ Endotracheal tube

    ❑ Oxygen cannula

    ❑ Suction

    ❑ Hepatitis B vaccine

Savannah needs an epidural anesthesia for surgery and so her IV fluids are increased.

Exercise 15-15: *Multiple Choice Question*

The nurse understands that increasing the patient's circulatory volume will assist in decreasing which of the following conditions?

    A. Hypertension

    B. Hypotension

    C. Vertigo

    D. Facial numbness

eResource 15-8: To learn more about epidural anesthesia,

    ■ Open a browser on your mobile device and go to: www.nlm.nih.gov to access MedlinePlus [Pathway: *nlm.nih.gov* → select "MedlinePlus → enter "epidural" into the search field → scroll down and select "Spinal and Epidural Anesthesia." Note: there are other items of interest related to epidural anesthesia → scroll down to "Causes."]

    ■ View a brief video from Medical Videos: *www.medicalvideos.us/videos/1241/combined-spinal-epidural-obstetric-anesthesia*

After the epidural is effective, Savannah is prepped for the Cesarean birth. Her mother is seated at the head of the bed in the OR next to the anesthesiologist, who constantly monitors her blood pressure.

Exercise 15-16: *Multiple Choice Question*

Savannah asks the nurse if she will feel any pain; the nurse's best reply is:

    A. "Some people describe it as pain when they pull the baby out."

    B. "No, the epidural will take care of everything."

The answers can be found on page 238.

C. "Yes, the epidural cannot take away all sensation."

D. "You may feel pressure when they take the baby out."

 eResource 15-9: To learn more about this procedure, you can view Medline media files [Pathway: *nlm.nih.gov* → select "MedlinePlus → select "Videos and Cool Tools" → enter "cesarean section" into the search field → select one of the following:]

■ A graphic tutorial from the National Library of Medicine explaining the common reasons for this procedure

■ a Cesarean section birth performed at Shawnee Mission Medical Center, Merriam, Kansas.

Once the baby is out the PCP tells Savannah and her mother that it is a boy. The baby is 3 pounds and 3 ounces. He cries right away and is taken to the NICU for care.

Exercise 15-17: *Multiple Choice Question*

Savannah's mother asks the nurse if it means the baby will not need a ventilator because he is crying and breathing on his own. The best answer for the nurse to give is:

A. "Yes, since he is doing so well I would expect him to be OK without a ventilator."

B. "No, at this gestational age they all need ventilators."

C. "Yes, the two doses of Betamethasone matured his lungs."

D. "No, very often they get tired and stressed and need respiratory assistance."

After the Cesarean birth recovery period, Savannah is taken to her postpartum room and is encouraged to visit the NICU as often as possible. The mother-baby nursing staffs also assist Savannah to pump her breasts so her breast milk can be stored for her infant.

Exercise 15-18: *Select All That Apply*

Advantages of providing breast milk to preterm infants include:

❑ Faster growth

❑ Increased immunity

❑ Increased sleep time

❑ Decreased necrotizing enterocolitis

❑ Decreased retinopathy of prematurity

After three hospital days Savannah is discharged and her mom then drives her back and forth to the NICU each day.

The answers can be found on page 239.

Answers

Exercise 15-1: *Matching*

Match the term with its definition.

    B   Rupture of membranes before the onset of true labor.

    A   Rupture of membranes before 37 weeks' gestation and before the true onset of labor.

    C   Rupture of membranes for more than 24 hours.

  A. Preterm premature rupture of membranes (PPROM)

  B. Preterm rupture of membranes (PROM)

  C. Prolonged rupture of membranes

Exercise 15-2: *Multiple Choice Question*

The nurse understands that an elevation in FHR is an indication of:

  A. Fetal distress—NO, not necessarily, it may be related to fetal movement.

  B. **Possible maternal infection—YES, one of the first signs of an infection is fetal tachycardia.**

  C. Lack of amniotic fluid—NO, this many cause cord compression related to lack of fluid to protect the cord, but this would result in bradycardia.

  D. Onset of true labor—NO, this should not change the FHR baseline.

Exercise 15-3: *Select All That Apply*

The known risk factors for preterm rupture of membranes are:

❑ Oligohydramnios—NO, actually hydramnios (polyhydramnios) is a risk factor because the uterus is overdistended.

☑ **Multiple gestation—YES, due to over distention.**

❑ SGA (small for gestational age)—NO.

☑ **Uterine anomalies—YES, anomalies can decrease the uterine space needed for the fetus to grow such as a bicornate uterus.**

☑ **Fetal anomalies—YES, this is a risk factor.**

☑ **Incompetent cervix—YES, this to can initiate ROM.**

☑ **Smoking—YES, this causes vasoconstriction and decreases the hemodynamic needed to keep the pregnancy healthy.**

☑ **STIs (sexually transmitted infections)—YES infection can disrupt the integrity of the membranes.**

Exercise 15-4: *Multiple Choice Question*

The nurse would expect the nitrazine paper to be what color if positive for amniotic fluid?

A. Yellow—NO, this would be no change.

B. Orange—NO, this is not an indicator color.

C. **Blue—YES, this indicates an alkaline substance (>7.0 pH).**

D. Brown—NO, this is not an indicator color.

Exercise 15-5: *Multiple Choice Question*

Which picture indicates positive ROM?

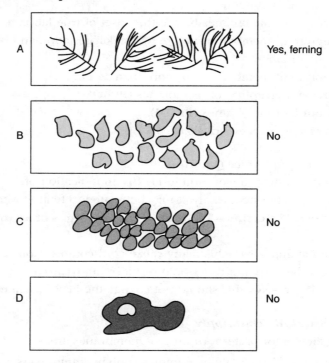

Exercise 15-6: *Multiple Choice Question*

ROM is confirmed by a transvaginal ultrasound that reveals:

A. **Oligohydramnios—YES, since much of the fluid has escaped.**

B. Hydramnios—NO, this would indicate that the membranes are intact.

C. Polyhydramnios—NO, this would indicate that the membranes are intact, and it is another name for excess amniotic fluid.

D. Multidramnios—NO such term.

Exercise 15-7: *Calculation*

The intravenous order is 1,000 mL Ringers Lactate at 100 mL/hr and the gtt factor is 12 gtts/mL. How many gtts/min should the nurse deliver?

100 mL/hr × 12 gtts/mL = 1,200 gtts/hr divided by 60 min = **20 gtts/min**

Exercise 15-8: *Multiple Choice Question*

The nurse knows that the indication for administering Betamethasone to a patient who may deliver preterm is to:

A. Decrease fetal infection—NO, this is not the action of the medication.

B. **Increase fetal surfactant production—YES, it increases surfactant production.**

C. Decrease fetal bowel ischemia—NO, this is not the action of the medication.

D. Increase glomerular filtration rate in the fetus—NO, this is not the action of the medication.

Exercise 15-9: *Ordering*

Put in order the nursing interventions for a patient with preterm, premature rupture of membranes:

_____**3**_____ Check bladder every 2 hours

_____**4**_____ Keep on bed rest

_____**1**_____ Temperature every 2 hours

_____**2**_____ Monitor vaginal discharge

_____**5**_____ Provide dimensional activity

Exercise 15-10: *Multiple Choice Question*

The best answer the nurse can provide as a response to the question about antibiotics is:

A. "Some PCPs do order antibiotics in this situation."—NO, this is not helpful and antibiotics are not recommended by ACOG (American College of Obstetricians and Gynecologists, 2003).

B. "Antibiotic reactions can kill the fetus."—NO, this is not true.

C. **"Antibiotics may mask an infection."—YES, this is the rationale.**

D. "Antibiotics can destroy the fetal immune system."—NO, this is not true.

Exercise 15-11: *Exhibit Question*

According to the following external fetal monitor strip, how far apart are the uterine contractions?

A. Every 1–2 minutes—NO, the UCs are not this close.

B. Every 2–3 minutes—NO, the UCs are not this close.

C. **Every 3–4 minutes—YES.**

D. Every 4–5 minutes—NO, the UCs are closer together.

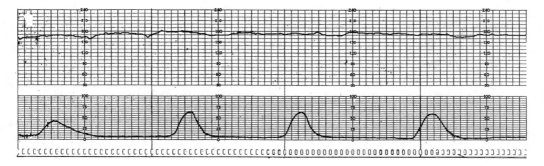

Exercise 15-12: *Exhibit Question*

The fetal heart baseline in the strip would be classified as:

A. Reassuring

B. Bradycardic

C. Sinusoidal

D. **Tachycardic**

Exercise 15-13: *Multiple Choice Questions*

The priority intervention for this fetal heart rate is to:

A. Turn the patient to the left side—NO, this is not acute fetal distress.

B. Increase IV fluids—NO, this is not acute fetal distress.

C. Place oxygen on the mother at 10L via mask—NO, this is not acute fetal distress.

D. **Call the PCP—YES, this indicates chorioamnionitis may be setting in.**

Exercise 15-14: *Select All That Apply*

What equipment should be ready for a preterm infant in the delivery room?

☑ **Warmed transport incubator—YES, this is needed to prevent cold stress.**

❑ Phototherapy—NO, this may be indicated in two to three days.

☑ **Endotracheal tube—YES, this should be in every delivery room in case positive pressure O$_2$ is needed.**

❑ Oxygen cannula—NO usually this is used as a weaning process not an initial oxygen intervention.

☑ **Suction—YES, the airway must be cleared.**

❑ Hepatitis B vaccine—NO, this is given before discharge.

Exercise 15-15: *Multiple Choice Question*

The nurse understands that increasing the patient's circulatory volume will assist in decreasing which of the following conditions?

A. Hypertension—NO.

B. **Hypotension—YES, increasing the volume will assist the blood pressure to remain normal and perfuse the placenta**

C. Vertigo—NO, this is prevented by positioning after the epidural is given.

D. Facial numbness—NO, this is prevented by positioning after the epidural is given.

Exercise 15-16: *Multiple Choice Question*

Savannah asks the nurse if she will feel any pain; the nurse's best reply is:

A. "Some people describe it as pain when they pull the baby out."—NO, this is reinforcing anxiety about pain.

B. "No, the epidural will take care of everything."—NO, epidurals do not take away pressure sensation.

C. "Yes, the epidural cannot take away all sensation,"—NO, this is true but not very informative or reassuring.

D. **"You may feel pressure when they take the baby out."—YES, this is true, informative and reassuring.**

Exercise 15-17: *Multiple Choice Question*

Savannah's mother asks the nurse if it means the baby will not need a ventilator because he is crying and breathing on his own The best answer for the nurse to give is:

A. "Yes, since he is doing so well I would expect him to be OK without a ventilator."—NO, this is not usually the course of preterm respiratory distress.

B. "No, at this gestational age they all need ventilators."—NO, although most do need ventilators this is not reassuring.

C. "Yes, the two doses of Betamethasone matured his lungs."—NO, the Betamethasone helps but does not "cure" respiratory distress of the preterm infant.

D. **"No, very often they get tired and stressed and need respiratory assistance."—YES, this is the most honest answer.**

Exercise 15-18: *Select All That Apply*

Advantages of providing breast milk to preterm infants include:

❑ Faster growth—NO, this is not usually the case.

☑ **Increased immunity—YES, IgA is passed in breast milk.**

❑ Increased sleep time—NO, this is not a usual claim.

☑ **Decreased necrotizing enterocolitis—YES, this is very important.**

❑ Decreased retinopathy of prematurity—NO, this has not been correlated to breast milk with research evidence.

16

Preterm Labor (PTL)

Case 16 ▮ Bonnie

Bonnie is sent up to the high-risk perinatal unit from the ED. She is in town visiting her sister and is at 25 weeks' gestation when she feels cramping. You take a full history on Bonnie since her prenatal records are not available.

HISTORY: Bonnie is a 25-year-old unmarried female of African American descent. She lives with her boyfriend, who is currently unemployed, of 3 years and works in a restaurant as a waitress. She is a G-3, T-0, P-1, A-1, L-1. She has a year-old daughter who was born at 32 weeks' gestation. She receives WIC (Women, Infant, and Children) benefits. She smokes on occasion but does not drink and is negative for IPV (intimate partner violence). She denies drug use. Bonnie completed high school and has family support for child care. She states she is negative for UTIs (urinary tract infections) and STIs. She has been seen in the clinic at home twice and has had no special testing. She missed an ultrasound appointment due to work. She has not been to a dentist since high school.

Exercise 16-1: *Fill-in*
List five risk factors identified for preterm labor (PTL) in the patient's history:

1. _____
2. _____
3. _____
4. _____
5. _____

Bonnie is placed on the external fetal monitor and uterine contractions are recorded every 5–7 minutes. They are mild and last 30–40 seconds. You call the covering primary care physician (PCP) and tell her the patient's history and current condition using the S-B-A-R format. The following orders are received:

1. Obtain a fetal fibronectin test.

2. Have a transvaginal ultrasound completed for cervical length and dilatation.

3. Notify NICU of impending delivery.

4. Type and X-match.

The answer can be found on page 249.

5. CBS with differential.

6. Obtain a GBS (*Group B streptococcus*) culture.

7. UA culture.

8. Start an IV of 1,000 mL R/L (Ringer's Lactate) at 120 mL/hr with 18 1-11/4 angiocatheter.

9. Start MgSO$_4$ (magnesium sulfate) at 2 gm per hour with a loading dose of 5 gm in 30 minutes.

10. Call if contractions become closer together or SROM (spontaneous rupture of membranes) occurs.

11. Give Betamethasone (Celestone) 12 mg IM now and in 12 hours.

12. Keep NPO.

13. Bed rest.

You assist Bonnie out of bed (OOB) to the bathroom (BR) to obtain the urinalysis (UA) before you draw the blood work and start the IV.

Exercise 16-2: *True/False*

Is it true or false to say that taking blood specimens from an IV site decreases specimen hemolysis? _____

Exercise 16-3: *Calculation*

How many gtts/min would you set the IV of R/L at 120 mL/hr if the gtt factor was 15 gtts/mL?

eResource 16-1:
- Go to *MedCalc.com* to use the online IV rate calculator [Pathway: *medcalc.com* → select "Fluids/Electrolytes" → select "IV Rate"] or
- On your mobile device, use Skyscape's Archimedes, to calculate the infusion rate [pathway: Archimedes → enter "IV" into the Main Index → scroll down to "IV Calc: Infusion rate mL/hr."]

Exercise 16-4: *Calculation*

For how many mL/hr would you set the IV of MgSO$_4$ in order to deliver 5 gms in the first 30 minutes?

Exercise 16-5: *Calculation*

For how many mL/hr would you set the IV of MgSO$_4$ in order to deliver 2 gms/hr for the remainder of the time?

eResource 16-2:
- Go to *MedCalc.com* to use the online IV rate calculator [Pathway: *medcalc .com* → select "Fluids/Electrolytes" → select "Dose Calculator"] or
- On your mobile device, use Skyscape's Archimedes, to calculate the infusion rate [pathway: Archimedes → enter "IV" into the Main Index → scroll down to "IV Calc: Infuse a dose."]

The answers can be found on page 249.

You are aware that $MgSO_4$ is not FDA approved as a tocolytic agent, but it is commonly used to decrease the impulses at the neuromuscular junctions in an attempt to stop preterm labor.

 eResource 16-3: To learn more about $MgSO_4$ and dosage:
- Open MerckMedicus on your mobile device and go to the Merck Manual [Pathway: Merck Manual → select "Topics" → enter "Magnesium sulfate" into the search field → scroll down to select "in preterm labor."]
- Go to Medscape from WebMD on your mobile device. [Pathway: Medscape → select "Magnesium Sulfate" → select "Adult Dosing and Uses." Note: the dosage and that use for treatment of Preterm Labor is off-label.]

Exercise 16-6: *Select All That Apply*
The nurse understands the following items should be at the patient's bedside once they are maintained on $MagSO_4$:
- ❑ Tongue blade
- ❑ Padded side rails
- ❑ Calcium gluconate
- ❑ Adult naloxone (Narcan)
- ❑ Reflex hammer
- ❑ Ophthalmoscope

A certified nurse midwife (CNM) is covering the L&D (labor and delivery) unit and comes to assist with the sterile speculum exam and feta fibronectin. The GBS test and the cultures are sent to the lab.

Exercise 16-7: *Hot Spot*
Betamethasone is given deep IM in the right ventrogluteal muscle. Put an X on the spot where it should be given.

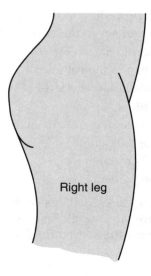

Right leg

The answers can be found on page 250.

In approximately 3 hours, Bonnie's UCs (uterine contractions) are less frequent and are irregular. She experiences a variable deceleration.

Exercise 16-8: *Hot Spot*

Place Xs on the variable deceleration.

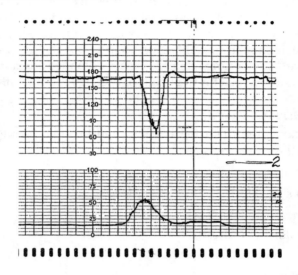

You turn Bonnie to the left side and the variable corrects itself. Bonnie has to urinate so you provide the bedpan as she is on bed rest. She cannot void on the bedpan so you call the PCP for a catheter order.

Exercise 16-9: *Ordering*

Number in order the steps required for a sterile catheterization procedure:

_____ Insert the catheter.

_____ Don sterile gloves.

_____ Explain the procedure to the patient.

_____ Secure the catheter to the patient's leg.

_____ Open the sterile package.

_____ Attach the bag to the catheter.

_____ Place the bag below the level of the bed.

_____ Prep the patient.

_____ Check the balloon is functional; blow up and deflate.

_____ Blow up the balloon.

_____ Lubricate the catheter.

_____ Position the patient.

(e) **eResource 16-3:** Open MerckMedicus on your mobile device and go to the Merck Manual [Pathway: Merck Manual → select "Topics" → enter "Magnesium sulfate" into the search field → scroll down to select "in preterm labor."]

The answer can be found on pages 250–251.

Bonnie is complaining about feeling "hot," "thirsty," and "agitated," and you know that this is a side effect of $MgSO_4$.

Exercise 16-10: *Multiple Choice Question*
The best nursing diagnosis to describe the patient at this point is:
- A. Activity intolerance
- B. Ineffective coping
- C. Decisional conflict
- D. Situational low self-esteem

Exercise 16-11: *Fill-in*
List three nursing interventions that would help the patient:
1. _____
2. _____
3. _____

Bonnie's lab results come back via the computer within 6 hours of admission.

Exercise 16-12: *Exhibit Question*
The lab report reads as follows: Circle the value that is of concern.

WBC	$5.7 \times 10E3/uL$
RBC	$4.23 \times 10E6/uL$
Hemoglobin	13.0 g/dL
Hematocrit	37.1%
Platelets	$330 \times 10E3/uL$
Neutrophils	$3.0 \times 10E3/uL$
Lymphs	$1.9 \times 10E3/uL$
Monocytes	$0.5 \times 10E3/uL$
Eosinophils	$0.2 \times 10E3/uL$
Basophils	$0.1 \times 10E3/uL$
Fetal fibronectin	0.02 ug/dL

The ultrasonographer finds that Bonnie's external cervical os is closed, but her internal cervical os is slightly (1cm) dilated. Bonnie settles down and sleeps for the night. Assessments are done every two hours while she is on $MgSO_4$.

Exercise 16-13: *Multiple Choice Question*
Focused assessments priorities for a patient on $MgSO_4$ include:
- A. Pulse and DTR (deep tendon reflexes)
- B. DTR and blood pressure
- C. Blood pressure and respirations
- D. Respirations and DTR

The answer can be found on pages 251–252.

The next morning Bonnie is no longer contracting and the $MgSO_4$ is decreased to 1 g/hr.

Exercise 16-14: *Calculation*

The $MgSO_4$ is now ordered at 1 g/hr $\times$ 12 hours. It is still in 40 gms/500 mL. At what level would you set the IV pump?

 eResource 16-4: IV Infusion Calculations (see eResource 16-2)
- Go to *MedCalc.com* to use the online IV rate calculator; or
- Use Skyscape's Archimedes, to calculate the new infusion rate.

The second dose of Betamethasone is given in the other ventrogluteal muscle. Discharge plans are being made for Bonnie. Since she lives 100 miles away, she agrees that it would be best for her to stay with her sister for the rest of the pregnancy since she will be on modified bed rest. Bonnie will be sent home with a home uterine activity monitor.

Exercise 16-15: *Fill-in*

List five other discharge instructions for the patient on modified bed rest for PTL:

1. _____
2. _____
3. _____
4. _____
5. _____

Bonnie is also sent home on Nifedipine (Procardia) because it blocks calcium from going into muscle cells and inhibits muscle activity.

 eResource 16-5:
- Open a browser and go to Epocrates online [Pathway: *online.epocrates.com* → tap on the "Drug" tab → enter "nifedipine" into the search field → select "Procardia" → read information. Note: be sure to tap on the Patient Education tab on the right.]
- Go to *MerckManuals.com* and select the "The Merck Manual for healthcare professionals" [Pathway: *merckmanuals.com* → select "Manual for healthcare professionals" → enter "hypertension in pregnancy" into the search field to view information regarding management of hypertension in pregnancy.]
- Go to the National Guidelines Clearinghouse (NGC) to view established practice guidelines for management of hypertension in pregnancy [Pathway: *guideline.gov* → enter "hypertension in pregnancy" into search field → tap to select the guideline to view.]
- On your mobile device, open MerckMedicus and go to the Merck Manual [Pathway: Merck Manual → Topics → enter "Nifedipine" into the search field → scroll down and select "in pregnancy" to read about treatment of hypertension in pregnancy.]

The answers can be found on page 252.

Exercise 16-16: *Multiple Choice Question*

Because of the side effect of Nifedipine (Procardia), patients should learn the signs of:

    A. Hypotension

    B. Hypertension

    C. Heart block

    D. Stroke

The answer can be found on page 252.

Answers

Exercise 16-1: *Fill-in*

List five risk factors identified for preterm labor (PTL) in the patient's history:

1. **African American (double the risk for PTL)**
2. **Low socioeconomic group**
3. **Maternal periodontal disease**
4. **Cigarette smoking**
5. **History of PTL (triples the risk)**
6. **Late prenatal care**
7. **Short interval between birth of children**

Exercise 16-2: *True/False*

Is it true or false to say that taking blood specimens from an IV site decreases specimen hemolysis? **False—it increases hemolysis.**

Exercise 16-3: *Calculation*

How many gtts/min would you set the IV of R/L at 120 mL/hr if the gtt factor was 15 gtts/mL?

120 mL $\times$ 15 gtt/mL = 1,800 gtts divided by 60 minutes = **30 gtts/min**

Exercise 16-4: *Calculation*

For how many mL/hr would you set the IV of $MgSO_4$ at in order to deliver 5 gms in the first 30 minutes?

500 mL divided by 40 = 1 gm in each 12.5 mL

12.5 mL $\times$ 5 gms = 62.5 mL

$\dfrac{\textbf{62.5 mL in 30 min}}{60 \text{ min}}$ = **125 mL/hr**

Exercise 16-5: *Calculation*

For how many mL/hr would you set the IV of $MgSO_4$ at in order to deliver 2 gms/hr for the remainder of the time?

2 gms = 25 mL or 12.5 $\times$ 2

so the answer is 25 mL/hr after the first 30 minutes

Exercise 16-6: *Select All That Apply*

The nurse understands the following items should be at the patient's bedside once they are maintained on MagSO$_4$:

❑ Tongue blade—NO, she does not have PIH (pregnancy induced hypertension).

❑ Padded side rails—NO, she does not have PIH (pregnancy induced hypertension).

☑ **Calcium gluconate—YES, this is the antidote.**

❑ Adult naloxone (Narcan)—NO, this is an antagonist for narcotics.

☑ **Reflex hammer—YES, MgSO$_4$ dulls reflexes.**

❑ Ophthalmoscope—NO, this is not needed.

Exercise 16-7: *Hot Spot*

Betamethasone is given deep IM in the right ventrogluteal muscle. Put an X on the spot where it should be given.

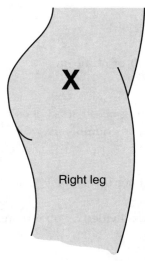

Right leg

Exercise 16-8: *Hot Spot*

Place Xs on the variable deceleration.

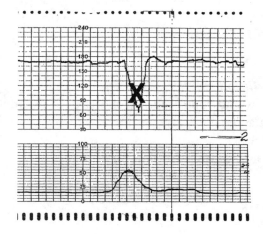

Exercise 16-9: *Ordering*

Number in order the steps required for a sterile catheterization procedure.

___7___ Insert the catheter.

___4___ Don sterile gloves.

___1___ Explain the procedure to the patient.

___10___ Secure the catheter to the patient's leg.

___3___ Open the sterile package.

___9___ Attach the bag to the catheter.

___11___ Place the bag below the level of the bed.

___4___ Prep the patient.

___5___ Check the balloon is functional—blow up and deflate.

___8___ Blow up the balloon.

___6___ Lubricate the catheter.

___2___ Position the patient.

Exercise 16-10: *Multiple Choice Question*

The best nursing diagnosis to describe the patient at this point is:

A. Activity intolerance—NO, this may occur later if the patient remains on bed rest.

B. **Ineffective coping—YES, she is having trouble coping with the side effects.**

C. Decisional conflict—NO, she has not been given a decision to make.

D. Situational low self-esteem—No, this has not been verbalized as a problem.

Exercise 16-11: *Fill-in*

List three nursing interventions that would help the patient:

1. **Provide ice chips and mouth care.**

2. **Provide a cool bath.**

3. **Decrease the environmental stimuli.**

4. **Change sheets.**

5. **Encourage her to verbalize.**

Exercise 16-12: *Exhibit Question*

The lab report reads as follows:

Circle the value that is of concern. **Fetal fibronectin should be negative. This indicates PTL and a value over 0.05 ug/dL is a strong indicator for PTL within 7–14 days.**

WBC	5.7 × 10E3/uL
RBC	4.23 × 10E6/uL
Hemoglobin	13.0 g/dL
Hematocrit	37.1%
Platelets	330 × 10E3/uL
Neutrophils	3.0 × 10E3/uL

Lymphs	$1.9 \times 10E3/uL$
Monocytes	$0.5 \times 10E3/uL$
Eosinophils	$0.2 \times 10E3/uL$
Basophils	$0.1 \times 10E3/uL$
Fetal fibronectin	0.02 ug/dL

Exercise 16-13: *Multiple Choice Question*

Focused assessments priorities for a patient on $MgSO_4$ include:

A. Pulse and DTR (deep tendon reflexes)—NO, pulse rate should not be affected.

B. DTR and blood pressure—NO, blood pressure should not be greatly affected.

C. Blood pressure and respirations—NO, blood pressure should not be greatly affected.

D. **Respirations and DTR—YES, both respirations and DTR are affected by $MgSO_4$.**

Exercise 16-14: *Calculation*

The $MgSO_4$ is now ordered at 1 g/hr $\times$ 12 hours. It is still in 40 gms/500 mL. At what level would you set the IV pump?

12.5 mL = 1 gm so the answer is **12.5 mL/hr**

Exercise 16-15: *Fill-in*

List five other discharge instructions for the patient on modified bed rest for PTL:

1. **Drink 8–10 glasses of water a day to prevent a UTI.**
2. **Do not lift heavy objects, including your toddler.**
3. **Visit the dentist—periodontal disease is directly related to PTL**
4. **No sexual activity—prostaglandins in sperm can set off labor.**
5. **Recognize the signs of PTL.**
6. **Do not smoke.**
7. **Avoid traveling.**

Exercise 16-16: *Multiple Choice Question*

Because of the side effect of Nifedipine (Procardia), patients should learn the signs of:

A. **Hypotension—YES, it can produce hypotension.**

B. Hypertension—NO, this is not the effect.

C. Heart block—NO, this is not the effect.

D. Stroke—NO, this is not the effect.

17

Cardiac Disease

Case Study 17 ▬ Maggie

Maggie is a 26-year-old gravida 1 who is at 32 weeks' gestation. Like 1% of women in this country, Maggie has a cardiac condition. She was born with a congenital heart defect and had corrective treatment for Tetralogy of Fallot and an artificial mitral valve replacement. In years past, Maggie would never have survived to childbearing age, but now, with improved technology and antibiotics, she is doing well. To understand the implications of pregnancy on heart disease your mentor reviews the hemodynamics of pregnancy with you in anticipation of Maggie's arrival on the high-risk perinatal unit.

 eResource 17-1: To learn more about Tetralogy of Fallot, go to:
- Medscape on your mobile device [Medscape → enter "Tetralogy" into the search field → select "Tetralogy of Fallot" and review content; be sure to click on "Workup" and "Treatment" to learn more and view images.]
- WebMD on your mobile device [Pathway: WebMD → enter "Tetralogy" into the search field → select "Tetralogy of Fallot" and review content; be sure to click on links to learn more.]

Exercise 17-1: *Fill-in*
Blood volume increases by _____ % during pregnancy.

Exercise 17-2: *Select All That Apply*
Other hemodynamic changes during pregnancy include:
- ❑ Increased cardiac output by 30–50%
- ❑ Decreased stroke volume
- ❑ Increased intravascular resistance
- ❑ Decreased pulmonary resistance
- ❑ Increased coagulability
- ❑ Increase in systolic and diastolic blood pressures

The answers can be found on page 259.

Although Maggie's heart defect was surgically repaired as a child she still has some cardiac decomposition. She is classified as a Class II cardiac by the New York Heart Association (1994), which is the most widely used classification.

Exercise 17-3: *Matching*
Match the classification with the degree of cardiac decomposition.

_____ Asymptomatic with no limitations

_____ Symptomatic at rest or with any activity

_____ Symptomatic with increased activity

_____ Symptomatic with normal activity

A. Class I

B. Class II

C. Class III

D. Class IV

Exercise 17-4: *Multiple Choice Question*
The nurse understands that symptoms of cardiac decomposition include:

A. Dyspnea, chest pain, and fatigue

B. Alertness, palpitations, and dyspnea

C. Palpitations, alertness, and fatigue

D. Decreased pulse, fatigue, dyspnea

eResource 17-2:
- To learn more about the NYHA Cardiac Classifications, go to: *www.abouthf.org/questions_stages.htm*
- To view established practice guidelines for Tetralogy of Fallot, go to the National Guidelines Clearinghouse (NGC) [*guideline.gov* → enter "Tetralogy of Fallot" into search field → tap to select a current guideline to review.]

Exercise 17-5: *Multiple Choice Question*
One reason the women who are pregnant experience dyspnea in their second trimester may be:

A. Uterus pushing on the diaphragm

B. Increased fetal growth

C. Increase oxygen consumption by 20–30%

D. Decreased lung capacity

Exercise 17-6: *Multiple Choice Question*
One of the important physical assessments to determine on a cardiac patient is:

A. Hemoglobin

B. Pedal edema

C. Pedal pulses

D. Visual disturbances

The answers can be found on pages 259–260.

eResource 17-3: To review information regarding management of heart disease in pregnancy, go to MerckMedicus and open the Merck Manual [Pathway: Merck Manual → Topics → enter "pregnancy" into the search field → select "Pregnancy" → scroll down and select "heart disorders in . . ." → select "Heart Disorders in Pregnancy" → tap on the drop-down menu in the upper right corner of the screen to navigate the content; be sure to read "Symptoms and Signs."]

Exercise 17-7: *Hot Spot*

Place a mark on the four areas affected by Tetralogy of Fallot.

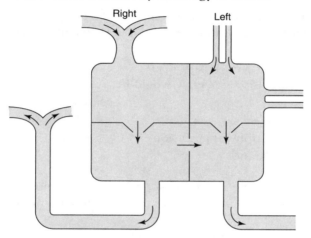

As more women with cardiac conditions decide to start families, the perinatal nurse must become increasingly aware of the types of cardiac anomalies in order to understand the underlying pathophysiology that complicates pregnancy.

 eResource 17-4: Staying in the Merck Manual [Pathway: Merck Manual → Topics → enter "pregnancy" into the search field → select "Pregnancy" → scroll down and select "heart disorders in . . ." → select "Approach to the Cardiac Patient" to review assessment of the cardiac patient; be sure to tap on the drop-down menu in the upper right corner of the screen to navigate the content containing all assessment parameters.]

Exercise 17-8: *Matching*

Match the condition with its description.

_____ Opening between the atria producing a left to right shunt and may cause arrhythmias.

_____ Opening between the ventricles causing a left to right shunt with possible symptoms of arrhythmias, heart failure, and pulmonary hypertension.

_____ Communication between the aorta and the pulmonary artery causing pulmonary hypertension.

_____ The valve opening is narrower than normal and obstructs left ventricular ejection of blood.

The answers can be found on pages 260–261.

      A. Patent ductus arteriosus (PDA)

      B. Aortic stenosis

      C. Ventricle septal defect (VSD)

      D. Atrial septal defect (ASD)

Exercise 17-9: *Fill-in*

In addition to congenital heart defects, the nurse is aware that 50% of heart defects in pregnant women are acquired. The most commonly acquired heart defect in this age group is: _____.

While taking Maggie's history and collecting your data, you notice that she prefers to sit while speaking to you and takes her time between sentences.

Exercise 17-10: *Multiple Choice Question*

A priority nursing diagnosis for Maggie would be:

      A. Fatigue

      B. Fluid volume excess

      C. Ineffective peripheral perfusion

      D. Activity intolerance

You receive orders from the cardiologist and the primatologist. A 12-lead EKG is ordered and is completed; it shows a rate of 210 beats per minute (Exercise 17-11).

Exercise 17-11: *Exhibit Question*

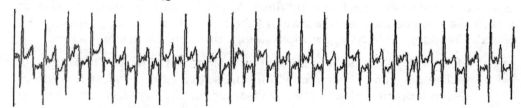

The above EKG is displaying what type of cardiac pattern? _____.

 eResource 17-5: To learn more about EKG interpretation, view:
■ Video tutorial reviewing the basics of EKG interpretation: *youtu.be/ex1k_MPF-w4;* or go to
■ The EKG Library: *www.ecglibrary.com*

Propranolol (Inderal) is ordered for Maggie to 40 mg po b.i.d. Maggie is kept for 2 days to assess her tolerance to the medication. She does well with no further complaints of a "fast heart beat." On the second morning you prepare Maggie for discharge. She is to return to the high-risk perinatal clinic every 2 weeks for evaluation.

 eResource 17-6: For patient education material regarding Maggie's medication and follow-up care, go to Epocrates online [Pathway: *online.epocrates.com* → tap on the "Drugs" tab → enter "inderal" in the search field to view content → be sure to select "Patient Education."]

The answers can be found on page 261.

Exercise 17-12: *Select All That Apply*

Discharge teaching for Maggie should include:

❑ Increasing rest periods

❑ Medication administration

❑ Medication side effects

❑ Increasing exercise

❑ Using weights once a week

❑ Daily fetal kick counts

❑ Fluid restriction

❑ Decreasing fiber in her diet

Maggie tells you during the discharge teaching session that she knows a woman who was diagnosed with a heart disease who she needed a heart transplant after she had her baby and that the baby caused the heart disease. Maggie is concerned that this is going to happen to her.

Exercise 17-13: *Multiple Choice Question*

An appropriate response to Maggie's statement is:

A. "You may be describing peripartum cardiomyopathy, which is a rare occurrence and unrelated to your diagnosis."

B. "You could also get peripartum cardiomyopathy with your heart disease."

C. "Peripartum cardiomyopathy happens very rarely."

D. "Peripartum cardiomyopathy will be prevented if you adhere to your medication and rest schedule."

Maggie asks you if they will automatically schedule a Cesarean section for her since she is high risk.

Exercise 17-14: *Multiple Choice Question*

The nurse would base her answer about the type of delivery for a cardiac patient based on the knowledge that:

A. General anesthesia provides the best control for the surgeon.

B. Local anesthesia is needed for a Cesarean delivery.

C. Decreasing intrathoracic pressure by a low forceps delivery is preferred.

D. Cardiac patients are a surgical risk and should push their babies out.

 eResource 17-7: To supplement your patient teaching, you can provide Maggie with the Mayo Clinic's patient pamphlet: "Heart Problems and Pregnancy." To access, open a browser on your mobile device and go to the National Library of Medicine to access MedlinePlus [Pathway: *nlm .nih.gov* → select "MedlinePlus" → enter "heart problems and pregnancy" into the search field → scroll down and select "Heart Problems and Pregnancy" to review. Note: information regarding delivery options is included.]

The answers can be found on page 262.

Answers

Exercise 17-1: *Fill-in*

Blood volume increases by **50**% during pregnancy.

Exercise 17-2: *Select All That Apply*

Other hemodynamic changes during pregnancy include:

☑ **Increase cardiac output by 30–50%—YES.**

☐ Decreased stroke volume—NO, stroke volume is increased to compensate for the increase in blood volume.

☐ Increased intravascular resistance—NO, resistance is decreased to accommodate the increased blood volume and progesterone (smooth muscle relaxer) plays a part in this physiological change.

☑ **Decreased pulmonary resistance—YES, this helps increased blood volume get to the lungs because there is increased oxygen consumption.**

☑ **Increased coagulability—YES, pregnancy is a hypercoagulability state to prevent postpartum hemorrhage.**

☐ Increase in systolic and diastolic blood pressures—NO, it is decreased due to decreased resistance.

Exercise 17-3: *Matching*

Match the classification with the degree of cardiac decomposition:

_____**A**_____ Asymptomatic with no limitations

_____**D**_____ Symptomatic at rest or with any activity

_____**B**_____ Symptomatic with increased activity

_____**C**_____ Symptomatic with normal activity

A. Class I

B. Class II

C. Class III

D. Class IV

Exercise 17-4: *Multiple Choice Question*
The nurse understands that symptoms of cardiac decomposition include:
  A. **Dyspnea, chest pain, and fatigue—YES.**
  B. Alertness, palpitations, and dyspnea—NO, alertness is not a usual symptom.
  C. Palpitations, alertness, and fatigue—NO, alertness is not a usual symptom.
  D. Decreased pulse, fatigue, dyspnea—NO pulse is increased.

Exercise 17-5: *Multiple Choice Question*
One reason the women who are pregnant experience dyspnea in their second trimester may be:
  A. Uterus pushing on the diaphragm—NO, this is a third trimester symptom.
  B. Increased fetal growth—NO, most of the fetal weight is added in the third trimester.
  C. **Increase oxygen consumption by 20–30%—YES.**
  D. Decreased lung capacity—NO, it is actually increased during pregnancy.

Exercise 17-6: *Multiple Choice Question*
One of the important physical assessments to determine on a cardiac patient would be:
  A. Hemoglobin—NO, this is a lab diagnosis, not a physical assessment.
  B. **Pedal edema—YES, this is a sign of cardiac decompensation.**
  C. Pedal pulses—NO, this should not be affected.
  D. Visual disturbances—NO, this should not be affected.

Exercise 17-7: *Hot Spot*
Place a mark on the four areas affected by Tetralogy of Fallot.

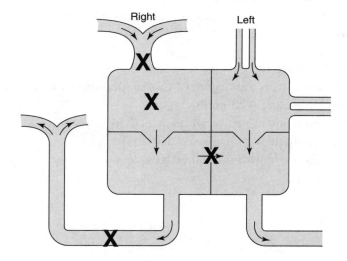

Exercise 17-8: *Matching*

Match the condition and description

_____**D**_____ Opening between the atria producing a left to right shunt; may cause arrhythmias.

_____**C**_____ Opening between the ventricles causing a left to right shunt with possible symptoms of arrhythmias, heart failure, and pulmonary hypertension.

_____**A**_____ Communication between the aorta and the pulmonary artery causing pulmonary hypertension.

_____**B**_____ The valve opening is narrower than normal and obstructs left ventricular ejection of blood

A. Patent ductus arteriosus (PDA)
B. Aortic stenosis
C. Ventricle septal defect (VSD)
D. Atrial septal defect (ASD)

Exercise 17-9: *Fill-in*

Besides congenital heart defects, the nurse is aware that 50% of heart defects in pregnant women are acquired. The most commonly acquired heart defect in this age group is: **rheumatic heart disease.**

Exercise 17-10: *Multiple Choice Question*

A priority nursing diagnosis for Maggie would be:

A. Fatigue—NO, she has not complained of tiredness at this point.
B. Fluid volume excess—NO, you have not assessed her edema currently.
C. Ineffective peripheral perfusion—NO, you have not assessed pulses as of yet.
D. **Activity intolerance—YES, she is displaying signs of normal activity intolerance.**

Exercise 17-11: *Exhibit Question*

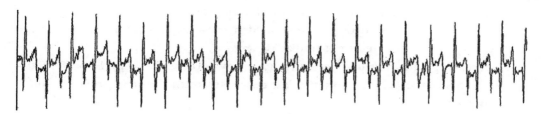

The above EKG is displaying what type of cardiac pattern? **Supraventricular Tachycardia**

Exercise 17-12: *Select All That Apply*

Discharge teaching for Maggie should include:

☑ **Increasing rest periods—YES, this will conserve energy.**

☑ **Medication administration—YES, she must understand how to accurately take her Inderal.**

❑ Medication side effects—YES, she should contact her PCP if she experiences side effects.

❑ Increasing exercise—NO, this is contraindicated for a cardiac patient who is symptomatic.

❑ Using weights once a week—NO, they should be done every day.

☑ **Daily fetal kick counts—YES, this is for fetal wellbeing.**

❑ Fluid restriction—NO, this is not done unless there are signs of congestive heart failure.

❑ Decreasing fiber in her diet—NO, fiber should be increased to reduce straining and reduce the chance of a vagal response.

Exercise 17-13: *Multiple Choice Question*

An appropriate response to Maggie's statement would be:
A. **"You may be describing peripartum cardiomyopathy, which is a rare occurrence and unrelated to your diagnosis."—YES, this is the best answer.**
B. "You could also get peripartum cardiomyopathy with your heart disease."—NO, this will increase anxiety.
C. "Peripartum cardiomyopathy happens very rarely."—NO, this is false reassurance.
D. "Peripartum cardiomyopathy will be prevented if you adhere to your medication and rest schedule."—NO, this is unrelated and not based on evidence.

Exercise 17-14: *Multiple Choice Question*

The nurse would base her answer about the type of delivery for a cardiac patient based on:
A. General anesthesia provides the best control for the surgeon—NO, general anesthesia is a risk to the patient with a cardiac disease.
B. Local anesthesia is needed for a Cesarean delivery—NO, this is true, but a Cesarean delivery is not preferred for a cardiac patient.
C. **Decreasing intrathoracic pressure by a low forceps delivery is preferred— YES, this is the preferred method; it decreases intra thoracic pressure and is controlled.**
D. Cardiac patients are a surgical risk and should push their babies out—NO, pushing is discouraged because of the pressure changes it produces.

18

Asthma

Case Study 18 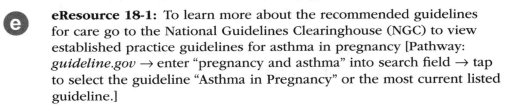 Rachel

Rachel is a 24-year-old who is in the clinical for preconceptual counseling due to her asthma. She has had a history of asthma since she was a child and has allergies to pollen, dust mites, and mold. She was on allergy shots until college and then discontinued them. She has two inhalers: a maintenance inhaler of albuterol (Proventil) and an "emergency" inhaler of prednisone (Deltasone). If her asthma attack is severe she takes po prednisone also.

e **eResource 18-1:** To learn more about the recommended guidelines for care go to the National Guidelines Clearinghouse (NGC) to view established practice guidelines for asthma in pregnancy [Pathway: *guideline.gov* → enter "pregnancy and asthma" into search field → tap to select the guideline "Asthma in Pregnancy" or the most current listed guideline.]

Exercise 18-1: *Multiple Choice Question*
The nurse understands that the therapeutic effect of albuterol (Proventil) is:

    A. Antispasmodic

    B. Bronchodilator

    C. Antiallergic

    D. Antihistamine

e **eResource 18-2:** To learn more about Rachel's medications, go to Epocrates online [Pathway: *online.epocrates.com* → tap on the "Drugs" tab → enter "proventil" and "prednisone" in the search field to review information.]

The answer can be found on page 267.

According to her history, Rachel's asthma attacks are induced by seasonal variations as well as environmental triggers. Rachel asks about her risks as well as the best method of preventing complications. In order to best answer her questions you review the effects of pregnancy on the respiratory system.

Exercise 18-2: *Select All That Apply*
The changes that are normal for the respiratory system during pregnancy include:

❑ Increased respiratory rate.
❑ Elevated diaphragm.
❑ Increase in hyperventilation near term.
❑ Increase in residual lung capacity.

e   **eResource 18-3:** To learn more about women and asthma and the effects of pregnancy on asthma control, listen to this podcast from National Jewish Health featuring Esther Langmack, MD *www.nationaljewish.org/ healthinfo/multimedia/podcasts/asthma-women-podcast.aspx*

Exercise 18-3: *Multiple Choice Question*
The fetal side effects of woman who have uncontrolled asthma include:

A. Increased infant death, large for gestational age, preterm birth.
B. Postterm birth, intrauterine growth restriction, prolonged labor.
C. Prolonged labor, postterm birth, increased infant death.
D. Preterm birth, increased infant death, intrauterine growth restriction.

Rachel also inquires if her asthma will become worse during pregnancy.

Exercise 18-4: *Multiple Choice Question*
What percent of women with asthma experience a worsening of the condition?

A. 1/8
B. 1/4
C. 1/3
D. 1/2

Rachel also asks about complications to herself.

Exercise 18-5: *Select All That Apply*
Maternal complications of uncontrolled asthma during pregnancy include:

❑ Pregnancy-induced hypertension
❑ Postdate
❑ Placenta abruption
❑ Hemorrhage

Her physical assessment reveals no wheezing in her lungs, but she does have a dry nonproductive cough. The nurse asks Rachel some further questions related to her living conditions and if she has recently traveled outside the country or

The answers can be found on pages 267–268.

experiences a fever or night sweats. What other respiratory condition, which is rising in incidence, is the nurse screening for?

Exercise 18-6: *Multiple Choice Question*

What other respiratory condition, which is rising in incidence, is the nurse screening for?

 A. Whooping cough or pertussis

 B. Pneumonia

 C. Severe acute respiratory syndrome (SARS)

 D. Tuberculosis (TB)

 eResource 18-4: To learn more about the risks associated with asthma and pregnancy:

 ■ View the Pregnancy Show's video "Risks of Maternal Asthma" by going to: *www.thepregnancyshow.com/Risks_Of_Maternal_Asthma.html*

 ■ Open a browser on your mobile device and go to: *nlm.nih.gov* to access MedlinePlus [Pathway: *nlm.nih.gov* → select "MedlinePlus → enter "asthma and pregnancy" into the search field → scroll down and select "Asthma Management in Pregnancy."]

You investigate reasons for Rachel's anemia and find out that she is a vegetarian. She is asked to keep a 24-hour diet history for a week and then return with it. Her diet history reveals a lack of iron-rich foods.

Exercise 18-7: *Multiple Choice Question*

The best dietary suggestions for the patient are:

 A. Green leafy vegetables, meats, iron-fortified cereal.

 B. Dried fruit, high-fiber food, iron-fortified cereal.

 C. Green leafy vegetables, legumes, dried fruit.

 D. Legumes, peanut butter, high-fiber cereal.

A purified protein derivative (PPD) test is done on Rachel as well as a rubella titer and some routine blood work. She is instructed to continue her maintenance inhaler and return to the clinic in two days for her one-step PPD to be read. Rachel does return in two days and although her PPD is negative, she has a hematocrit result of 30.6%, which places her in the anemic category.

 eResource 18-5: To review the procedure for administering a PPD test and reading the results, view this video: *youtu.be/bR86G-itrTQ*

Exercise 18-8: *Select All That Apply*

The nurse should include which of the following suggestions when teaching the anemic patient?

 ❑ Take iron supplements with meals.

 ❑ Avoid taking iron supplements with chocolate.

 ❑ Increase high-fiber foods.

 ❑ Increase exercise.

The answers can be found on page 268.

Rachel is not only ordered an iron supplement but also prenatal vitamins to ensure that preconceptually she is receiving plenty of folic acid as well as vitamins.

Exercise 18-9: *Fill-in*

Folic acid is needed for iron absorption and to prevent _____ in the fetus.

eResource 18-6: To supplement patient teaching regarding the healthy benefits of folic acid,

- how Rachel this March of Dimes video "Healthy Pregnancy, Healthy Baby: Folic Acid for Women" *youtu.be/kg2xqK0Zy5c*
- To learn more about folic acid and to supplement your patient teaching, go to Epocrates online [Pathway: *online.epocrates.com* → tap on the "Drugs" tab → enter "folic acid" in the search field to review information; be sure to refer to the "Patient Education" section.]

Exercise 18-10: *Fill-in*

Which vitamin should be given with iron to increase absorption? _____

In three months Rachel returns to the clinic because she has missed her period and has had a positive result on an at-home pregnancy test. The pregnancy is confirmed at the clinic.

The answer can be found on page 269.

Answers

Exercise 18-1: *Multiple Choice Question*

The nurse understands that the therapeutic effect of albuterol (Proventil) is:

A. Antispasmodic—NO.

B. **Bronchodilator—YES.**

C. Antiallergic—NO.

D. Antihistamine—NO.

Exercise 18-2: *Select All That Apply*

The changes that are normal for the respiratory system during pregnancy include:

❑ Increase respiratory rate—NO, the rate does not change.

☑ **The diaphragm is elevated—YES, it is pushed up by the uterus.**

☑ **Increase in hyperventilation near term—YES, this is experienced by 48% of women.**

❑ Increase in residual lung capacity—NO, this is decreased.

Exercise 18-3: *Multiple Choice Question*

The fetal side effects of women who have uncontrolled asthma include:

A. Increased infant death, large for gestational age, preterm birth—NO, they are small for gestational age.

B. Postterm birth, intrauterine growth restriction, prolonged labor—NO, preterm birth is more frequent.

C. Prolonged labor, postterm birth, increased infant death—NO, they do not have prolonged labor.

D. **Preterm birth increased infant death, intrauterine growth restriction—YES.**

Exercise 18-4: *Multiple Choice Question*

What percent of women with asthma experience a worsening of the condition?

A. 1/8

B. 1/4

C. **1/3**

D. 1/2

Exercise 18-5: *Select All That Apply*

Maternal complications of uncontrolled asthma during pregnancy include:

☑ **Pregnancy-induced hypertension—YES, this is a complication more frequent in women with asthma.**

❑ Postdate—NO, women with asthma more frequently have preterm births.

❑ Placenta abruption—NO, placenta previa is associated with women with asthma.

☑ **Hemorrhage—YES, this is a perinatal complication experienced more frequently by women with asthma.**

Exercise 18-6: *Multiple Choice Question*

What other respiratory condition, which is rising in incidence, is the nurse screening for?

❑ Whooping cough or pertussis—NO, this is on the rise, but night sweats are not a classic symptom.

❑ Pneumonia—NO, this is on the rise, but night sweats are not a classic symptom.

❑ Severe acute respiratory syndrome (SARS)—NO, this is on the rise, but night sweats are not a classic symptom.

☑ **Tuberculosis (TB)—YES, these are the screening questions for TB.**

Exercise 18-7: *Multiple Choice Question*

The best dietary suggestions for the patient are:

A. Green leafy vegetables, meats, iron-fortified cereal—NO, vegetarians do not eat meat.

B. Dried fruit, high-fiber food, iron-fortified cereal—NO, high-fiber foods decrease the absorption of iron.

C. **Green leafy vegetables, legumes, dried fruit—YES, these all contain iron.**

D. Legumes, peanut butter, high-fiber cereal—NO, high-fiber foods decrease the absorption of iron.

Exercise 18-8: *Select All That Apply*

The nurse should include which of the following suggestions when teaching the anemic patient?

❑ Take iron supplements with meals—NO, it should be taken between meals.

☑ **Avoid taking iron supplements with chocolate—YES, avoid taking it with coffee, tea, or chocolate; caffeine decreases absorption.**

☑ **Increase high-fiber foods—YES, now high fiber is needed because iron will constipate the patient.**

❑ Increase exercise—NO, rest is needed for anemic patients.

Exercise 18-9: *Fill-in*

Folic acid is needed for iron absorption and to prevent **neural tube defects (NTD)** in the fetus.

Exercise 18-10: *Fill-in*

Which vitamin should be given with iron to increase absorption? **Vitamin C**

19

Sickle Cell Anemia

Case Study 19 Maria

Maria is a 28-year-old gravida 2 who is at 34 weeks' gestation and is being admitted to the high-risk perinatal unit with sickle cell crises. Maria is known to the perinatal staff because she had crises with her first pregnancy also. Maria is reporting severe pain in her right knee, which is observed to be edematous, tender, and warm to the touch.

Exercise 19-1: *Multiple Choice Question*
The nurse knows that the abnormal HbS in sickle cell disease replaces:

    A. HbA

    B. HbB

    C. HbC

    D. HbD

Exercise 19-2: *Multiple Choice Question*
The nurse understands that a patient with sickle cell disease inherited:

    A. A dominant gene from his/her father

    B. A dominant gene from his/her mother

    C. A sex-linked gene from his/her mother

    D. Recessive genes from both parents

 eResource 19-1: To review information regarding sickle cell disease, go to
- The National Library of Medicine's Genetics Home Resource [Pathway: *ghr.nlm.nih.gov* → enter "sickle cell" into the search field → select "sickle cell disease" to view information.
- MerckMedicus on your mobile device and open the Merck Manual [Pathway: Merck Manual → enter "sickle cell" into the search field → select "Sickle Cell Disease" → select "pregnancy and . . ." and review the Basics;
- On your mobile device, open WebMD [Pathway: WebMD → enter "sickle cell" into the search field → select "Sickle cell Disease" to read an overview and about pain management.]

The answers can be found on page 275.

Exercise 19-3: *Fill-in*

The nurse understands that the normal life span of a red blood cell (RBC) is _____ days.

Exercise 19-4: *Multiple Choice Question*

Sickle cells have a shorter life span than normal RBCs; it is:

    A. 10–20 days

    B. 30–40 days

    C. 50–60 days

    D. 70–80 days

Exercise 19-5: *Multiple Choice Question*

A priority nursing assessment for a sickle cell patient complaining of pain in the right knee would be:

    A. Examine the left knee

    B. Check vital signs

    C. Pedal pulse on the right side

    D. Femoral pulse on the right side

Maria is given an analgesic that also has an anti-inflammatory effect. Her knee is immobilized and an IV is started to increase hydration.

 eResource 19-2: For additional information regarding the management of sickle cell disease, go to:

    ■ Epocrates Online [Pathway: *online.epocrates.com* → tap on the "Diseases" tab → enter "sickle" in the search field → select "sickle cell disease" and then "Treatment" to review information.]

    ■ View the recommended guidelines for care for Maria, go to the National Guideline Clearinghouse to view the established guidelines [Pathway: *guideline.gov* → enter "sickle cell and pregnancy" into the search field → scroll down and select "Hemoglobinopathies in pregnancy" or other relevant guidelines.]

    ■ Listen to the CDC podcast "A Century of Sickle Cell": *www2c.cdc.gov/ podcasts/player.asp?f=3162007*

Exercise 19-6: *Calculation*

An IV is ordered Normal Saline at 150 mL/hr. The tubing has a gtt factor of 12. For how many gtts/min should the IV run?

Antibiotics are also ordered for Maria to prevent secondary infection at the inflamed site. She is ordered 1,000 mg of amoxicillin IB piggyback (IVPB) to run for 30 min t.i.d.

Exercise 19-7: *Calculation*

Amoxicillin comes in IVPB of 100 mL and is to run for 30 minutes. How many gtts/ min is that?

The answers can be found on pages 275–276.

eResource 19-3: To use a medication calculator:
- Go to *MedCalc.com* to use the online IV Rate calculator [Pathway: *medcalc.com* → select "Fluids/Electrolytes" → select "IV Rate"] or
- On your mobile device, use Skyscape's Archimedes, to calculate the infusion rate [pathway: Archimedes → enter "IV" into the Main Index → scroll down to "IV Calc: Infusion rate mL/hr"]
- To learn more about Maria's medications, go to Epocrates online [Pathway: *online.epocrates.com* → tap on the "Drugs" tab → enter "amoxicillin" in the search field to review information; be sure to review "Adverse Reactions" and "Safety and Monitoring."]

Weekly NSTs are ordered for fetal surveillance.

Exercise 19-8: *Exhibit*

The following fetal monitor strip is Maria's NST.

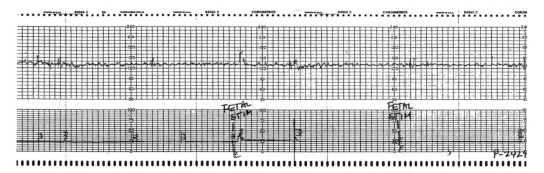

Is the above strip:

    A. Equivocal

    B. Reactive

    C. Nonreactive

    D. Positive

 eResource 19-4: Let's review again how to interpret a fetal heart rate strip,
- Go to *Fetalmonitorstrips.com* [Pathway: *fetalmonitorstrips.com* → click on "Learn more about monitor patterns and fetal distress" located at the top of the screen] or
- Go to *Monitorart.org* [Pathway: *monitorart.org* → scroll down and select "How to interpret the fetal heart monitor tracing" from the menu on the left.]

The answer can be found on page 276.

Maria is given some cold water to drink to stimulate the fetus. After three days of bed rest, extra hydration, and analgesics Maria is discharged to home.

Exercise 19-9: *Select All That Apply*

Discharge instructions for Maria should include:

❏ Exercise

❏ Nutritional counseling

❏ Increased hydration

❏ Infection prevention

Maria is told to increase her clinic visits to weekly at this point for monitoring her condition and for fetal surveillance.

Exercise 19-10: *Multiple Choice Question*

Another hematological concern for sickle cell patients is:

A. Hyperbilirubinemia

B. Elevated WBCs

C. Mediterranean anemia

D. Iron deficiency anemia

 eResource 19-5: To supplement patient teaching, you may elect to show Maria the following:

■ A video from the National Heart, Lung and Blood Institute: *www.nhlbi .nih.gov/health/dci/videos/sca/video_sca.html* or

■ For another patient education video about sickle cell anemia disease, go to the Health Science Channel: *www.healthsciencechannel .com/?video_id=504*

■ For additional information to share with Maria about sickle cell and pregnancy, go to:

■ March of Dimes [Pathway: *marchofdimes.com* → enter "sickle cell disease" into the search field → scroll down and review information; or

■ The U.S. Preventative Services Task Force: [Pathway: *www .uspreventiveservicestaskforce.org* → enter "sickle cell screening" into the search field → select "Screening: Sickle Cell Disease in Newborns" to review screening recommendations for the newborn as well as other relevant materials listed.]

The answers can be found on page 276.

Answers

Exercise 19-1: *Multiple Choice Question*

The nurse knows that the abnormal HbS in sickle cell disease replaces:

A. **HbA—YES, it is HbA that is replaced with HbS.**

B. HbB—NO.

C. HbC—NO.

D. HbD—NO.

Exercise 19-2: *Multiple Choice Question*

The nurse understands that a patient with sickle cell disease inherited:

A. A dominant gene from his/her father—NO.

B. A dominant gene from his/her mother—NO.

C. A sex-linked gene from his/her mother—NO.

D. **Recessive genes from both parents—YES, both parents are carriers.**

Exercise 19-3: *Fill-in*

The nurse understands that the normal life span of a red blood cell (RBC) is __120__ days.

Exercise 19-4: *Multiple Choice Question*

Sickle cells have a shorter life span than normal RBCs; it is:

A. **10–20 days—YES, the life span is very short.**

B. 30–40 days—NO.

C. 50–60 days—NO.

D. 70–80 days—NO.

Exercise 19-5: *Multiple Choice Question*

A priority nursing assessment for a sickle cell patient complaining of pain in the right knee would be:

A. Examine the left knee—NO, this is a needed assessment but not the priority.

B. Check vital signs—NO, this is a needed assessment but not the priority.

C. **Pedal pulse on the right side—YES, this is below the vaso-occlusion and there is always the concern of lack of circulation to any body part below the occlusion.**

D. Femoral pulse on the right side—NO, this is a needed assessment but not the priority.

Exercise 19-6: *Calculation*

An IV is ordered Normal Saline at 150 mL/hr. The tubing has a gtt factor of 12. For how many gtts/min should the IV run?

150 mL/hr $\times$ 12 gtts/ mL = <u>1,800 gtts/hr</u> = **30 gtts/ min**
60 min/hr

Exercise 19-7: *Calculation*

Amoxicillin comes in IVPB of 100 mL and is to run for 30 minutes. How many gtts/min is that?

100 mL/ 30 min $\times$ 12 gtts/ mL = 1,200 gtts/ 30 min = **40 gtts/min**

Exercise 19-8: *Exhibit*

Is the above strip:
  A. Equivocal—NO, this is for some accelerations.
  B. Reactive—NO, this is two accelerations in 20 minutes.
  C. **Nonreactive—YES, there are no accelerations with the fetal movements, which is why Maria is given cold water to drink. It stimulates the fetus to increase movements.**
  D. Positive—NO, this is a term used for contraction stress tests (CSTs).

Exercise 19-9: *Select All That Apply*

Discharge instructions for Maria should include:

❑ Exercise—NO, resting the joint is more beneficial.

☑ **Nutritional counseling—YES, high iron diets are needed.**

☑ **Increased hydration—YES, to decrease blood viscosity.**

☑ **Infection prevention—YES, to decrease stress on the immune and circulatory system.**

Exercise 19-10: *Multiple Choice Question*

Another hematological concern for sickle cell patients is:
  A. Hyperbilirubinemia—NO, adult livers can reduce this amount of bilirubin.
  B. Elevated WBCs—NO, this will only happen with an infection.
  C. Mediterranean anemia—NO, this is a different condition.
  D. **Iron deficiency anemia—YES, HbS does not carry as much Fe.**

20

Human Immunodeficiency Virus (HIV)

Case Study 20 ▬ Kendall

Kendall is a 26-year-old gravida 1 who is HIV positive for the past 3 years and is now pregnant with her first child. You are the nurse in the perinatal unit and do the intake history on Kendall.

Exercise 20-1: *Multiple Choice Question*
The nurse understands that the HIV virus attacks the:

    A. T3 cells
    B. T4 cells
    C. WCBs
    D. Lymphocytes

Kendall's history includes an uneventful childhood, with no major illness. She had a tonsillectomy and adenoidectomy (T&A) at age 5. After high school she went to a community college for a year to study becoming an X ray technician. She dropped out of school when she met her boyfriend who was a recovered IV drug addict. She stayed with him for 3 years, during which time he became severely immuno-suppressed and had AIDS (acquired immunodeficiency syndrome). He has since died and Kendall has finished school. She is in a healthy relationship with a man who is aware that she is HIV positive. They have protected sex with condoms and to conceive she was artificially inseminated with his sperm.

Exercise 20-2: *Multiple Choice Question*
Partners of HIV-positive individuals should understand that the latent phase be-fore HIV antibodies can be detected in an enzyme-linked immunosorbent assay (ELISA) is:

    A. 2–3 weeks
    B. 4–8 weeks
    C. 6–12 weeks
    D. 6 months

The answers can be found on page 281.

Kendall takes antiretroviral drugs to decrease the progression of the disease. Efavirenz (Atripla) 100 mg a day in combination with azidothymidine (AZT). She is advised to continue taking them during her pregnancy.

Exercise 20-3: *Multiple Choice Question*

The nurse understands that the primary rationale for continuing a woman's antiretroviral therapy during pregnancy is to:

    A. Slow the disease.

    B. Stop the progression of the disease during pregnancy.

    C. Decrease perinatal transmission.

    D. Increase the mother's immune status.

 eResource 20-1:
- Go to AIDSinfo (*www.aidsinfo.nih.gov*) to download PDA Tools containing treatment guidelines onto your mobile device (Palm and Pocket PC)
- Open another browser and go to the Trip Database: [Pathway: *tripdatabase.com* → enter "HIV in Pregnancy" into the search field → scroll down and if available, select a result from the Cochran Database of Systematic Review.]

Kendall asks many questions about her condition.

Exercise 20-4: *Fill-in*

The nurse explains that the fastest growing population of people contracting HIV are:

    A. Homosexual males

    B. Heterosexual males

    C. Homosexual females

    D. Heterosexual females

 eResource 20-2: For Patient Educational Material regarding HIV and Pregnancy go to: *www.merckmedicus.com* [Pathway: *merckmedicus.com* → select the "Patient Education" tab → enter "HIV and Pregnancy" into the search field to locate relevant patient education material.]

Kendall knows that taking her antiretroviral therapy decreases the chance of perinatal transmission from 35 to 5%. Should a child contract HIV by perinatal transmission, 80% have symptoms within 3–5 years of life.

Exercise 20-5: *Fill-in*

The HIV virus _____ be transmitted by breast milk.

 eResource 20-3: On your mobile device, open MerckMedicus and go to the Merck Manual [Pathway: Merck Manual → enter "Human immunodeficiency" into the search field → select "Human immunodeficiency virus (HIV) infection" → scroll down and select "Transmission of" → select "mother-to-child" and scroll down to "Transmission."]

The answers can be found on pages 281–282.

Exercise 20-6: *Select All That Apply*

Fetal and newborn risks associated with HIV are:

- ❑ Premature birth
- ❑ Postdate births
- ❑ Large for gestation age
- ❑ Small for gestational age

Exercise 20-7: *Multiple Choice Question*

The nurse knows from working in the high-risk clinic that it is recommended by the U.S. Public Health Service that HIV screening should be done prenatally on:

- A. Underprivileged women
- B. Women of African American decent
- C. Women who admit to drug use
- D. All women

 eResource 20-4:

- ■ For more information regarding recommended treatment for Kendall, go to the National Guideline Clearinghouse (NGC) *guideline.gov* [Pathway: NGC Home → enter "HIV and Pregnancy" into the search field → enter "recommendations" into the search field.]
- ■ Open Harrison's Practice on your mobile device to review PEARLS (practice guidelines) related to the care of HIV-positive pregnant women [Pathway: Mobile MerckMedicus → Harrison's Practice → Topics → enter "HIV" into the search field → select "during pregnancy" → tap on the menu bar on the upper right corner of the screen and select "PEARLS."]

Exercise 20-8: *Fill-in*

Should a woman have a positive ELISA test, what would be the next test to confirm the diagnosis? _____

 eResource 20-5: Refer to Harrison's Practice on your mobile device to learn more about diagnostic procedures associated with HIV [Pathway: MerckMedicus → Harrison's Practice → Topics → enter "HIV" into the search field → select "HIV, AIDS" → tap on the menu bar on the upper right corner of the screen and select "Diagnosis" → scroll down to "Laboratory Tests."]

Kendall asks if her baby will need treatment.

The answers can be found on page 282.

Exercise 20-9: *Multiple Choice Question*

The normal treatment for infants born to an HIV-positive mother include:

    A. Blood tests for the virus every month for a year

    B. Antibiotics immediately after birth

    C. AZT for 6 months IV

    D. AZT 6 months po

You discuss delivery options with Kendall also.

Exercise 20-10: *Multiple Choice Question*

A goal of delivery for an HIV-positive patient is:

    A. Cesarean birth before rupture of membranes

    B. Low forceps to decrease pushing during labor

    C. Episiotomy assisted to decrease length of labor

    D. Vacuum-assisted delivery

 eResource 20-6: Refer to Pocket Guide to Diagnostic Tests in MerckMedicus on your mobile device to learn more about CD4 cell count [Pathway: MerckMedicus → Pocket Guide to Diagnostic Tests → enter "CD4" into the search field].

Kendall's viral load and CD4 cell count are done periodically during her pregnancy in order to know if the disease is progressing. Kendall does not reach the level of less than 200 cells per micro liter at which point the disease is diagnosed as AIDS.

Exercise 20-11: *Fill-in*

Normal levels of CD4 are _____ cells per micro liter.

Kendall comes to the clinic every two weeks for prenatal care in order to monitor both her HIV condition and the pregnancy.

The answers can be found on page 282.

Answers

Exercise 20-1: *Multiple Choice Question*

The nurse understands that the HIV virus attacks the:

A. T3 cells—NO.

B. **T4 cells—YES.**

C. WCBs—NO.

D. Lymphocytes—NO.

Exercise 20-2: *Multiple Choice Question*

Partners of HIV-positive individuals should understand that the latent phase before HIV antibodies can be detected in an enzyme-linked immunosorbent assay (ELISA) is:

A. 2–3 weeks—NO.

B. 4–8 weeks—NO.

C. **6–12 weeks—YES, sometimes it takes 6–12 weeks to convert.**

D. 6 months—NO.

Exercise 20-3: *Multiple Choice Question*

The nurse understands that the primary rationale for continuing a woman's antiretroviral therapy during pregnancy is to:

A. Slow the disease—NO, although this is a goal, it is not the main issue during pregnancy.

B. Stop the progression of the disease during pregnancy—NO, the disease can be treated not cured.

C. **Decrease perinatal transmission—YES, this is the goal.**

D. Increase the mother's immune status—NO, although this is a goal, it is not the main issue during pregnancy.

Exercise 20-4: *Fill-in*

The nurse explains that the fastest growing population of people contracting HIV are:

A. Homosexual males—NO.

B. Heterosexual males—NO.

C. Homosexual females—NO.

D. **Heterosexual females—YES, the disease incidence is rising fastest in this group.**

Exercise 20-5: *Fill-in*

The HIV virus ____can____ be transmitted by breast milk.

Exercise 20-6: *Select All That Apply*

Fetal and newborn risks associated with HIV are:

☑ **Premature birth—YES.**

❑ Postdate births—NO.

❑ Large for gestation age—NO.

☑ **Small for gestational age—YES.**

Exercise 20-7: *Multiple Choice Question*

The nurse knows from working in the high-risk clinic that it is recommended by U.S. Public Health Service that HIV screening should be done prenatally on:

 A. Underprivileged women—NO.

 B. Women of African American decent—NO.

 C. Women who admit to drug use—NO.

 D. **All women—YES.**

Exercise 20-8: *Fill-in*

Should a woman have a positive ELISA test, what would be the next test to confirm the diagnosis? **Western Blot or Immunofluorescence assay**

Exercise 20-9: *Multiple Choice Questions*

The normal treatment for infants born to an HIV-positive mother include:

 A. Blood tests for the virus every month for a year—NO.

 B. Antibiotics immediately after birth—NO, it is viral not bacterial.

 C. AZT for 6 months IV—NO, you would have to maintain a line too long.

 D. **AZT 6 months po—YES.**

Exercise 20-10: *Multiple Choice Question*

A goal of delivery for an HIV-positive patient would be:

 A. **Cesarean birth before rupture of membranes—YES, this is the recommended mode of delivery to decrease transmission.**

 B. Low forceps to decrease pushing during labor—NO, this runs the risk of tearing skin and opening portals of entry.

 C. Episiotomy assisted to decrease length of labor—NO, this opens portals of entry.

 D. Vacuum assisted delivery—NO, this runs the risk of tearing skin and opening portals of entry.

Exercise 20-11: *Fill-in*

Normal levels of CD4 are **500–1,200** cells per micro liter.

21

Preterm Infant Care

Case Study 21 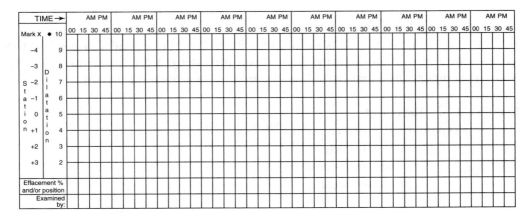 Preterm Multiples

Isabella starts having uterine contractions (UCs) and is very excited. An ultrasound is done and determines that baby A or the fetus closest to the cervix is vertex. Isabella's labor starts approximately 11 p.m. with mild UCs at 5–10 minutes lasting 30 seconds. Isabella is dilating as expected 1 cm every 1–2 hours during the latent phase.

Exercise 21-1: *Exhibit Question*

Plot Isabella's labor progress. At 12:45 she is 3 cms dilated, 2+ station. At 1,400 she is 4 cms and 1+ station and becoming uncomfortable. At 1,500 she is 6 cms and 0 station and at 1,600 she is 9 cms dilated. Finally at 1,700 she is fully dilated and starts to push.

Is this a normal labor curve for a nullipara? YES/NO

The answer can be found on page 297.

eResource 21-1: To supplement your understanding of the normal labor curve,

- open a browser and go to MerckMedicus Online [Pathway: *merckmedicus.com* → select Merck Manual Professional Edition → enter "stages of labor" into the search field].
- On your mobile device, open Merckmedicus and select the Merck Manual [Pathway: → Merck Manual → enter "labor" into the search field → select "Labor and delivery" → scroll down to select "stages of . . ." to review content].
- Go to March of Dimes to obtain a free professional resource: Pre-term Labor Assessment toolkit [Pathway: *marchofdimes.com* → select category: "Professionals" → select "Medical Resources" → scroll down and select "Pre-term Labor Assessment toolkit"].

Isabella pushes for 45 minutes and baby A is crowning. No episiotomy is made since the infants are only 32 weeks' gestation; they are expected to not be extremely large. Baby A is born and placed on the warmed infant table for assessment and evaluation. Baby A is a girl. Isabella complains of severe lower back discomfort as baby B is descending.

Exercise 21-2: *Multiple Choice Question*

When a patient in labor complains of lower back or sacral pain, the nurse suspects that the fetus is in what position?

A. Brow presentation

B. Shoulder presentation

C. Vertex

D. Occiput posterior

Twenty minutes later baby B is born and is placed on the second warmer bed for assessment and evaluation. Baby B is also a girl. Baby A has been taken to the NICU. It is determined that baby C is descending in a breech position.

Exercise 21-3: *Matching*

Match the type of breech presentation with its picture (opposite page).

_____ Frank breech

_____ Complete breech

_____ Footling breech

The answers can be found on page 298.

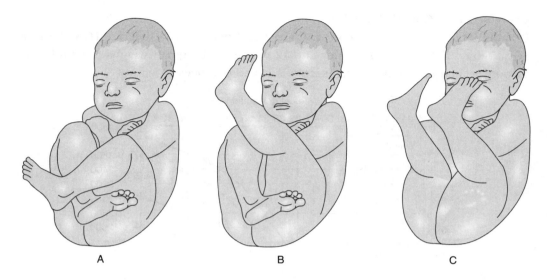

A   B   C

To supplement your understanding of the breech presentation:

- Open a browser and go to MerckMedicus Online [Pathway: *merckmedicus.com* → select "Merck Manual Professional Edition → enter "breech" into the search field → select "breech presentation"].
- On your mobile device, open Merckmedicus and select the Merck Manual [Pathway: → Merck Manual → enter "breech" into the search field → select "Breech presentation" → select "Fetal Dystocia" to review content].

It was decided to do a cesarean birth for the third baby due to the dangers of extracting a breech presentation for both the mother and infant.

eResource 21-3: Supplement your understanding by viewing videos depicting the following:

- Management and considerations of a breech birth: *www.medicalvideos .us/videos/2789/spontaneous-breech-delivery-childbirth*
- Cesarean section surgical procedure: *www.medicalvideos.us/ videos/236/cesarean-section*

Baby B is taken to NICU and Isabella is prepared for the cesarean. NICU staff awaits the delivery. Twenty-six minutes later, baby C is delivered and is in distress. Baby C is a boy. He is intubated in the delivery room and bagged for transport to the NICU.

The triplets are identified before they leave the delivery room, given a quick assessment, and provided with the appropriate oxygen mechanism. Once in the NICU unit they are weighed and measured.

The answer can be found on page 298.

Exercise 21-4: *Exhibit Question*

Plot the infants' weight on the growth chart and determine if they are LGA, AGA, or SGA. Baby girl A weighs 3 pounds and 12 ounces, baby girl B weighs 3 pounds and 11 ounces, and baby boy C weighs 2 pounds and 6 ounces.

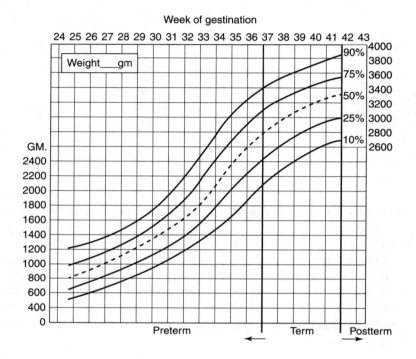

eResource 21-4:
- Go to *www.infantchart.com* or *www.medcalc.com/growth* to utilize an interactive growth chart.
- Use STAT GrowthCharts™ WHO you downloaded to your iPod/iPhone/iPad in eResource 2-3.

Baby girl A is breathing at 66 breaths per minute with mild intercostal retractions. She is placed on nasal cannula at 2 liters to see if her retractions decrease.

Exercise 21-5: *Multiple Choice Question*

A priority assessment for baby A is:

    A. CBC

    B. Otaloni's sign

    C. Pulse oximetry

    D. Cardiac monitor

The answers can be found on pages 298–299.

eResource 21-5:

■ On your mobile device, open the Merck Manual to view information regarding the management of respiratory distress in neonates and infants [Pathway: Merck Manual → Topics → enter "respiratory distress" into the search field → select "Respiratory distress syndrome" → select "Premature Infant" on the drop-down menu in the upper right corner, select "Prognosis and Treatment"].

■ View video clips provided by *NICU.org*, depicting respiratory distress in a neonate *youtu.be/J2R8MOoQtd8*

Baby girl B is breathing on her own at 52 breaths per minute with very mild intercostals retractions. She is placed on the cardio-respiratory (C-R) monitor for continuous readings of her vital signs and pulse oxygenation.

Exercise 21-6: *Fill-in*

The first symptoms that a newborn is experiencing respiratory distress are _____ and _____.

eResource 21-6:

■ To verify normal vital signs for a newborn, go to Medscape from WebMD on your mobile device. [Pathway: Medscape → select "Procedures & Protocols" → select "Pediatric and Neonatal" → select "Normal Vital Signs."]

■ Using the Web browser on your mobile device, go to MerckMedicus online (*merck.ubmed.com*) to learn more about newborn respiratory distress. In the search field, enter "newborn respiratory distress" → scroll down to locate and select "Respiratory Disorders in Neonates, Infants and Young Children."

Baby C is a boy and is given surfactant therapy and placed on continuous positive airway pressure (CPAP) to facilitate lung expansion. Baby girls A and B are placed in incubators with temperature probes attached to their abdomens on the left side (not to be over the liver border), and the incubators are set on servo temperature at 37° Celsius. Baby boy C is maintained on an infant warming bed until an umbilical catheterization is placed for access. Babies A and B have peripheral vein intravenous started for parenteral fluids.

eResource 21-7:

■ Using the Web browser on your mobile device, go to MerckMedicus online (*merck.ubmed.com*) to learn more about the treatment of newborn respiratory distress. In the search field, enter "surfactant," → scroll down to locate and select "Respiratory Distress Syndrome."

■ View the *New England Journal of Medicine*'s video which provides an in-depth overview of the procedure: *youtu.be/8ChhAt0Fcj8* (Anderson, Lenard, Braner, Lai, & Tegtmeyer, October 9, 2008).

The answer can be found on page 299.

Isabella and Christopher come to the NICU after the postanesthesia recovery room. Isabella is on a stretcher and is shown each baby one at a time.

Exercise 21-7: *Multiple Choice Question*

A nursing intervention used to promote initial mother-infant interaction in the NICU is to:

    A. Encourage the mother to hold the baby.

    B. Encourage the mother to read to the baby.

    C. Encourage the mother to massage the baby.

    D. Encourage the mother to get eye level with the baby.

 eResource 21-8: For patient educational material regarding mother-infant interaction, go to MerckMedicus online [Pathway: *merckmedicus.com* → select "Patient Education" tab → "Searchable Patient Handouts" → enter "bonding" into search field → scroll down and select "Pediatric Advisor: Infant Massage"].

Exercise 21-8: *Multiple Choice Question*

Babies A and C have similar facial features and the parents ask if they are twins. The best answer is:

    A. "It is possible they are fraternal twins."

    B. "It is possible they are monozygotic twins."

    C. "It is possible they are identical twins."

    D. "It is possible but not likely."

Isabella is overwhelmed with the situation and begins to cry when she sees that baby C needs help to breathe. She asks how long the babies will be in the NICU.

Exercise 21-9: *Multiple Choice Question*

The most appropriate nursing diagnosis for Isabella at this time is:

    A. Anxiety related to situation.

    B. Defensive coping related to situation.

    C. Post-traumatic syndrome related to situation.

    D. Impaired religiosity related to situation.

Exercise 21-10: *Fill-in*

The goal of oxygen therapy for preterm infants is to keep their peripheral saturation level of oxygen between 92% and _____ %.

Exercise 21-11: *Hot Spot*

Isabella and Christopher are taken to their postpartum room and told that they are welcome to visit any time. Isabella and Christopher want the baby's crib cards to identify their names as Natalie, Olivia, and Connor.

The answers can be found on pages 299–300.

Baby girl A, Natalie, is fully assessed at this point. Her face is symmetrical and her fontanels are open and flat. Her ear pina have some recoil and she has an intact palate. Her neck is supple and clavicles intake. There are slight intercostals, and supraclavicular retractions on her chest but her lung sounds are clear. Her pulse oximeter is in place as well as her nasal cannular at 2 liters 21% oxygen. Her heart rate is regular with no murmurs.

Identify with an X where you would assess supraclavicular retractions.

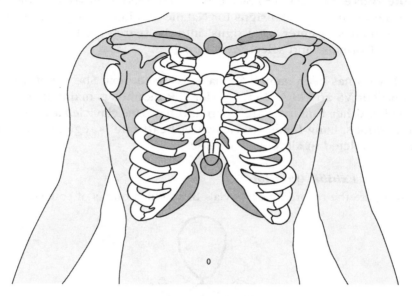

eResource 21-9: To see an example of an infant with stridor and retractions, view: *youtu.be/-rqSsVceu3I*

Both of Natalie's arms are in a semi-flexed position. Her hands appear normal with five fingers on each and no simian creases. Her IV site on her right arm is intact and clean. Her abdomen is normal with two nipples and a prominent xiphoid process. She has bowel sounds in all four quadrants and her umbilical site looks clean and moist.

Exercise 21-12: *Multiple Choice*

Evidence supports the use of which agent to clean infant umbilical cords?

     A. Alcohol three times a day

     B. Soap and water daily

     C. Peroxide twice a day

     D. Triple blue dye four times a day

Natalie's hips do not have any clicks. Her legs are semi-flexed and she has five toes on each foot. She has one crease along the sole of her foot. Her spin is straight, no dimple, and her gluteal folds are symmetrical. Her vital signs (VS) at this point are 97.8 A, 166, 62. Her IV is set at 10 mL/hr on the pump and is infusing well. She has had a meconium stool. Natalie's temperature probe is maintained so the incubator regulates her temperature to decrease her expenditure of energy.

The answer can be found on page 300.

Exercise 21-13: *Fill-ins*

Name three physical assessment findings that indicate that Natalie has been born preterm.

A. _____

B. _____

C. _____

 eResource 21-10: Go to Skyscape's Archimedes on your mobile device to see the normal vital signs for Natalie and her siblings [Pathway: Archimedes → enter "vital signs" into the search field → select "Vital Signs Normals" and select "newborn"].

Baby girl B who has been named Olivia is assessed next. She is not using oxygen support and her VS are 98 A, 154, 56. Her C-R monitor is maintained. Her face is symmetrical and her fontanels are open and flat. Her clavicles are intact and she has no retractions. Lung fields are clear. Her heart rate is regular with a murmur, so BPs are completed in all four extremities.

Exercise 21-14: *Exhibit Question*

The following are the recording of Olivia's BPs. Which one is of concern?

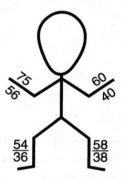

Her abdomen is soft and BS are positive in all four quadrants. Her umbilicus is moist and clean. She has no hip clicks and her feet are in line and symmetrical. Olivia's spine is intact and she has a small pilonidal dimple, but there is no opening and she is moving both legs well. Her labia majora and minora are both viable the same size. Her IV site is in her left foot and is infusing well via the pump at 10 mL/hr maintenance dose. Olivia has voided twice since her admission but has not yet had a meconium stool.

Exercise 21-15: *Multiple Choice Question*

In lieu of Olivia's physical assessment findings, the nurse would expect what diagnostic test to be ordered?

A. EEG (electroencephalogram)

B. MRI (magnetic resonance imaging)

C. CT or CAT scan (computed axial tomography)

D. Echocardiogram

The answers can be found on pages 300–301.

Connor or baby boy C is on the warmer table attached also to a temperature probe. His CPAP is maintained nasally at 2 cm of H$_2$O, and blood gases have been completed twice. He has a protective film over his nose to protect his nares from the pressure of the CPAP. His face is symmetrical and his fontanels are open and flat. His clavicles are intact and his respirations are 50 breaths per minute with the assistance of the CPAP. His nipples are appropriately placed and his abdomen is soft. He has an umbilical line that is clean and intact and TPN (total parenteral nutrition) has been started. His spine is straight with no dimple. His testicles are undescended and his meatus is on the tip of his penis. He has voided once so far but has not had a meconium.

 eResource 21-11: Two videos highlight the use and impact of Bubble CPAP on neonates at Texas Health Harris Methodist Hospital, Fort Worth, can be viewed by going to:
- *youtu.be/kcytHfT9gmo* and
- *youtu.be/36Ndn0UZWgg*

Exercise 21-16: *Multiple Choice Question*
The nurse knows that the concern for cryptorchidism is that:
- A. There will be an aesthetic consequence for a male.
- B. There is no way to know when it will resolve by itself.
- C. It is normal for all infants.
- D. If it is not corrected within the first couple of years, male infertility may ensue.

The following day (day 2) all three infants are stable except Natalie, who has been having some apnea and bradycardia spells. Her vital signs are 97.4 A, 166, 72 and she is requiring an increase in oxygen to keep her pulse oximeter above 92%. A CBC with differential is ordered and a blood specimen is taken from her heel.

Exercise 21-17: *Exhibit Question*
The WBC results are:
- **Total WBC: 15,000**
- **Bands or stabs: 9%**
- **Granulocytes** (or polymorphonuclears)
  - **Neutrophils** (or segs): **55% relative value**
  - **Eosinophils: 3% relative value**
  - **Basophils: 1% relative value**
- **Agranulocytes** (or mononuclears)
  - **Lymphocytes: 26% relative value**
  - **Moncytes: 6% relative value**

The value that indicates that the newborn may be having an immunological response is _____.

The answers can be found on page 301.

Antibiotics are ordered for Natalie.

Exercise 21-18: *Calculation*

Today Natalie weighs 3 pounds and 6 ounces. The correct dose for Ampicillin is 50–100 mg/kg/day. What are the upper and lower limits of the dose she should receive?

 eResource 21-12: On your mobile device, use Skyscape's Archimedes, to first do the conversion from pounds to kilogram, then calculate the drug dose:
- [Pathway: Archimedes → enter "weight" into the Main Index → scroll down to select "Weight conversion (kg ⇔ lbs)"].
- [Pathway: Archimedes → enter "dose" into the Main Index → scroll down to "Drug dosing (mg/kg/day)."]

Natalie's incubator temperature is increased slightly (1° Celsius) in order to offset the mild decrease in body temperature that sometimes accompanies sepsis.

Exercise 21-19: *Multiple Choice Question*

The nurse understands that maintaining an environment that is too warm for an infant is likely to:

    A. Decrease metabolic needs.

    B. Increase metabolic needs.

    C. Increase immunological response.

    D. Decrease immunological response.

A strict record of the number of apnea and bradycardia spells experienced by Natalie is maintained.

Exercise 21-20: *Fill-in*

Apnea is defined as a condition in which the neonate stops spontaneous respirations for a period of _____ sec.

    Olivia is doing well today and small continuous po feedings are going to begin. An NG tube is inserted.

The answers can be found on page 302.

Exercise 21-21: *Hot Spot*

Draw the path used to measure an NG tube

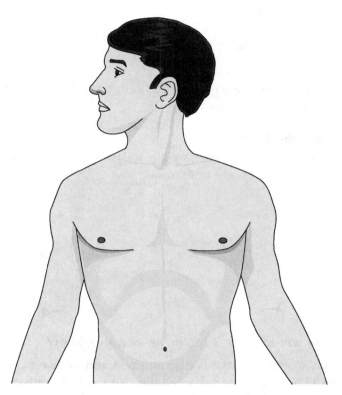

The order is to provide Olivia with 1 mL of formula per hour on a continuous pump. If she is tolerating it (less than 10% residual) in 3 hours then her IV can be decreased 1 mL per hour.

Connor is doing well and tolerating his CPAP.

Exercise 21-22: *Exhibit Exercise*

Connor's blood gases show the following:

> pH 7.40
> H^+ 40 nmol/L (nM)
> PaO_2 90 mmHg
> $PaCO_2$ 40 mmHg
> HCO_3 24 mmol/L.
> SBC_e 23 mmol/L (sodium bicarbonate)
> Base excess 1 mmol/L

The answers can be found on pages 302–303.

This would be interpreted as:

    A. Metabolic acidosis

    B. Metabolic alkalosis

    C. Respiratory acidosis

    D. Respiratory alkalosis

    E. Normal

Connor's I & O is calculated for the last 24 hours also. He has had eight wet diapers and two small meconium stools.

Exercise 21-23: *Exhibit Exercise*

A dry diaper weighs 8 gms. Connor's weight today is 2 pounds and 3 ounces. The weight of Connor's wet diapers are as follows:

1. 10 gms
2. 14 gms
3. 9 gms
4. 10 gms
5. 15 gms
6. 13 gms
7. 20 gms
8. 9 gms

Is Connor's output within the 1–3 mL/hr/kg as it should be?

The following day Connor's CPAP is discontinued and he is on room air. His IV is maintained with TPN. The second day Natalie's apnea and bradycardia spells have decreased and she is back down to 2 liters of oxygen by nasal cannula.

Exercise 21-24: *Calculation*

Natalie's intake for the past 24 hours has been 10 mL/hr. Today she weighs 3 pounds and 4 ounces. How many mL/kg/day is she receiving? _____

    Natalie is placed on caffeine to decrease her apnea and bradycardia spells.

Exercise 21-25: *Calculation*

The order is 2.2 mg/kg of caffeine every day. How much should Natalie receive today?

    eResource 21-13:
- To review the effects of caffeine on Natalie, go to Epocrates online [Pathway: *online.epocrates.com* → tap on the "Drugs" tab → enter "caffeine" in the search field → select "caffeine citrate."]
- To do the calculations, turn to your mobile device and use Skyscape's Archimedes; see eResource 21-12.

The answers can be found on pages 303–304.

Olivia is being weaned off of her IV the second day, and she is tolerating her po feedings via the NG tube well.

Exercise 21-26: *Multiple Choice Question*
The nurse knows that Olivia's NG tube must be checked for placement with each feed so she should:

     A. Get an X-ray each feed.

     B. Replace the NG tube each feed.

     C. Put saline down first.

     D. Listen for air bolus.

All three babies are placed under the bili lights because they are all starting to look slightly jaundiced, and most preterm babies have difficulty excreting bilirubin. Day four po feedings are begun on Natalie now that she is off CPAP. Olivia is totally po fed and her IV is maintained as a heplock for her antibiotics.

Exercise 21-27: *Calculation*
The heplock flush order is 1 mL of flush, which is premixed 10 mL of 10 U/mL in 250 mL bag of NNS (normal saline). If the nurse flushes her IV with 1 mL, how much heparin is the nurse administering? _____

    Olivia is being weaned to an open crib. She is starting to gain weight and tolerates her po feedings well. Isabella visits regularly and provides Kangaroo maternal care (KMC) to the infants often.

Exercise 21-28: *Multiple Choice Question*
Evidence shows that KMC provides the following physiological benefits to the infant:

     A. Decreases metabolism

     B. Stabilizes temperature

     C. Increases food intake

     D. Increases bonding

Olivia's murmur is due to a patent ductus arteriosus (PDA), which is still present and Indomethecin (Indocin) is ordered in an attempt to close the PDA.

 eResources 21-14: Go to Epocrates to look up information regarding this medication [Pathway: *online.epocrates.com* → select the "Drug" tab → enter "Indomethecin" and select "Indocin" → select "Peds Dosing," focusing on potential complications and safety monitoring.]

Exercise 21-29: *Calculation*
Indomethicin (Indocin) is given in three doses 12 hours apart. Each dose is 0.2 mg/kg. Currently Olivia is back to birth weight 3 pounds and 11 ounces. What should each dose be? _____

The answers can be found on page 304.

eResources 21-15:
- Go to *medcalc.com* for an online dose calculator offered by MedCalc.com. [Pathway: Top on 'General'→Tap on 'Weights and Measures' → Tap on "Pediatrics" → "Dose Calculator" to access the calculator.]
- On your mobile device, use Skyscape's Archimedes, to calculate the drug dose. [Pathway: Archimedes → enter "dose" into the Main Index → scroll down to "Drug dosing (mg/kg/day)."]

The drug therapy is successful in closing the PDA; in 48 hours, the murmur is no longer heard. Natalie is done with her antibiotics although the caffeine therapy continues, and she is tolerating all her feeds well, including po feeding. Connor is still being weaned off of his IV, but is tolerating his po feedings. Isabella is pumping for the babies and each of them is receiving some breast milk along with the formula. At 34 weeks post-conceptual age, they are introduced to the bottle once a day and progressed as they tolerate it.

Exercise 21-30: *Multiple Choice Question*
The nurse should be aware of the metabolic consequences of spending too much time trying to po or bottle-feed preterm infants. The length of each feeding should be generally done within how many minutes?
    A. 10 minutes
    B. 15 minutes
    C. 20 minutes
    D. 30 minutes

As the babies grow and wean to open cribs, Isabella and Christopher become more and more comfortable taking care of them. Discharge planning is begun and they are infant CPR certified and C-R monitor certified.

Exercise 21-31: *Select All That Apply*
The following referrals are appropriate for preterm infants:
- ❏ Ophthalmologist
- ❏ Optometrist
- ❏ Developmental clinic
- ❏ Rheumatologist
- ❏ Pediatrician
- ❏ Obstetrician
- ❏ Neurologist

The answers can be found on pages 304–305.

Answers

Exercise 21-1: *Exhibit Question*

Plot Isabella's labor progress. At 12:45 she is 3 cms dilated, 2+ station. At 1,400 she is 4 cms and 1+ station and becoming uncomfortable. At 1,500 she is 6 cms and 0 station and at 1,600 she is 9 cm dilated. Finally at 1,700 she is fully dilated and starts to push.

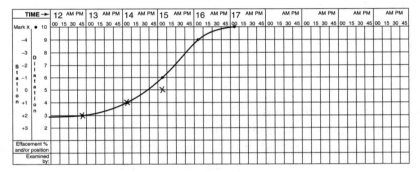

Composite normal dilatation curves

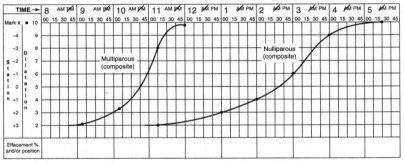

Composite normal of abnormal labor progress - Multiparous

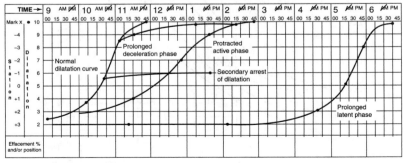

Is this a normal labor curve for a nullipara? **YES**, it has the shape of a normal labor curve.

Exercise 21-2: *Multiple Choice Question*
When a patient in labor complains of lower back or sacral pain, the nurse suspects that the fetus is in what position?
A. Brow presentation—NO.
B. Shoulder presentation—NO.
C. Vertex—NO.
D. **Occiput posterior—YES, this is an indication that the fetal occiput is pressing on the sacrum as the fetus descends.**

Exercise 21-3: *Matching*
Match the type of breech presentation with its picture.
_____**C**_____ Frank breech
_____**A**_____ Complete breech
_____**B**_____ Footling breech

Exercise 21-4: *Exhibit Question*
Plot the infant's weight on the growth chart and determine if they are LGA, AGA, or SGA. Baby girl A weighs 3 pounds and 12 ounces, baby girl B weighs 3 pounds and 11 ounces, and baby boy C weighs 2 pounds and 6 ounces.
Baby girl A weighs 3 pounds and 12 ounces = 1.70 kg
Baby girl B weighs 3 pounds and 11 ounces = 1.67 kg
Baby boy C weighs 2 pounds and 6 ounces = 1.08 kg

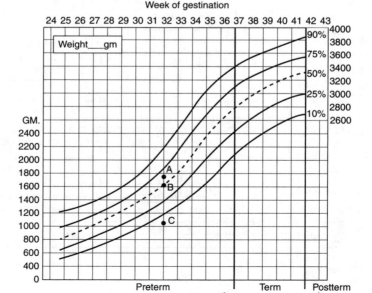

Exercise 21-5: *Multiple Choice Question*

A priority assessment for baby A is:

A. CBC—NO, the nurse does not want to wait for these results, and they will not reveal the oxygen concentration of the blood.

B. Otaloni's sign—NO, this is to test for hip dysplasia.

C. **Pulse oximetry—YES, this is to assess oxygen concentration in the blood.**

D. Cardiac monitor—NO, this will not assess respiratory status.

Exercise 21-6: *Fill-in*

The first symptoms that a newborn is experiencing respiratory distress are **nasal flaring** and **grunting.**

Exercise 21-7: *Multiple Choice Question*

A nursing intervention used to promote initial mother-infant interaction in the NICU is to:

A. Encourage the mother to hold the baby—NO, the infants are being stabilized.

B. Encourage the mother to read to the baby—NO, this may be done at a later date but is not appropriated initially.

C. Encourage the mother to massage the baby—NO, this may be done at a later date but is not appropriated initially.

D. **Encourage the mother to get to eye level with the baby—YES, this is important so the mother sees the infant's face and the infant starts to build a memory of her.**

Exercise 21-8: *Multiple Choice Question*

Babies A and C have similar facial features and the parents ask if they are twins. The best answer is:

A. **"It is possible they are fraternal twins"—YES, this is possible.**

B. "It is possible they are monozygotic twins"—NO, they are different genders.

C. "It is possible they are identical twins"—NO, they are different genders.

D. "It is possible but not likely"—NO, this is not a good answer to the question.

Exercise 21-9: *Multiple Choice Question*

The most appropriate nursing diagnosis for Isabella at this time is:

A. **Anxiety related to situation—YES, this is anxiety related to such an unfamiliar situation.**

B. Defensive coping related to situation—NO, this is not defensive at all.

C. Post-traumatic syndrome related to situation—NO, even though NICU parents experience this, it is too soon.

D. Impaired religiosity related to situation—NO, there is no mention of an omnipotent being referred to in this situation at this time.

Exercise 21-10: *Fill-in*

The goal of oxygen therapy for preterm infants is to keep their peripheral saturation level of oxygen between 92% and ___**95%**___.

Exercise 21-11: *Hot Spot*

Identify with an X where you would assess supraclavicular retractions.

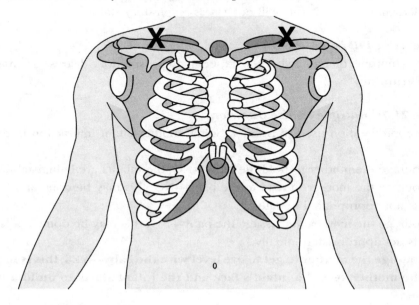

Exercise 21-12: *Multiple Choice*

Evidence supports the use of which agent to clean infant umbilical cords?

A. Alcohol three times a day—NO, this is not necessary and is very drying.

B. **Soap and water daily—YES, this is all that is needed to keep it clean.**

C. Peroxide twice a day—NO, this is not recommended.

D. Triple blue dye four times a day—NO, even if this is used, this is too often.

Exercise 21-13: *Fill-in*

Name three physical assessment findings that indicate that Natalie has been born preterm.

A. **Slow recoil on the pina.**

B. **Semi-flexed extremities.**

C. **Lack of sole creases.**

Exercise 21-14: *Exhibit Question*

The following are the recording of Olivia's BPs. Which one is of concern?

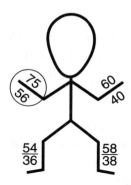

Exercise 21-15: *Multiple Choice Question*

In lieu of Olivia's physical assessment findings, the nurse would expect what diagnostic test to be ordered?

A. EEG (electroencephalogram)—NO, this is a brain analysis.

B. MRI (magnetic resonance imaging)—NO, this is not usually the first cardiac test.

C. CT or CAT scan (computed axial tomography)—NO, this is not usually the first cardiac test.

D. **Echocardiogram—YES, this will provide the best information.**

Exercise 21-16: *Multiple Choice Question*

The nurse knows that the concern for cryptorchidism is that:

A. There will be an aesthetic consequence for a male—NO, this is not the main concern.

B. There is no way to know when it will resolve by itself—NO, it may resolve but should not be left untreated for more than 24 months.

C. It is normal for all infants—NO, it is more common in premature infants.

D. **If it is not corrected within the first year, male infertility may ensue—YES, it should be corrected within the first couple of years.**

Exercise 21-17: *Exhibit Question*

The WBC results are:

- **Total WBC: 15,000**
- **Bands or stabs: 9%**
- **Granulocytes** (or polymorphonuclears)
    - **Neutrophils** (or segs): **55% relative value**
    - **Eosinophils: 3% relative value**
    - **Basophils: 1% relative value**
- **Agranulocytes** (or mononuclears)
    - **Lymphocytes: 26% relative value**
    - **Moncytes: 6% relative value**

The value that indicates that the newborn may be having an immunological response is: **Elevated bands–the body is sending out immature cells.**

Exercise 21-18: *Calculation*
Today Natalie weighs 3 pounds and 6 ounces. The correct dose for Ampicillin is 50–100 mg/kg/day. What are the upper and lower limits of the dose she should receive?
3 pounds 6 ounces = 1.5 kg 1.5 × 50 = **75 mg (lower dose)**
1.5 × 100 = **150 mg (upper dose)**

Exercise 21-19: *Multiple Choice Question*
The nurse understands that maintaining an environment that is too warm for an infant is likely to:
  A. Decrease metabolic needs—NO.
  B. **Increase metabolic needs—YES, it will increase metabolic needs.**
  C. Increase immunological response—NO.
  D. Decrease immunological response—NO.

Exercise 21-20: *Fill-in*
Apnea is defined as a condition in which the neonate stops spontaneous respirations for a period of _____**20**_____ seconds.

Exercise 21-21: *Hot Spot*
Draw the path used to measure an NG tube.

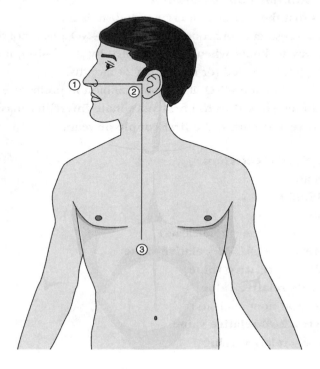

Exercise 21-22: *Exhibit Exercise*

Connor's blood gases show the following:

pH 7.40

H^+ 40 nmol/L (nM)

PaO_2 90 mmHg

$PaCO_2$ 40 mmHg

HCO_3 24 mmol/L.

SBC_e 23 mmol/L (sodium bicarbonate)

Base excess 1 mmol/L

This would be interpreted as:

A. Metabolic acidosis—NO, this is a low pH, low **$\underline{SBC_e}$**, and low $PaCO_2$.
B. Metabolic alkalosis—NO, this is a high pH, high **$\underline{SBC_e}$**, and high $PaCO_2$.
C. Respiratory acidosis—NO, this is a low pH, high **$\underline{SBC_e}$**, and high $PaCO_2$.
D. Respiratory alkalosis—NO, this is a high pH, low **$\underline{SBC_e}$**, and low $PaCO_2$.
E. **Normal—YES.**

Exercise 21-23: *Exhibit Exercise*

A dry diaper weighs 8 gms. His weight today is 2 pounds and 3 ounces. The weight of Connor's wet diapers are as follows:

1. 10 gms
2. 14 gms
3. 9 gms
4. 10 gms
5. 15 gms
6. 13 gms
7. 20 gms
8. 9 gms

Is Connor's output within the 1–3 mL/hr/kg as it should be? **Total diapers weights = 100 gms minus the dry diaper weight (8 gms × 8 = 64 gms) = 36 gms Conner weighs 1 kg so 36 gms divided by 1 = 36 gms divided by 24 hours = 1.5 gm/hr or 1.5 mL (it is a direct correlation 1 gm = 1 mL) per hr. It is adequate.**

Exercise 21-24: *Calculation*

Natalie's intake for the past 24 hours has been 10 mL/hr. Today she weighs 3 pounds and 4 ounces. How many mL/kg/day is she receiving? Natalie weighs 1.5 kg **10 mL × 24 hours = 240 mL/24 hours divided by 1.5 × 160 mg/kg/day, which is above the recommended amount.**

Exercise 21-25: *Calculation*
The order is 2.2 mg/kg of caffeine every day. How much should Natalie receive today?
2.2 mg × 1.5 kg = **3.3 mg/day**

Exercise 21-26: *Multiple Choice Question*
The nurse knows that Olivia's NG tube must be checked for placement with each feed so she should:
  A. Get an X-ray each feed—NO, usually one is gotten initially.
  B. Replace the NG tube each feed—NO, this is too irritating to the infant.
  C. Put saline down first—NO, if it is not in place this will cause aspiration.
  D. **Listen for air bolus—YES, this is the method still used in NICUs.**

Exercise 21-27: *Calculation*
The heplock flush order is 1 mL of flush, which is premixed 10 mL of 10 U/mL in 250 mL bag of NNS (normal saline). If the nurse flushes her IV with 1 mL how much heparin is the nurse administering?
There is 100 U of heparin in 250 mL bag = **0.4 units/mL**

Exercise 21-28: *Multiple Choice Question*
Evidence shows that KMC provides the following physiological benefits to the infant:
  A. Decreases metabolism—NO, this may be an effect but it is not the one that there has been evidence gathered on.
  B. **Temperature stabilization—YES, it is known to stabilize their temperature.**
  C. Increases food intake—NO, this may be an effect but it is not the one that there has been evidence gathered on.
  D. Increases bonding—NO, this may be an effect but it is not the one that there has been evidence gathered on.

Exercise 21-29: *Calculation*
Indomethicin (Indocin) is given in three doses 12 hours apart. Each dose is 0.2 mg/kg. Currently Olivia is back to birth weight 3 pounds and 11 ounces. What should each dose be?
Olivia is 1.7 kg.
1.7 kg × 0.2 mg = **0.34 mg for each dose**

Exercise 21-30: *Multiple Choice Question*
The nurse should be aware of the metabolic consequences of spending too much time trying to po or bottle-feed preterm infants. The length of each feeding should be generally done within how many minutes?
  A. 10 minutes—NO, many infants take longer.
  B. 15 minutes—NO, many infants take longer.
  C. **20 minutes—YES, this is the standard limit.**
  D. 30 minutes—NO, this is too long.

Exercise 21-31: *Select All That Apply*

The following referrals are appropriate for preterm infants:

☑ **Ophthalmologist—YES, preterm infants must be checked for retinopathy of prematurity.**

❑ Optometrist—NO, this specialist makes eye glasses.

☑ **Developmental clinic—YES, preterm infants are at high risk for developmental delays.**

❑ Rheumatologist—NO, this is a diseases that is not diagnosed in childhood.

☑ **Pediatrician—YES, a pediatrician schedule should be established for checkups and immunizations.**

❑ Obstetrician

❑ Neurologist

References

Anderson, J., Leonard, D., Braner, D. A. V., Lai, S., & Tegtmeyer, K. (October 9, 2008). Umbilical vascular catheterization. *New England Journal of Medicine, 359*:e18. Retrieved from: *http://www.nejm.org/doi/full/10.1056/NEJMvcm0800666.*

MedCalc.com, Created by: Charles Hu, Ron Kneusel, & Gary Barnas M.D. Created: January 15, 2000; last modified: January 27, 2010.

22

Retinopathy of Prematurity and Bronchopulmonary Dysplasia (BPD)

Case Study 22 ▰ Robert

Robert is Tamiko's baby boy that was born at 29 weeks' gestation. Her preterm labor was unexpected and by the time she arrived at the hospital she was already 6 cms dilated. Robert was born vaginally and was 1,200 gms, which is AGA for 29 weeks' gestation. His Apgar scores were 4, 6, and 8 at 10 minutes and he was intubated immediately and given surfactant therapy. Initially he was maintained on mechanical ventilation and then graduated to CPAP the second week of his life.

Robert remained on CPAP until 21 days and then was weaned off. He had one round of antibiotics for possible sepsis and was maintained on TPN for the first 2 weeks as po feeds were introduced gradually through the NG tube. Currently Robert is 4 weeks old and 33 weeks postconceptual age. He is 1,600 gms on nasal cannula at 1.4 liter 21% oxygen. He has an NG tube but is taking every other feed po. He is in an open crib, dressed for warmth, and is on caffeine because he still has occasional apnea and bradycardia spells. He is maintained on the C-R monitor with audible limits set. Today Robert will be seen by the ophthalmologist to be screened for retinopathy of prematurity (ROP).

Exercise 22-1: *Multiple Choice Question*

The current theory behind the etiology of retinopathy of prematurity is that one risk factor may be:

    A. Lack of oxygen.

    B. Excessive oxygen.

    C. Unstable oxygen.

    D. Humidified oxygen.

(e)   **eResource 22-1:** To learn more about the cause of ROP, open Medscape on your mobile device [Pathway: Medscape → enter "retinopathy" into the search field → select "Retinopathy of Prematurity" → tap on "Overview" → read "Pathophysiology" and "Epidemiology."]

The answer can be found on page 311.

Exercise 22-2: *Multiple Choice Question*

The nurse would expect orders to prepare a preterm infant for an ophthalmologist's exam to focus on:

    A. Keeping the infant NPO.

    B. Medicating the infant.

    C. Having the parents present.

    D. Dilating eye pupils.

 eResource 22-2: Remain in Medscape on your mobile device [Pathway: Medscape → enter "retinopathy" into the search field → select "Retinopathy of Prematurity" → tap on "Treatment" → read "Consultation."]

Exercise 22-3: *Select All That Apply*

Robert has the following risk factors for developing ROP:

    ❑ Gestational age above 32 weeks.

    ❑ Birth weight under 1,500 gms.

    ❑ Prolonged exposure to oxygen.

    ❑ Prolonged exposure to intense lighting.

After Robert's examination the ophthalmologist discusses the results with the family. Robert is diagnosed with stage I ROP and will be followed up in 2 weeks.

 eResource 22-3: To learn more about the ROM standards of care for the premature infant, go to the National Guideline Clearinghouse [Pathway: *guideline.gov* → enter "retinopathy of prematurity" into the search field → select "Best evidence statement (BESt). Screening for retinopathy of prematurity (ROP)" or another current standard of care.]

Exercise 22-4: *Multiple Choice Question*

The nurse understands that Robert's parents need more education when they say:

    A. "He is going to be blind."

    B. "There is treatment for this."

    C. "There is abnormal vessel development in his eye."

    D. "Follow-up is the most important thing."

Exercise 22-5: *Fill-in*

The nurse explains to the parents that if treatment is needed it is called _____.

 eResource 22-4: To learn more about the early treatment of ROP and to supplement patient teaching, go to the National Eye Institute's Web site:

    ■ [Pathway: *nei.nih.gov* → select "Health Information" → scroll down and select "retinopathy of prematurity" → select "Facts about Retinopathy of Prematurity (ROP)."]

    ■ In that same area, you will see an overview of "Cryotherapy for Retinopathy of Prematurity."]

The answers can be found on pages 311–312.

■ For more information, listen to Dr. Steven Rosenberg provide a brief overview of ROP: *youtu.be/tV0NkWK9Yl4*

■ In addition, you decide that you want to learn more about some of the other treatments utilized for more severe cases of ROP. To view an overview of the surgical repair, go to: *youtu.be/k4DN3LK3OBQ*; you can show these videos to supplement patient teaching.

Two weeks later Robert is 35 weeks' gestation (corrected age) and is still on his nasal cannula at 1/8 liter and is taking all of his feedings po. He is steadily gaining weight, so is being prepared for discharge. The ophthalmologist examines his eyes again in preparation for discharge and notes that Robert's ROP has progressed to stage II ROP zones I and II; he needs to be seen in 1 week.

Exercise 22-6: *Multiple Choice Question*

The nurse understands that it is her responsibility to:

    A. Tell the parents to call the ophthalmologist's office for an appointment when they can.

    B. Give the parents the phone number to the ophthalmologist's office and tell them to call.

    C. Provide transportation for the ophthalmologist office visit even if they have transportation.

    D. Make the appointment for the ophthalmologist office visit before Robert leaves the NICU.

Another discharge issue that needs to be taken care of is Robert's continuing need for oxygen.

Exercise 22-7: *Fill-in*

The nurse understands that BPD is diagnosed when oxygen is needed after _____ weeks' gestational age.

A home care company that supplies oxygen is contacted and company representatives will meet Robert's parents at the house in order to assess the environment for safe oxygen setup.

Exercise 22-8: *Multiple Choice Question*

The nurse explains to the parents that BPD causes a(n):

    A. Overuse of oxygen.

    B. Noncompliance of lung tissue.

    C. Overcompliance of lung tissue.

    D. Inadequate use of oxygen.

The answers can be found on page 312.

Exercise 22-9: *Multiple Choice Question*

While teaching the parents about ROP it is correct to tell them that:

    A. Robert will be treated on an outpatient basis.

    B. Robert will be readmitted to the hospital for treatment if it is needed.

    C. Robert will have to go to a larger hospital or tertiary center for treatment.

    D. Robert can be treated at home with mediation.

 eResource 22-5: To learn more about BPD, open MerckMedicus on your mobile device and tap on Merck Manual [Pathway: Merck Manual → enter "Bronchopulmonary" into the search field → scroll down and select "Bronchopulmonary Dysplasia" → read "General Overview" → Tap on the menu in the upper right corner of the screen and select "Treatment" from the drop-down menu.]

Along with the need for oxygen in the home, Robert's parents will use a home monitoring system. The monitor will detect a fall in oxygenation or an apnea spell.

Exercise 22-10: *Multiple Choice Question*

A priority for parents taking a child home on a monitor is:

    A. Monitor training.

    B. CPR training.

    C. Developmental care training.

    D. Aseptic technique training.

The discharge plans are made and reviewed in detail with the parents. They are provided with a list of the discharge plans plus a medication reconciliation list. Robert's mother says to you, "I am overwhelmed; this is too much responsibility for me."

Exercise 22-11: *Multiple Choice Question*

A priority nursing diagnosis for Robert's family is:

    A. Decisional conflict

    B. Powerlessness

    C. Ineffective coping

    D. Impaired individual resilience

The answers can be found on pages 312–313.

Answers

Exercise 22-1: *Multiple Choice Question*

The current theory behind the etiology of retinopathy of prematurity is that one risk factor may be:

A. Lack of oxygen—NO, it is due to unstable O2.

B. Excessive oxygen—NO, it is due to unstable O2.

C. **Unstable oxygen—YES, the current theory is that it is due to unstable O2.**

D. Humidified oxygen—NO, it is due to unstable O2.

Exercise 22-2: *Multiple Choice Question*

The nurse would expect orders to prepare a preterm infant for an ophthalmologist's exam to focus on:

A. Keeping the infant NPO—NO, this is not necessary.

B. Medication the infant—NO, this is not necessary.

C. Having the parents present—NO, this is not necessary.

D. **Dilating eye pupils—YES, medication is instilled in each eye every 5 minutes × 3.**

Exercise 22-3: *Select All That Apply*

Robert has the following risk factors for developing ROP:

❑ Gestational age above 32 weeks—NO, below 32 weeks.

☑ **Birth weight under 1,500 gms—YES.**

☑ **Prolonged exposure to oxygen—YES.**

☑ **Prolonged exposure to intense lighting—YES, other risk factors include being male and having a bout of sepsis.**

Exercise 22-4: *Multiple Choice Question*

The nurse understands that Robert's parents need more education when they say:

A. **"He is going to be blind"—YES, this is not true if it is caught and treated early.**

B. "There is treatment for this"—NO, this is true.

C. "There is abnormal vessel development in his eye"—NO, this is true.

D. "Follow-up is the most important thing"—NO, this is true.

Exercise 22-5: *Fill-in*

The nurse explains to the parents that if treatment is needed it is called **cryotherapy or laser therapy.**

Exercise 22-6: *Multiple Choice Question*

The nurse understands that it is her responsibility to:

A. Tell the parents to call the ophthalmologist's office for an appointment when they can—NO, this is not conclusive enough.

B. Give the parents the phone number to the ophthalmologist's office and tell them to call—NO, this is not conclusive enough.

C. Provide transportation for the ophthalmologist office visit even if they have transportation—NO, this is not conclusive enough.

D. **Make the appointment for the ophthalmologist office visit before Robert leaves the NICU—YES, it is imperative the appointment is made and the parents know when it is before the infant leaves the NICU.**

Exercise 22-7: *Fill-in*

The nurse understands that BPD is diagnosed when oxygen is needed after ___**36**___ weeks' gestational age.

Exercise 22-8: *Multiple Choice Question*

The nurse explains to the parents that BPD causes a(n):

A. Overuse of oxygen—NO, this is not the etiology.

B. **Noncompliance of lung tissue—YES, this is the reason for BPD.**

C. Overcompliance of lung tissue—NO, this is not the etiology.

D. Inadequate use of oxygen—NO, this is not the etiology.

Exercise 22-9: *Multiple Choice Question*

While teaching the parents about ROP it is correct to tell them that:

A. **Robert will be treated on an outpatient basis—YES, treatment can now be completed as an outpatient.**

B. Robert will be readmitted to the hospital for treatment if it is needed—NO.

C. Robert will have to go to a larger hospital or tertiary center for treatment—NO.

D. Robert can be treated at home with mediation—NO.

Exercise 22-10: *Multiple Choice Question*

A priority for parents taking a child home on a monitor is:

A. Monitor training—NO, this is important but not the priority.

B. **CPR training—YES, this is the priority since the infant is high risk for respiratory and cardiac complications.**

C. Developmental care training—NO, this is important but not the priority.

D. Aseptic technique training—NO, this is important but not the priority.

Exercise 22-11: *Multiple Choice Question*

A priority nursing diagnosis for Robert's family is:

A. Decisional conflict—NO, there is no decision involved currently.

B. Powerlessness—NO, she has not verbalized that she feels someone or the situation is overpowering her.

C. **Ineffective coping—YES, she is verbalizing difficulty coping right now.**

D. Impaired individual resilience—NO, this situation in family driven not individually driven.

23

Anemia and Polycythemia

Case Study 23 ▨ Twin-to-Twin Transfusion Syndrome (TTTS)

Admitted to the NICU the same day as Robert was discharged were a set of 33-week gestational-age twins. Both infants are girls and one is much larger than the other. Baby A is 5 pounds and 2 ounces and baby B is 3 pounds and 4 ounces.

Exercise 23-1: *Multiple Choice Question*

The nurse would expect the smaller twin to appear:

    A. Mottled

    B. Pale

    C. Ruddy

    D. Cyanotic

Exercise 23-2: *Select All That Apply*

The nurse understands that TTTS occurs because in utero the twins share:

    ❑ The amnion

    ❑ The chorion

    ❑ The placenta

    ❑ The umbilical cord

ⓔ **eResource 23-1:** To learn more about TTTS, go to:

    ■ The National Library of Medicine's MedlinePlus [Pathway: *nlm.nih .gov* → select "MedlinePlus" → enter "twin to twin" into the search field →

        ■ Select "Twin-to-Twin Transfusion Syndrome" and review content.

        ■ Be sure to tap on the video providing an overview of "Twin-to-Twin Transfusion Syndrome."

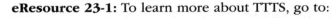

The answers can be found on page 319.

■ On your mobile device, open Medscape [Pathway: Medscape → enter "Twin" into the search field → select "Twin-to-Twin Transfusion Syndrome" → select "Overview."]

CBCs are drawn on the infants and the results are as follows:

Baby A	Baby B
Hct 30%	70%

Exercise 23-3: *Matching*

Match the risk factors with the correct infant.

_____ Lack of organ perfusion

_____ Cerebral vascular accident

_____ Severe jaundice

_____ Excessive sleepiness

A. Baby A

B. Baby B

Baby A is scheduled for an exchange transfusion in order to decrease the chances of complications. Whole blood will be replaced with plasma in order to decrease the cellular concentration of RBCs. Baby B is scheduled for a transfusion to boost her Hct.

e **eResource 23-2:** Remaining in Medscape on your mobile device [Pathway: Medscape → enter "Twin" into the search field → select "Twin-to-Twin Transfusion Syndrome" → select "Treatment" → "Medical."]

Exercise 23-4: *Ordering*

Place in order the steps to blood administration:

_____ Connect the blood product to the pump.

_____ Administer slowly and observe for reactions.

_____ Check doctor's order for blood product, time, date, & time to be infused.

_____ Establish patency of the IV site.

_____ Verify parents signed the inform consent.

_____ Check baseline VS.

_____ With two licensed people, check the blood product to the doctors order, the blood type of the patient in the chart or on the computer, the expiration date, and the blood product bag to the label.

_____ Dispose of blood bag properly and send end of transfusion tag back to blood bank.

_____ Retrieve the blood product from the blood bank.

The answers can be found on page 319.

_____ 15 minute VS.

_____ Two licensed people check the blood product to the patient's ID band.

_____ Verify that the baby has at least 2 ID bands on with name, date of birth, and hospital number.

_____ Double check the type and cross match results for blood type.

_____ Check the appearance of the blood product.

_____ Stay with patient for first 15 minutes.

Exercise 23-5: *Fill-in*

Pyrexia is a temperature of _____ Celsius or over.

eResource 23-3: To learn more about pyrexia, open MerckMedicus on your mobile device and tap on Harrison's Practice [Pathway: Harrison's Practice → enter "pyrexia" into the search field → scroll down and select "pyrexia of unknown origin" → read "Basics" to learn about pyrexia.]

The twin's mother comes to the NICU to see them. She tells you that baby A is named Addison and baby B is named Farrah. The twin's mother also tells you that besides being worried about her babies, she is "petrified to bring them home because her first baby died of SIDS (sudden infant death) at 1 month of age."

Exercise 23-6: *Multiple Choice Question*

The nurse understands that parents need further education about SIDS when they say:

A. "I will keep the infants' room at a comfortable temperature, not too warm."

B. "I will take all the stuffed animals out of the crib."

C. "I will put the infants to sleep only on their backs."

D. "I will sleep with the infants to make sure they are breathing."

You set up a teaching session for at-home monitors for the twins because there is a family history of SIDS. Some of the other social behaviors that are important to find out about are smoking in the home and using a pacifier.

Exercise 23-7: *Select All That Apply*

To decrease the incidence of SIDS the parents should:

❑ Provide a soft mattress.

❑ Sleep near but not with parents.

❑ Consider using a pacifier.

❑ Cover with blankets up to the neck.

The answers can be found on page 320.

eResources 23-4:
- To supplement new parent teaching regarding SIDS, you can show the mother this brief tutorial developed by South Carolina's Healthy Start Program. To view, go to *youtu.be/t-Q9qfOKUNE*
- Listen to this brief audio clip about the "Back to Sleep" initiative from the American Academy of Pediatrics: *www.aap.org/audio/mfk/011408.mp3*
- For more teaching material regarding a safe sleeping environment for the infant, go to: *www.cdc.gov/SIDS*

Both twins are doing well after their blood transfusions and baby A is receiving phototherapy. Discharge teaching has begun and home monitoring has been established.

eResources 23-5:
- To guide your patient education intervention, review the American Academy of Pediatrics Subcommittee on Hyperbilirubinemia issued Clinical Practice Guideline: *www.aap.org/qualityimprovement/quiin/SHB/Hyperbili.pdf*

Answers

Exercise 23-1: *Multiple Choice Question*

The nurse would expect the smaller twin to appear:

A. Mottled—NO, this should not be the case—only if hypoxic.

B. **Pale—YES, due to lack of RBCs.**

C. Ruddy—NO, this is how they look with too many RBCs (sometimes called plethoric).

D. Cyanotic—NO, this should not be the case—only if anoxic.

Exercise 23-2: *Select All That Apply*

The nurse understands that TTTS occurs because in utero the twins share:

❏ The amnion—NO, there are two amnions.

☑ **The chorion—YES, they share chorions.**

☑ **The placenta—YES, the share one placenta.**

❏ The umbilical cord—NO, they each have their own cord.

Exercise 23-3: *Matching*

Match the risk factors with the correct infant.

_____**A**_____ Lack of organ perfusion

_____**B**_____ Cerebral vascular accident

_____**B**_____ Severe jaundice

_____**A**_____ Excessive sleepiness

A. Baby A

B. Baby B

Exercise 23-4: *Ordering*

Place in order the steps to blood administration:

_____**13**_____ Connect the blood product to the pump.

_____**10**_____ Administer slowly and observe for reactions.

_____**1**_____ Check doctor's order for blood product, time, date, & time to be infused.

_____**4**_____ Establish patency of the IV site.

_____**3**_____ Verify parents signed the inform consent.

___6___ Check baseline VS.

___12___ With two licensed people, check the blood product to the doctors order, the blood type of the patient in the chart or on the computer, the expiration date, and the blood product bag to the label.

___15___ Dispose of blood bag properly and send end of transfusion tag back to blood bank.

___8___ Retrieve the blood product from the blood bank.

___14___ 15 minute VS.

___2___ Two licensed people check the blood product to the patient's ID band.

___5___ Verify that the baby has at least 2 ID bands on with name, date of birth, and hospital number.

___9___ Double check the type and cross match results for blood type.

___11___ Check the appearance of the blood product.

___7___ Stay with patient for first 15 minutes.

Exercise 23-5: *Fill-in*

Pyrexia is a temperature of ___38___ Celsius or over.

Exercise 23-6: *Multiple Choice Question*

The nurse understands that parents need further education about SIDS when they say:

A. "I will keep the infants room at a comfortable temperature, not too warm."—NO, this is correct; overheating increases the incidence of SIDS.

B. "I will take all the stuffed animals out of the crib."—NO, this is correct.

C. "I will put the infants to sleep only on their back."—NO, this is correct.

D. **"I will sleep with the infants to make sure they are breathing."—YES, co-bedding is not recommended.**

Exercise 23-7: *Select All That Apply*

To decrease the incidence of SIDS the parents should:

❑ Provide a soft mattress—NO, it should be firm.

☑ **Sleep near but not with parents—YES, in close proximity.**

☑ **Consider using a pacifier—YES, studies show that it decreases SIDS.**

❑ Cover with blankets up to the neck—NO, cover only to the chest.

24

Transient Tachypnea
of the Newborn (TTN)

Case Study 24 ▨ Aaron

Aaron is a 36 gestational-age infant that has just been brought into the nursery for evaluation. He was born by Cesarean section 4 hours ago and his respirations are 76 per minute. His lung sounds are moist. Aaron has a lag on inspiration, just visible retractions, no xyphoid retractions, minimal nasal flaring, and audible grunting.

Exercise 24-1: *Fill-in*
The next priority nursing interventions would be: _____.

 eResource 24-1: To supplement your understanding of this disorder, go to:
- ▨ on your mobile device, to learn more about TTN, open MerckMedicus on your mobile device and tap on Merck Manual [Pathway: Merck Manual → enter "transient tachypnea" into the search field → scroll down and select "Transient tachypnea of the newborn" → select "Transient Tachypnea of the Newborn."]
- ▨ You can also view a short video clip depicting an infant with TTN: *youtu.be/INAfjCcPFZY.*

Aaron is placed in an oxygen hood with humidified oxygen at 100%. His pulse oximetry rises from 88 to 96% and his retractions decrease. A chest X-ray is taken and it shows classic signs of TTN, which shows over aeration and streaking or retained fetal fluid.

 eResource 24-2: To learn more about the standards of care for Aaron, go to the National Guideline Clearinghouse [Pathway: *guideline.gov* → enter "Transient Tachypnea of the Newborn" into the search field → select "Prevention, Diagnosis and Treatment of Pediatric Bronchiolitis" or another current standard of care.]

The answer can be found on page 329.

Exercise 24-2: *Select All That Apply*

Select the risk factors for TTN:

❑ Under 35 weeks' gestation

❑ Small for gestational age (SGA)

❑ Cesarean birth

❑ Maternal smoking

❑ Maternal asthma

❑ Maternal hypertension

 eResource 24-3: To supplement patient teaching, you can go to KidsHealth.org [Pathway: kidshealth.org → select "For Parents" → enter "Transient Tachypnea of the Newborn" into the search field → tap on "Transient Tachypnea of the Newborn" to review available teaching material.]

Exercise 24-3: *Multiple Choice Question*

Aaron's mother asks if she could breast-feed him as she planned. The best answer would be:

    A. "He is too sick to breast–feed."

    B. "He will need to bottle-feed until his respirations are slower."

    C. "He will need to have nothing until we stabilize him."

    D. "He will need intravenous fluid until his respirations are slower."

Exercise 24-4: *Fill-in*

The nurse knows that an infant should not be po fed if respirations are above 60 per minute because it increases the risk for _____.

Exercise 24-5: *Multiple Choice Question*

The nurse understands that Aaron's parents need further information when they state:

    A. "I know he will be here for the entire week."

    B. "I know this is more common with babies born by Cesarean."

    C. "I know that he may only need oxygen for a couple of days."

    D. "I know he may not be discharged with me."

Aaron does well on his oxygen hood and his pulse oxygen is maintaining at 95–98%. An IV is ordered for him at 20 mL/hr to keep him hydrated. He is given prophylactic antibiotics because of the TTN, and his mom did not have a Group B streptococcus (GBS) done due to her early delivery. His mom is taught to pump her breasts to stimulate milk production for when he is able to take nourishment po. He is rooting so a pacifier is provided to him for when he is in the oxygen hood. His mother is concerned about the pacifier interfering with breast-feeding. You explain that it can be discontinued once he can breast or bottle-feed. During the night the oxygen level is decreased little by little and Aaron is tolerating it

The answers can be found on pages 325–326.

well. By the afternoon the following day he is removed from the oxygen hood. His pulse oximeter reads 96% on room air and his respiratory rate is 54 per minute.

Exercise 24-6: *Multiple Choice Question*

Aaron's mother is breast-feeding him for the first time. What instruction is a priority?

A. Let him nurse as long as he wants.

B. Provide rest periods during the feeding.

C. Hold him as upright as possible.

D. Keep him on one breast the entire time.

Aaron does well for the first feed. He still has his IV running and is still on the C-R monitor. It is decided that he will be discharged to the newborn nursery in the morning if he continues to breast-feed well and his respirations remain below 60 per minute. In the newborn nursery they will be able to accommodate his mother's request to have him circumcised. He also needs his hepatitis B vaccine.

Exercise 24-7: *Hot Spot*

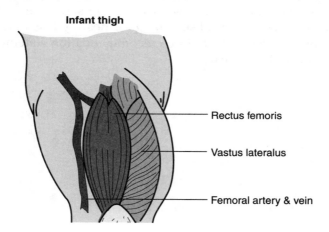

Infant thigh

- Rectus femoris
- Vastus lateralus
- Femoral artery & vein

Place an X on the spot where the hepatitis B vaccine should be given:

Exercise 24-8: *Fill-in*

Another consideration for Aaron is to have his newborn screen tests for metabolic and hereditary disorders. This test has to be completed after the infant is _____ hours old.

 eResource 24-4: To learn more about newborn screening tests, go to MerckMedicus on your mobile device and open Merck Manual [Pathway: Merck Manual → select "Topics" → enter "neonate" into the search field → scroll down and select "screening tests for . . ." → tap on the drop-down menu on the upper right corner of the screen → review recommended screening tests for "the first few hours" as well as those recommended for the "first few days."]

The answers can be found on page 330.

Exercise 24-9: *Multiple Choice Question*

Aaron has a universal newborn hearing screen (UNHS) done with a "pass," but a repeat should be ordered for a later date if what antibiotic is used?

    A. Ampicillin (Principen)

    B. Clindamycin (Cleocin)

    C. Gentamicin (Garamycin)

    D. Vancomycin (Vancocin)

Aaron is discharged without further complications.

eResource 24-5: To learn more about practices standards associated with UNHS:

- go to the Agency for Health Research and Quality's (AHRQ) Electronic Preventive Services Selector (ePSS) application on your mobile device [Pathway: ePSS → tap on "Browse" → tap on "Screening" → scroll down to select "Universal Newborn Hearing Screen" to review the recommendation.]
- Also go to the National Guideline Clearinghouse [Pathway: *guideline .gov* → enter "Universal Newborn Hearing Screen" into the search field → select "Universal screening for hearing loss in newborns: U.S. Preventive Services Task Force recommendation statement" or another current standard of care.]

The answer can be found on page 325.

Answers

Exercise 24-1: *Fill-in*

The next priority nursing interventions would be: **apply the pulse oximeter to obtain a reading.**

Exercise 24-2: *Select All That Apply*

Select the risk factors for TTN:

☐ Under 35 weeks' gestation—NO, TTN usually affects infants over 35 weeks gestational age.

☐ Small for gestational age (SGA)—NO, TTN affects AGA or LGA babies also.

☑ **Cesarean birth—YES, they miss the effect of some of the fetal fluid being squeezed out.**

☑ **Maternal smoking—YES, this increases the prevalence of TTN.**

☑ **Maternal asthma—YES, this increases the prevalence of TTN.**

☐ Maternal hypertension—NO, this is not correlated.

Exercise 24-3: *Multiple Choice Question*

Aaron's mother asks if she could breast-feed him as she planned. The best answer would be:

A. "He is too sick to breast feed"—NO, this is a dismissive answer.

B. "He will need to bottle-feed until his respirations are slower"—NO, he will be able to breast feed.

C. "He will need to have nothing until we stabilize him"—NO, this is true but does not provide the parent with a full rationale.

D. **"He will need intravenous fluid until his respirations are slower"—YES, this is the best answer.**

Exercise 24-4: *Fill-in*

The nurse knows that an infant should not be fed if respirations are above 60 per minute because it increases the risk for **aspiration**.

Exercise 24-5: *Multiple Choice Question*

The nurse understands that Aaron's parents need further information when they state:
A. **"I know he will be here for the entire week"—YES, TTN usually resolves in 72 hours.**
B. "I know this is more common with babies born by Cesarean"—NO, this is true.
C. "I know that he may only need oxygen for a couple of days"—NO, this is true.
D. "I know he may not be discharged with me"—NO, this is true.

Exercise 24-6: *Multiple Choice Question*

Aaron's mother is breast-feeding him for the first time. What instruction is a priority?
A. Let him nurse as long as he wants—NO, this will exhaust him.
B. **Provide rest periods during the feeding—YES, this is most important for an infant who has had compromised respiratory status.**
C. Hold him as upright as possible—NO, this is not necessary.
D. Keep him on one breast the entire time—NO, this is not effective feeding.

Exercise 24-7: *Hot Spot*

Place an X on the spot where the hepatitis B vaccine should be given:

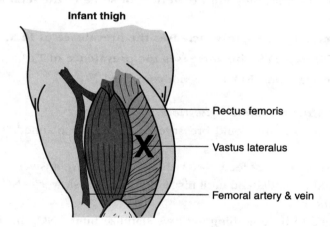

Infant thigh

—— Rectus femoris

X —— Vastus lateralus

—— Femoral artery & vein

Exercise 24-8: *Fill-in*

Another consideration for Aaron is to have his newborn screen tests for metabolic and hereditary disorders. This test has to be completed after the infant is ___**24**___ hours old.

Exercise 24-9: *Multiple Choice Question*

Aaron has a universal newborn hearing screen (UNHS) done with a "pass," but a repeat should be ordered for a later date if what antibiotic is used?
A. Ampicillin (Principen)—NO, this is not ototoxic.
B. Clindamycin (Cleocin)—NO, this is not ototoxic.
C. **Gentamicin (Garamycin)—YES, this is ototoxic.**
D. Vancomycin (Vancocin)—NO, this is not ototoxic.

25

Meconium Aspiration Syndrome (MAS)

Case Study 25 ▰ Benjamin

Paulette is a 24-year-old gravida II para I who came into the ED in active labor. She was quickly transported to the labor and delivery (L&D) suite and placed in the bed just in enough time for the baby to be born. She was 40 2/7 weeks' gestation and was scheduled for an nonstress test (NST) this afternoon. Thick meconium was presenting as the baby was delivering.

Exercise 25-1: *Fill-in*
A precipitous delivery is one in which contractions start and finish within _____ hours.

The baby cries before his mouth and nose can be suctioned with a meconium aspirator. He is taken to the warmer table and intubated. His vocal cords are visualized and he is suctioned below the cords. His respirations are strong and he is pink without oxygen at this time. The baby boy weighs 8 pounds and 10 ounces. He is ID'ed and taken to the newborn nursery for a full assessment.

 eResource 25-1: On your mobile device, open Medscape [Pathway: Medscape → enter "meconium" into the search field at the top of the screen → select "Meconium Aspiration, Prevention and Management" → tap on "Positioning" tab → tap on "View Image" to see proper positioning of the infant for intubation; tap on "Technique" tab, to view images of intubation and suctioning technique.]

Exercise 25-2: *Select All That Apply*
What are the risk factors for meconium aspiration?
- ❑ Postdates
- ❑ LGA (large for gestational age)
- ❑ Maternal hypertension
- ❑ Placental insufficiency
- ❑ Vertex delivery

The answers can be found on page 331.

eResource 25-2:
- Remain in Medscape on your mobile device [Pathway: Medscape → enter "meconium" into the search field at the top of the screen → this time select "Meconium Aspiration Syndrome" → select "Overview" → select "Epidemiology."]
- Go to the National Guidelines Clearinghouse (NGC) to view established practice guidelines for management of MAS [*guideline.gov* → enter "meconium aspiration syndrome" into search field → tap to select the guideline "Management of meconium at birth."]

In the newborn nursery the baby (named Ben) is doing fine after his initial bath and is in the first deep sleep pattern. While you are caring for the infant next to Ben, you notice that he is grunting with each exhalation. You check his pulse oximeter reading and it is 93%.

Exercise 25-3: *Multiple Choice Question*

The first intervention the nurse should do on an infant with a history of meconium at delivery who is grunting during deep sleep with a pulse oximeter reading of 92% is to:

    A. Call the pediatrician.

    B. Wake him up and stimulate to breathe.

    C. Do nothing and check every 15 minutes.

    D. Provide oxygen.

The oximeter reading does not improve and Ben is placed under the oxygen hood at 100% and the NICU is called. He is taken to the NICU after he is shown to his mom. In the NICU, he is placed on CPAP (continuous positive airway pressure) because his O2 keeps decreasing.

Exercise 25-4: *Multiple Choice Question*

In the case of meconium aspiration, the nurse would expect to see which findings on the chest X-ray?

    A. Streaking

    B. Ground glass

    C. Air outside the lung

    D. Hyperaeration

eResource 25-3: Review the two videos that highlight the use and impact of Bubble CPAP on neonates at the Texas Health Harris Methodist Hospital Fort Worth (see eResource 21-11).

An IV is started and antibiotics are ordered.

The answers can be found on page 331.

Exercise 25-5: *Multiple Choice Question*

The rationale for starting antibiotics on an infant with meconium aspiration is:

      A. They will probably get sepsis.

      B. The access lines are a ripe area for infection.

      C. Meconium is a rich medium for growth.

      D. They will help dissolve the meconium.

Arterial blood gases are done on Ben.

Exercise 25-6: *Exhibit*

The results of the arterial blood gases are:

  1. pH = 7.23

  2. PaCO2 = 60 mmHg

  3. PaC2 = 50 mmHg

  4. PhCO2 = 21 mEq/L

The infant is experiencing which condition?

      A. Respiratory acidosis

      B. Respiratory alkalosis

      C. Metabolic acidosis

      D. Metabolic alkalosis

 eResource 25-4: On your mobile device, use Skyscape's Outlines in Clinical Medicine (OCM), to see normal values and learn more about "Alkalosis" and "Acidosis."

    ■ [pathway: OCM → enter "ABG" into the "Main Index" search field → select "ABG."]

    ■ [pathway: OCM → enter "acidosis" into the "Main Index" search field → select "acidosis" → select "acidosis" again and peruse outline.]

    ■ [pathway: OCM → enter "alkalosis" into the "Main Index" search field → select "alkalosis" → select "alkalosis" again and peruse outline.]

A heart murmur is also heard on Ben indicating that shunting is still present. Ben is diagnosed with persistent pulmonary hypertension (PPHN) secondary to meconium aspiration. An echocardiogram shows the foremen ovale and the PDA are open.

Exercise 25-7: *Multiple Choice Question*

The diagnosis of PPHN would indicate that there is:

      A. Pulmonary vascular vasodilatation

      B. Pulmonary vascular vasoconstriction

      C. Cardiac vasoconstriction

      D. Cardiac vasodilatation

The decision is made to intubate Ben and place him on mechanical ventilation.

The answers can be found on page 332.

Exercise 25-8: *Multiple Choice Question*

For an infant of 40+ weeks' gestational age, what is the proper size endotracheal (ET) tube?

    A. 2.0-mm internal diameter

    B. 2.5-mm internal diameter

    C. 3.0-mm internal diameter

    D. 3.5-mm internal diameter

Exercise 25-9: *Calculation*

To prevent a term infant from "fighting" the ventilator, morphine (0.05–0.1 mg/kg q3-4h) is ordered at an initial dose. Ben is 8 pounds and 10 ounces. What is the upper and lower dose?

Ben is experiencing a gradual fall in PaO_2 and an increase in $PaCO_2$. The decision is made to place him on extracorporeal membrane oxygenation (ECMO).

Exercise 25-10: *Multiple Choice Question*

The nurse understands that ECMO works by:

    A. Increasing pressure in the left side of the heart to close shunts.

    B. Decreasing pressure in the pulmonary system.

    C. Bypassing the heart.

    D. Bypassing the lungs.

 eResource 25-5: To learn more about the ECMO and view images, open Medscape on your mobile device [Pathway: Medscape → enter "extracorporeal" into the search field at the top of the screen → select "Extracorporeal Membrane Oxygenation."]

Ben's parents are brought in and the procedure explained to them. They are visibly upset and choose to stay in the ECMO room most of the time. After 48 hours on ECMO, Ben's pulmonary system is becoming less vasoconstricted and perfusion is started slowly. After another 24 hours he is removed from the ECMO and is extubated and maintained on CPAP. Ben improves over the next few days and is discharged the following week.

The answers can be found on pages 332–333.

Answers

Exercise 25-1: *Fill-in*

A precipitous delivery is one in which contractions start and finish within ____3____ hours.

Exercise 25-2: *Select All That Apply*

What are the risk factors for meconium aspiration?

☑ **Postdates—YES.**

☐ LGA (large for gestational age)—NO, usually it is increased in small for gestational age (SGA) infants.

☑ **Maternal hypertension—YES, decreased oxygenation to the fetus is thought to increase adrenaline release causing a "fight or flight reaction" that shunts blood away from the GI tract to the major organs (i.e., heart and brain); therefore the GI tract relaxes and expels meconium.**

☑ **Placental insufficiency—YES, same as above.**

☐ Vertex delivery—NO, actually breech because of pressure on the fetal rectum.

Exercise 25-3: *Multiple Choice Questions*

The first intervention the nurse should do on an infant with a history of meconium at delivery who is grunting during deep sleep with a pulse oximeter reading of 92% is to:

A. Call the pediatrician—NO, this may have to be done but it is not your first reaction.

B. **Wake him up and stimulate to breathe—YES, this is the first intervention.**

C. Do nothing and check every 15 minutes—NO, an infant can deoxygenate in 15 minutes.

D. Provide oxygen—NO, this is the second intervention if waking him up does not help.

Exercise 25-4: *Multiple Choice Question*

In the case of meconium aspiration, the nurse would expect to see which findings on the chest X-ray?

A. Streaking—NO, this is a sign of Transitional Tachypnea of the Newborn (TTN) in which lung fluid is not fully absorbed.

B. Ground glass—NO, this is a sign of respiratory distress syndrome (RDS).

C. Air outside the lung—NO, this is a sign of a pneumothorax.

D. **Hyperaeration—YES, air is trapped in the lungs by the meconium.**

Exercise 25-5: *Multiple Choice Question*
The rationale for starting antibiotics on an infant with meconium aspiration is:
A. They will probably get sepsis—NO.
B. The access lines are a ripe area for infection—NO, this is true but not the main reason.
C. **Meconium is a rich medium for growth—YES.**
D. They will help dissolve the meconium—NO.

Exercise 25-6: *Exhibit*
The results of the arterial blood gases are:
1. pH = 7.23
2. PaCO2 = 60 mmHg
3. PaC2 = 50 mmHg
4. PhCO3 = 21 mEq/L

The infant is experiencing which condition?
A. **Respiratory acidosis—YES.**
B. Respiratory alkalosis—NO, pH would be higher, PaCO2 lower, and increased PaO2.
C. Metabolic acidosis—NO, PaCO2 would be within normal limits (WNL), and PaO2 WNL, and increased PHCO3.
D. Metabolic alkalosis—NO, pH would be increased, PaCO2 WNL, PaO2 WNL, and inc4reased PHCO3.

Exercise 25-7: *Multiple Choice Question*
The diagnosis of PPHN would indicate that there is:
A. Pulmonary vascular vasodilatation—NO.
B. **Pulmonary vascular vasoconstriction—YES.**
C. Cardiac vasoconstriction—NO.
D. Cardiac vasodilatation—NO.

Exercise 25-8: *Multiple Choice Question*
For an infant of 40+ weeks' gestational age, what is the proper size endotracheal (ET) tube?
A. 2.0-mm internal diameter—NO, this is for an extremely low birth weight infant.
B. 2.5-mm internal diameter—NO, this is for an infant under 30 weeks' gestation.
C. 3.0-mm internal diameter—NO, this is for an infant 30–34 weeks' gestation.
D. **3.5-mm internal diameter—YES, this is used for an infant over 35 weeks' gestation.**

Exercise 25-9: *Calculation*

To prevent a term infant from "fighting" the ventilator, morphine is ordered at an initial dose of 0.05–0.1 mg/kg q3-4h. Ben is 8 pounds and 10 ounces. What is the upper and lower dose?

8 lbs, 10 oz = 3.9 kg

0.05 mg/ kg × 3.9 kg = 0.195 (0.2) mg lower dose

0.1 mg/kg × 3.9 kg = 0.39 (0.4) mg upper dose

Exercise 25-10: *Multiple Choice Question*

The nurse understands that ECMO works by:

A. Increasing pressure in the left side of the heart to close shunts—NO, the catheter is threaded into the heart.

B. Decreasing pressure in the pulmonary system—NO, it bypasses it.

C. Bypassing the heart—NO.

D. **Bypassing the lungs—YES, it provides the lungs time to reabsorb the meconium.**

26

Periventricular-Interventicular Hemorrhage

Case Study 26 Jason

Jason is 2 weeks old but was born at 26 weeks' gestational age. He is now on continuous positive airway pressure (CPAP) and total parenteral nutrition (TPN). Jason is maintained in an incubator on servo temperature control and intake and outputs. He is attached to a cardio-respiratory (C-R) monitor with audible alarms. His current weight is 960 gms. You are Jason's nurse and have been caring for him intermittently for the past two weeks. Today you notice that he is having apnea and bradycardia (A&B) episodes, more than usual. His rectal temperature is 97 °F despite the set temperature of 38 °C on the incubator.

e   **eResource 26-1:** Review CPAP videos in Chapter 21 (eResource 21-11) to review the long-term benefits to the neonate.

Exercise 26-1: *Multiple Choice Question*
A common reason for hypothermia in the neonate is:

     A. Drug withdrawal

     B. Seizures

     C. Sepsis

     D. Hypoglycemia

A complete blood count (CBC) is ordered and a C-reactive protein.

Exercise 26-2: *Multiple Choice Question*
The nurse knows that a C-reactive protein elevations would indicate:

     A. Inflammation

     B. Vasoconstriction

     C. Vasodilation

     D. Renal insufficiency

The answers can be found on page 341.

eResource 26-2:

■ Go to Merck Medicus online to view related publications for health care providers.

■ [Pathway: *merckmedicus.com* → enter "intraventricular hemorrhage" into search field to view recent publications → scroll down to locate "Pediatric Advisor: Intraventricular Hemorrhage (IVH) of the Newborn" to read a comprehensive overview of the condition.]

■ To learn more about intraventricular hemorrhage use your mobile device, open MerckMedicus and go to the Merck Manual [Merck Manual → Topics → enter "neonate" into the search field → scroll down and select "intracranial hemorrhage in . . ." → scroll down to "intraventricular and/or intraparenchymal hemorrhage" to read more about intraventricular hemorrhage, treatment and prognosis.]

Jason's blood work was within normal limits (WNL), but his A&B spells are 20% more today, so it is decided that he will be put back on mechanical ventilation—high frequency. You notice an occasional jerking motion of Jason's right arm. You understand that seizures in infants manifest differently than in adults and are of five types:

1. Subtle—repetitive eye movements, tonic posture, clonic chin movements, or sucking motions;

2. Tonic seizures—decorticate posturing, occasional clonic movements;

3. Multifocal clonic seizures—clonic movements that move from one limb to another;

4. Focal seizures—localized and consciousness is maintained; and

5. Myoclonic seizures—synchronous, multiple jerking in upper or lower limbs (rare in infants).

 eResource 26-3: To learn more about seizures in neonates, use your mobile device, open MerckMedicus and go to the Merck Manual [Merck Manual → Topics → enter "neonate" into the search field → scroll down and select "seizures in" → using the drop-down menu located in the upper right corner of the screen to peruse content related to s/s, prognosis and treatment of seizures in neonates.]

An ultrasound of Jason's head is ordered.

Exercise 26-3: *Hot Spot*

Place an X on the lateral ventricle:

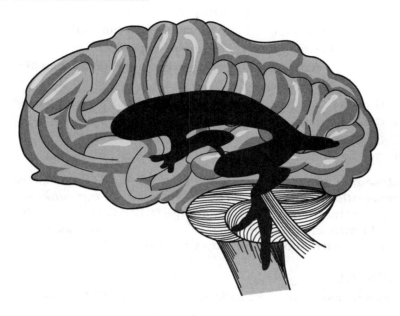

e   **eResource 26-4:** Open a browser and go to the Trip Database: [Pathway: *tripdatabase.com* → enter "Periventricular Hemorrhage (overview)" into the search field → scroll down and select Periventricular Hemorrhage—Intraventricular Hemorrhage" to read an overview, diagnosis, treatment, and follow-up as well as view radiology images.]

Exercise 26-4: *Multiple Choice Question*

The nurse understands that one of the suspected causative factors of periventricular-intraventricular hemorrhage is:

    A. Lack of cerebral oxygen.

    B. Aspiration of meconium.

    C. Vertex delivery of preterm infants.

    D. Rapid dilatation of cerebral blood vessels.

Jason is diagnosed with a grade III intraventricular hemorrhage.

The answers can be found on pages 341–342.

Exercise 26-5: *Matching*

Match the intraventricular hemorrhage grade with the area in which bleeding is present.

_____ Bleeding into the subependymal

_____ Bleeding into the ventricles, which causes distention

_____ Bleeding extended to the parenchymal

_____ Bleeding into the subependymal and ventricles without dilating the ventricles

A. Grade I

B. Grade II

C. Grade III

D. Grade IV

 eResource 26-5: Go to *AboutKidsHealth.com* to view a slideshow presentation of IVH grades I to IV [Pathway: *www.aboutkidshealth.ca* → Enter "Intraventricular Hemorrahge (IHV)" into the search field → scroll down and click on "Click to Start" to view the slide show (Note: you must have Adobe Flashplayer installed to view).]

Exercise 26-6: *Fill-in*

A priority nursing intervention for an infant with a grade III IVH is to _____.

Jason has more seizure activity so Phenobarbital is ordered.

Exercise 26-7: *Calculation*

Phenobarbital is ordered at 20 mg/kg. If Jason is 960 gms, how much should you administer? _____

The nurse knows that current evidence is being produced that head cooling of preterm infants with perinatal hypoxia is a new treatment to decrease rapidly dilating, fragile cerebral blood vessels during resuscitation efforts. This was not done in Jason's case because he was a precipitous delivery in the ED (emergency department). Jason does well on the phenobarbital and another head ultrasound is scheduled for the following week.

 eResource 26-6:
- To learn more about the drug prescribed, open Medscape from WebMD on your mobile device. [Pathway: Medscape → enter "phenobarbital" into the search field at the top of the screen → select "Phenobarbital."]
- To calculate the proper dosage:
  - Use Skyscape's Archimedes on your mobile device. [Pathway: Archimedes → enter "dose" into the Main Index → scroll down to "Drug dosing (mg/kg/day).]
  - Go to *MedCalc.com* to use the online dose calculator. [Pathway: *medcalc.com* → Tap on "Pediatrics" → "Dose Calculator".]

The answers can be found on page 342.

Exercise 26-8: *Select All That Apply*

Important environmental interventions for Jason are:

☐ Good lighting

☐ Soothing music

☐ Decreased handling

☐ Cluster care

☐ Bold pictures for him to view

The following week the head ultrasound shows no increase in the bleed. This is good news, and Jason's parents are happy.

Exercise 26-9: *Multiple Choice Question*

Jason's parents need further education when they state:

A. "I know Jason may grow up with some neurological deficits."

B. "I know handling him did not cause the bleed."

C. "I know they will check his head every week."

D. "I know there is no chance of his becoming hydrocephalic."

The answers can be found on pages 342–343.

Answers

Exercise 26-1: *Multiple Choice Question*

A common reason for hypothermia in the neonate is:

A. Drug withdrawal—NO, this usually produces increased metabolism and temperature rises.

B. Seizures—NO, this usually produces increased metabolism and temperature rises.

C. **Sepsis—YES, neonates many times get hypothermia instead of hyperthermia.**

D. Hypoglycemia—NO, this usually does not affect body temperature.

Exercise 26-2: *Multiple Choice Question*

The nurse knows that a C-reactive protein elevations would indicate:

A. **Inflammation—YES, it is a response to inflammation.**

B. Vasoconstriction—NO.

C. Vasodilation—NO.

D. Renal insufficiency—NO.

Exercise 26-3: *Hot Spot*

Place an X on the lateral ventricle:

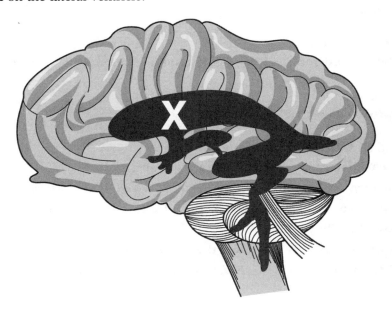

Exercise 26-4: *Multiple Choice Question*

The nurse understands that one of the suspected causative factors of periventricular-intraventricular hemorrhage is:

A. Lack of cerebral oxygen—NO, although this is partially true, the belief is that the leading causes is rapid administration of oxygen and dilatation of the cerebral veins.

B. Aspiration of meconium—NO.

C. Vertex delivery of preterm infants—NO, there is no evidence that states the type of delivery effects of a preterm outcome.

D. **Rapid dilatation of cerebral blood vessels—YES.**

Exercise 26-5: *Matching*

Match the intraventricular hemorrhage grade with the area in which bleeding is present.

____**A**____ Bleeding into the subependymal

____**C**____ Bleeding into the ventricles that causes distention

____**D**____ Bleeding extend to the parenchymal

____**B**____ Bleeding into the subependymal and ventricles without dilating the ventricles

A. Grade I

B. Grade II

C. Grade III

D. Grade IV

Exercise 26-6: *Fill-in*

A priority nursing intervention for an infant with a grade III IVH is to **measure head circumference**.

Exercise 26-7: *Calculation*

Phenobarbital is ordered at 20 mg/kg. If Jason is 960 gms, how much should you administer?

Jason weighs 0.96 kg

20 mg/kg × 0.96 kg = **19.2 mg**

Exercise 26-8: *Select All That Apply*

Important environmental interventions for Jason are:

❑ Good lighting—NO, dim lighting should be provided to decrease stimulation.

❑ Soothing music—NO, quiet should be provided to decrease stimulation.

☑ **Decreased handling—YES.**

☑ **Cluster care—YES, this will allow the infant to be disturbed once for all care.**

❑ Bold pictures for him to view—NO, this will not decrease stimulation.

Exercise 26-9: *Multiple Choice Question*

Jason's parents need further education when they state:

A. "I know Jason may grow up with some neurological deficits."—NO, this is true.

B. "I know handling him did not cause the bleed."—NO, this is true.

C. "I know they will check his head every week."—NO, this is true.

D. **"I know there is no chance of his becoming hydrocephalic."—YES, infants with IVH/PVH hemorrhage can develop hydrocephalus.**

27

Neonatal Abstinence Syndrome (NAS)

Case Study 27 ▨ Michael

Michael is a 38-week gestational age infant who has been exposed to tobacco, alcohol, and cocaine in utero. His mother is incarcerated for drug use and theft. He is in the newborn nursery presently and weighs 4 pounds, 6 ounces. Michael has some facial features that concern the nurses.

Exercise 27-1: *Hot Spot*
In this picture put an X on the facial features of fetal alcohol syndrome (FAS):

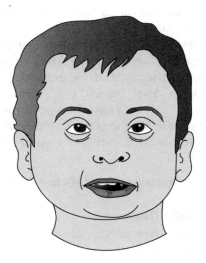

Fetal alcohol syndrome and fetal alcohol effects are among the most common causes of cognitive and social impairment in children. Michael's mother admits to drinking and taking drugs while she was pregnant.

The answer can be found on page 351.

eResource 27-1: Go to the Center for Disease Control (CDC) to view a video that provides a good overview of the long-term impact of FAS [pathway: *cdc.gov/fasd* → scroll down to locate and select the "View 'Story of Iyal' Video" link. (Note: there is considerable information on this Web site that can contribute to your understanding and support of patient education.]

Exercise 27-2: *Multiple Choice Question*

The nurse understands that FAS occurs when:

    A. A pregnant patient drinks in the first trimester.

    B. A pregnant patient drinks continuously throughout her pregnancy.

    C. A pregnant patient binge drinks.

    D. A pregnant patient drinks.

eResource 27-2:

- On your mobile device, open Medscape from WebMD. [Pathway: Medscape → enter "fetal" into the search field at the top of the screen → select "fetal alcohol syndrome."]

- To learn more about FAS and the clinical presentation, use your mobile device, open MerckMedicus and go to the Merck Manual. [Merck Manual → Topics → enter "neonate" into the search field → scroll down and select "drug withdrawal in" → select "Prenatal Drug Exposure" → tap on the menu icon on the upper right corner of the screen and select "Alcohol."]

- You can also listen to the CDC's podcast on pregnancy and alcohol. [Pathway: *cdc.gov/podcast* → scroll down to the bottom of the screen to locate and select the podcast "Search" tab → enter "Alcohol and Pregnancy" and tap "Start Search."]

- Additional material can be viewed on your mobile device. Go to: *nlm.nih.gov* to access MedlinePlus to learn more about FAS. [Pathway: nlm.nih.gov → select "MedlinePlus" → enter "fetal alcohol syndrome" into the search field.]

Besides being SGA (small for gestational age) Michael is also plethoric in appearance.

Exercise 27-3: *Multiple Choice Question*

The nurse understands that an infant with a ruddy or plethoric appearance:

    A. Had too many nutrients in utero.

    B. Was exposed to chemicals in utero.

    C. Was oxygen deprived in utero.

    D. Had an IgM reaction in utero.

The answers can be found on page 351.

Exercise 27-4: *Select All That Apply*

Other clinical signs the nurse would expect on an infant exposed to tobacco, alcohol, and drugs are:

❑ Small umbilical cord.

❑ Two-vessel umbilical cord.

❑ Small fontanels.

❑ Respiratory distress.

❑ Wakefulness.

At 36 hours' old, Michael is displaying signs of neonatal abstinence syndrome (NAS). For example,

1. He sleeps less than two hours after feeding.

2. He is mottled.

3. He has increased muscle tone .

4. He is feeding poorly with excessive sucking in between.

Use the following link to visualize the neonatal abstinence scale.

 eResource 27-3: *speciosum.curtin.edu.au/nas/ NeonatalAbstinenceScoreSheet.pdf*

 eResource 27-4:

■ On your mobile device, open Medscape provided by WebMD. [Pathway: Medscape → enter "neonatal" into the search field at the top of the screen → select "neonatal abstinence syndrome."]

■ Go to Merck Medicus Online to view related publications for health care providers. [Pathway: *merckmedicus.com* → enter "neonatal abstinence syndrome" into search field to view recent publications. Then repeat the process by entering "fetal alcohol syndrome" into the search field.]

■ Using the TripDatabase do a search for NAS treatment recommendations. [Pathway: *tripdatabase.com* → enter "neonatal abstinence syndrome" into the search field → scroll down and select "Neonatal Abstinence Syndrome (Treatment)."]

■ Or, go to: *nlm.nih.gov* to access MedlinePlus. [Pathway: nlm.nih.gov → select "MedlinePlus → enter "neonatal abstinence syndrome" into the search field → scroll down and select topic and images to view.]

For infants that are over the score of 8, pain medication is ordered to keep them comfortable. Paregoric (camphorated opium tincture) is ordered 1.5 mL q 6 hours.

The answer can be found on page 352.

Exercise 27-5: *Calculation*
Pediatric paregoric (camphorated opium tincture) normal dosage is 0.25–0.5 mL/ kg. Is Michael getting the proper amount?

eResource 27-5:
- To learn more about paregoric, open Medscape provided by WebMD on your mobile device. [Pathway: Medscape → enter "paregoric" into the search field at the top of the screen → select "paregoric."]
- Go to MedCalc.com for an online dose calculator. [Pathway: *medcalc.com* → Tap on "Pediatrics" → "Dose Calculator" to access the calculator.]
- On your mobile device, use Skyscape's Archimedes, to calculate the drug dose. [Pathway: Archimedes → enter "dose" into the main index → scroll down to "Drug dosing (mg/kg/day).]

Exercise 27-6: *Multiple Choice Question*
The priority nursing diagnosis for Michael would be:
    A. Acute pain
    B. Disturbed sleep pattern
    C. Ineffective infant feeding pattern
    D. Disorganized infant behavior

Michael has impaired skin integrity due to diarrhea. His buttock is raw from frequent stools.

Exercise 27-7: *Multiple Choice Question*
A nursing intervention effective for skin breakdown on infants is to:
    A. Keep the area covered.
    B. Expose the skin to air.
    C. Use cold compresses.
    D. Apply absorbing powder.

Exercise 27-8: *Select All That Apply*
Nursing interventions that are effective with infants with NAS are:
- [ ] Swings
- [ ] Swaddle
- [ ] Music
- [ ] Dim environment
- [ ] Horizontal rocking
- [ ] Pacifier

The answers can be found on pages 352–353.

Exercise 27-9: *Multiple Choice Question*

Michael is rubbing the skin raw on his elbows. An appropriate nursing intervention would be to:

    A. Turn him to a prone position.

    B. Cover his elbows with petroleum jelly.

    C. Place a transparent barrier film over his elbows.

    D. Use arm boards to keep his arms straight.

Michael's grandmother will be his caretaker as long as his mother is incarcerated.

Exercise 27-10: *Multiple Choice Question*

The nurse understands that Michael's caretaker needs more information about infant safety when she states:

    A. "I have a car seat with a 5-point restraint system."

    B. "I will put Michael to sleep on his back only."

    C. "I will keep Michael in my room at night."

    D. "I will put Michael to sleep in his mother's crib."

 eResource 27-6: To review follow-up recommendations for Michael, open Medscape on your mobile device. [Pathway: Medscape → enter "neonatal" into the search field at the top of the screen → select "neonatal abstinence syndrome" → click on the "Follow-up" tab and review material within.]

The answers can be found on page 353.

Answers

Exercise 27-1: *Hot Spot*

In this picture put an X on the facial features of fetal alcohol syndrome (FAS):

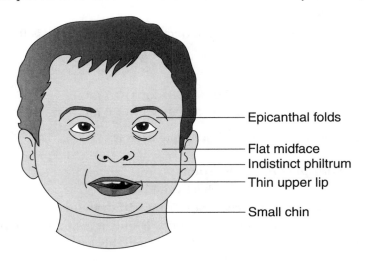

— Epicanthal folds

— Flat midface
— Indistinct philtrum

— Thin upper lip

— Small chin

Exercise 27-2: *Multiple Choice Question*

The nurse understands that FAS occurs when:

A. A pregnant patient drinks in the first trimester—NO, it may occur later in pregnancy.

B. A pregnant patient drinks continuously throughout her pregnancy—NO, it may be caused by one binge drinking episode.

C. A pregnant patient binge drinks—NO, it may also be constant drinking.

D. **A pregnant patient drinks—YES, the exact timing and amount of drinking that will cause FAS or fetal alcohol effects (FAE) is not known.**

Exercise 27-3: *Multiple Choice Question*

The nurse understands that an infant with a ruddy or plethoric appearance:

A. Had too many nutrients in utero—NO.

B. Was exposed to chemicals in utero—NO.

C. **Was oxygen deprived in utero—YES, the fetus produced more hemoglobin to compensate for oxygen deprivation.**

D. Had an IgM reaction in utero—NO.

Exercise 27-4: *Select All That Apply*

Other clinical signs the nurse would expect on an infant exposed to tobacco, alcohol, and drugs are:

☑ **Small umbilical cord—YES, this is due to oxygen deprivation.**

☐ Two-vessel umbilical cord—NO, this is a congenital malformation.

☐ Small fontanels—NO, they are usually large due to poor bone growth.

☐ Respiratory distress—NO, infants in constant stress in utero have less incidence of RDS. The stress increases lung surfactant production.

☑ **Wakefulness—YES, drug withdrawal makes infants hyperactive.**

Exercise 27-5: *Calculation*

Pediatric paregoric (camphorated opium tincture) normal dosage is 0.25–0.5 mL/ kg. Is Michael getting the proper amount?

Michael weigh 1.984 kg

$$0.25 \text{ mL/kg} \times 1.984 \text{ kg} = 0.5 \text{ mL}$$
$$0.5 \text{ mL/kg} \times 1.984 \text{ kg} = 1.0 \text{ mL}$$

The dose is too much; the nurse should question it.

Exercise 27-6: *Multiple Choice Question*

The priority nursing diagnosis for Michael would be:

A. **Acute pain—YES, he is in acute pain from withdrawing.**

B. Disturbed sleep pattern—NO, although this is true, it is not the priority.

C. Ineffective infant feeding pattern—NO, although this is true, it is not the priority.

D. Disorganized infant behavior—NO, although this is true, it is not the priority.

Exercise 27-7: *Multiple Choice Question*

A nursing intervention effective for skin breakdown on infants is to:

A. Keep the area covered—NO, this will contain the moisture from the diapers.

B. **Expose the skin to air—YES, this will dry it out.**

C. Use cold compresses—NO, this will chill the infant.

D. Apply absorbing powder—NO, powder is a respiratory irritant.

Exercise 27-8: *Select All That Apply*

Nursing interventions that are effective with infants with NAS are:

☑ **Swings—YES, the constant, steady motion helps.**

☐ **Swaddle—YES, it assists the infant to feel contained.**

☐ Music—NO, it overstimulates.

☑ **Dim environment—YES, it decreases stimulation.**

☐ Horizontal rocking—NO, vertical rocking works best for these infants.

☑ **Pacifier—YES, nutritive sucking decreases the pain.**

Exercise 27-9: *Multiple Choice Question*

Michael is rubbing raw the skin on his elbows. An appropriate nursing intervention would be to:

A. Turn him to a prone position—NO, this is not recommended due to SIDS; infants with NAS are high risk for SIDS.

B. Cover his elbows with petroleum jelly—NO, this will just rub off.

C. **Place a transparent barrier film over his elbows—YES, this will protect the skin.**

D. Use arm boards to keep his arms straight—NO, this is unnecessary restraining.

Exercise 27-10: *Multiple Choice Question*

The nurse understands that Michael's caretaker needs more information about infant safety when she states:

A. "I have a car seat with a 5-point restraint system."—NO, this is correct.

B. "I will put Michael to sleep on his back only."—NO, this is correct.

C. "I will keep Michael in my room at night."—NO, this is correct.

D. **"I will put Michael to sleep in his mother's crib."—YES, the crib probably doesn't not meet current safety standards.**

28

Inborn Errors of Metabolism

Case Study 28 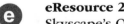 Frances

Frances is a 7-day-old newborn who is brought back to the ED by her parents because she is lethargic. She is admitted directly to the observation room in the NICU. Frances is the third child of a Mennonite family that lives on a farm. Her respirations are 60 and shallow, her heart rate is 98, and her temperature is 99.5 °F. Oxygen is applied at 3 liters via mask for a pulse oximeter reading of 90%. A CBC with differential and arterial blood gas (ABG) and cultures are done.

Exercise 28-1: *Exhibit Question*
The infant's ABGs show the following:

- pH 7.20
- $PaCO_2$ 58 mm Hg
- PaO_2 63 mm Hg
- $PHCO_3$ 37 mEq/L

What do the ABG results indicate?

    A. Metabolic acidosis
    B. Metabolic alkalosis
    C. Respiratory acidosis
    D. Respiratory alkalosis

e **eResource 28-1:** Review information on your mobile device using Skyscape's Outlines in Clinical Medicine (OCM), to see normal values and learn more about "Alkalosis" and "Acidosis" (eResource 25-4).

- [Pathway: OCM → enter "ABG" into the "Main Index" search field → select "ABG."]
- [Pathway: OCM → enter "acidosis" into the "Main Index" search field → select "acidosis" → select "acidosis" again and peruse outline.]
- [Pathway: OCM → enter "alkalosis" into the "Main Index" search field → select "alkalosis" → select "alkalosis" again and peruse outline.]

The answer can be found on page 359.

Exercise 28-2: *Multiple Choice Question*

Due to the ethnic background, what other test may be ordered for Frances?

    A. Stool

    B. Saliva

    C. Urine

    D. Vomit

Exercise 28-3: *Multiple Choice Question*

Blood tests show excess amino acid, and the following diagnosis is made:

    A. Hypothyroidism

    B. Galactosemia

    C. Phenylketonuria

    D. Maple syrup urine disease

 eResource 28-2: Go to *MerckManuals.com* and select the **Merck Manual for** healthcare professionals to view recent publications/ guidelines related to presenting s/s, physical assessment, diagnosis and treatment. [Pathway: *merckmanuals.com* → Heathcare Professionals → enter "inborn errors of metabolism" into search field.]

Frances is started on a formula that has low levels of the amino acids leucine, isoleucine, and valine. She will need a special diet free of branched-chain amino acids when she is older. Her amino acid blood levels are monitored.

Exercise 28-4: *Multiple Choice Question*

The diet you would expect Frances to be placed on is:

    A. Low calorie

    B. Low fat

    C. Low protein

    D. Low carbohydrate

Exercise 28-5: *Multiple Choice Question*

The nurse would expect that a child with maple syrup urine disease (MSUD) would be kept on a special diet:

    A. Until puberty

    B. Until young adulthood

    C. For life

    D. For infancy

The answers can be found on pages 359–360.

eResource 28-3:

■ Open a browser and go to the Trip Database: [Pathway: *tripdatabase .com* → enter "Maple Syrup Urine Disease (overview)" into the search field → scroll down and select topic to view. (Note: to learn more, scroll down to select segments about "diagnosis," "treatment," and "follow-up."]

■ On your mobile device, use Skyscape's Outlines in Clinical Medicine (OCM), to learn more about MSUD [pathway: OCM → enter "maple" into the main index search field → select "Maple Syrup Urine Disease" → tap on "Maple Syrup Urine Disease" again → scroll down to "F" and read 1–4].

Exercise 28-6: *Multiple Choice Question*

The nurse understands that Frances's parents need more education when they say:

    A. "If we don't stick to the diet there may be neurological damage."

    B. "If we don't stick to the diet there may be brain damage."

    C. "If we don't stick to the diet Frances may not be able to have children."

    D. "If we don't stick to the diet Frances could die."

eResource 28-4:

■ Using your mobile device, open MerckMedicus and go to the Merck Manual [Merck Manual → Topics → enter "maple" into the search field → select "Maple syrup urine disease."]

■ For educational material and support resources for the parents, go to the Genetics Home Reference provided by the National Library of Medicine. [Pathway: *ghr.nlm.nih.gov* → enter "maple syrup urine disease" into the search field to locate educational material.]

Exercise 28-7: *Hot Spot*

On the chart below, circle the offspring of the recessive carrier parents who have a chance of having the overt disease.

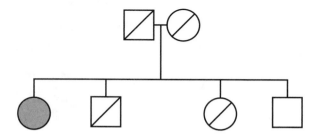

The answers can be found on page 360.

Answers

Exercise 28-1: *Exhibit Question*

The infant's ABGs show the following:

- ❏ pH 7.20
- ❏ PaCO2 58 mm Hg
- ❏ PaO2 63 mm Hg
- ❏ PHCO3 37 mEq/L

What do the ABG results indicate?

A. **Metabolic acidosis—YES, this is a low pH and high PHCO3.**

B. Metabolic alkalosis—NO, that is high pH and high PaCO2.

C. Respiratory acidosis—NO, that is low pH, high PaCO2, and

D. Respiratory alkalosis—NO, that is high pH and low PCO2.

Exercise 28-2: *Multiple Choice Question*

Due to the ethnic background what other test may be ordered for Frances?

A. Stool—NO.

B. Saliva—NO.

C. **Urine—YES.**

D. Vomit—NO.

Exercise 28-3: *Multiple Choice Question*

Blood tests show excess amino acid and the following diagnosis is made:

A. Hypothyroidism—NO.

B. Galactosemia—NO.

C. Phenylketonuria—NO.

D. **Maple syrup urine disease—YES.**

Exercise 28-4: *Multiple Choice Question*

The diet you would expect Frances to be placed on is:

A. Low calorie—NO.

B. Low fat—NO.

C. **Low protein—YES, it is an amino acid deficiency.**

D. Low carbohydrate—NO.

Exercise 28-5: *Multiple Choice Question*

The nurse would expect that a child with MSUD would be kept on a special diet:

A. Until puberty—NO.

B. Until young adulthood—NO.

C. **For life—YES, it is a diet for life.**

D. For infancy—NO.

Exercise 28-6: *Multiple Choice Question*

The nurse understands that Frances's parents need more education when they say:

A. "If we don't stick to the diet there may be neurological damage."—NO, this is true.

B. "If we don't stick to the diet there may be brain damage."—NO, this is true.

C. **"If we don't stick to the diet Frances may not be able to have children."—YES, the damage is neurological.**

D. "If we don't stick to the diet Frances could die."—NO, this is true.

Exercise 28-7: *Hot Spot*

On the chart below—circle the offspring of the recessive carrier parents who have a chance of having the overt disease.

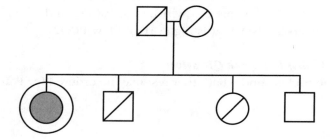

References

Anderson, J., Leonard, D., Braner, D. A. V., Lai, S., & Tegtmeyer, K. (2008, October 9). Umbilical vascular catheterization. *New England Journal of Medicine, 359*, e18. Retrieved from http://www.nejm.org/doi/full/10.1056/NEJMvcm0800666

Dunham, K. S. (2008). *How to survive and maybe even love nursing school*. Philadelphia, PA: F. A. Davis.

Gloe, D. (1999). Study habits and test-taking tips. *Dermatology Nurses' Association, 11*(6), 439–443, 447–449.

Hermann, J. W., & Johnson, A. N. (2009). From beta blockers to boot camp: Preparing students for the NCLEX-RN. *Nursing Education Perspectives, 30*(6), 384–388.

Hu, C., Kneusel, R., & Barnas, G. MedCalc.com. Created January 15, 2000; last modified January 27, 2001.

Landsberger, J. (1996). Overcoming test anxiety. Retrieved from http://www.studygs.net/tstprp8.htm

McDowell, B. M. (2008). KATTS: A framework for maximizing NCLEX-RN performance. *Journal of Nursing Education, 47*(4), 183–186.

Ricci, S. S. (2008). *Essentials of maternity, newborn, and women's health*. Philadelphia, PA: Lippincott, Williams & Wilkins.

Russell, S., & Triola, M. (1995–2006). *The precise neurological exam*. New York University School of Medicine. Retrieved from http://cloud.med.nyu.edu/modules/pub/neurosurgery/index.html

Sherin, K. M., Sinacore, J. M., Li, X. Q., Zitter, R. E., & Shakil, A. (1998). HITS: A short domestic violence screening tool for use in a family practice setting. *Family Medicine, 30*(7), 508–512.

Springhouse Review. (2006). *Lippincott manual of nursing practice pocket guides: Maternal-neonatal nursing*. Philadelphia, PA: Lippincott, Williams & Wilkins.

Wittmann-Price, R. A. (2009). Chapter 19: Caring for the newborn at risk. In S. L. Ward & S. M. Hisley (Eds.), *Maternal-child nursing care: Optimizing outcomes for mothers, children, and families*. Philadelphia, PA: F. A. Davis.

Wittmann-Price, R. A., & Thompson, B. R. (2010). *NCLEX-RN excel*. New York, NY: Springer.

Index

ABO incompatibility
  bilirubin test, 219, 221, 224, 225
  Coombs test, 218, 223
  exchange transfusion for, 221, 226
  jaundice and, 219, 220, 224, 225
  nursing diagnosis, 219, 224
  nursing intervention, 220, 225
  patient education, 221, 226
  Rh negative factor in, 217, 223
  Rh$_o$(D) Immune Globulin (RhoGAM),
      217, 218, 223
Abortion, 151, 160. *See also specific*
      abortions
  spontaneous. *See* Spontaneous
      abortion
  therapeutic, 180, 185
Abruption, 84–85, 101, 181, 186
Activated partial thromboplastin time
      (aPTT), 58
Acute pain, 348, 352
Advanced reproductive technology
      (ART), 80
AGA (appropriate for gestational age),
      14, 33
Albumin, 193, 201
Albuterol, 263, 267
Alpha fetal protein (AFP), 86, 101
Amenorrhea, 74, 95
Amethopterin. *See* Methotrexate
Amino acid deficiency, 356, 359
Amnion structure, 82, 99
Amoxicillin, 272, 276
Ampicillin, 292, 302
Anchors and lifesavers, 1, 7–9
Anemia and polycythemia, 315–320.
      See also Twin-to-twin transfusion
      syndrome (TTTS)
Angiomas, 86–87, 102
Anovulation, 75, 96

Anterior fontanel shape, 17, 35
Antibiotics, 230, 237
Anxiety
  avoiding, 3
  causes of, 2–3
  mild, 219, 224
  moderate, 91, 106, 129, 141
Aortic stenosis, 255–256, 261
Apgar score, 138, 147, 156, 164
Apnea, 292, 294, 302
Apresoline. *See* Hydrazaline
Arterial blood gas (ABG), 329, 332,
      355, 359
Artificial reproductive therapies, 80, 98
Aspiration, risk for, 322, 325
Asthma
  dietary suggestions, 265, 268
  fetal side effects of woman, 264, 267
  folic acid and, 266, 269
  maternal complications, during
      pregnancy, 264, 268
  pregnancy effects, on respiratory
      system, 264, 267
  screening, 265, 268
  suggestions for anemic patient,
      265, 268
  therapeutic effects, 263, 267
  vitamin C and, 266, 269
  worsening during pregnancy, 264, 267
Atrial septal defect (ASD), 255–256, 261
Atripla. *See* Efavirenz
Authorization to Test (ATT), 4
AVA (Artery, vein, artery). *See* Umbilical
      cords
Azidothymidine (AZT), 278, 280, 282

B-U-B-B-L-E-H-E format, 47
Babinski reflex, 23–24, 40–41

Bacterial vaginosis, 120–121, 125
Betamethasone, 230, 237, 243, 250
Bilirubin test, 28, 29, 44, 219–221,
    225–226
Birth control (BC) methods, 51–53, 66–67
Birth plan, 129, 141
Birth trauma incidence, increasing,
    19, 37
Blood administration, steps to
    first trimester bleeding and previa,
        157, 165
    twin-to-twin transfusion syndrome
        (TTTS), 316–317, 319–320
Blurred vision, 192, 201
Body heat loss methods, of infants, 24, 41
Body mass index (BMI) within normal
    limits (WNL), 73, 95
Bottle-feeding, 49, 64–65
    duration of, 296, 304
Bowel movement postpartum, 56, 70
Bowel sounds, for infants, 21
Brachial plexus injury, 22, 39
Bradley method, 91, 106
Breast engorgement, therapeutic
    intervention for, 59, 71
Breast-feeding, 25, 31, 41, 45, 49, 59,
    64–65, 71, 322, 323, 325, 326
Breast milk
    advantages of providing, 233, 239
    HIV transmitting by, 278, 282
Breech presentation, 284–285, 298
Brethine. See Terbutaline
Bronchodilator, 263, 267
Bronchopulmonary dysplasia (BPD),
    retinopathy of prematurity
    (ROP) and, 309, 312. See also
    Retinopathy of prematurity (ROP)
Brown fat, 87, 103
Butorphanol, 134

C-reactive protein, 335, 341
Caffeine, 294, 304
Calcium gluconate, 243, 250
Calcium leucovorin, 169, 172
Camphorated opium tincture. See
    Paregoric (camphorated opium
    tincture)
Caput succidarium, 17, 35

Carbohydrate count, 215
Cardiac disease
    classification with, 254, 259
    discharge teaching, 257, 262
    drug dosage, 256
    dyspnea, in second trimester, 254, 260
    EKG interpretation, 256, 261
    hemodynamic changes during
        pregnancy, 253, 259
    nursing diagnosis, 256, 261
    peripartum cardiomyopathy, 257, 262
    physical assessments determination
        on, 254, 260
    rheumatic heart disease, 256, 261
    symptoms of, 254, 260
    Tetralogy of Fallot and, 255, 260
Cardio-respiratory (C-R) monitor, 287,
    307, 335
Carpal tunnel syndrome, in pregnancy,
    88, 104
CD4, normal levels of, 280, 282
Cephalohematoma, 17, 35
Cephalosporins, 131, 142
Cerebral signs with gestational
    hypertension, 192, 201
Cervical cap, 52, 66–67
Cervical mucosa ferns, 75, 96
Cesarean birth, 54, 56, 68, 70
    preparation for, 154–155, 163
Chadwick's sign, 81, 99
Childbirth preparation classes, 91, 106
Chlamydia, 119, 120–121, 122, 125, 126
Chloasma, 86–87, 102
Choline, 114, 118
Choriocarcinoma, 174, 177–178
Chorion, 82, 99, 315, 319
Clavicle, palpation of, 19
Cleocin, 133, 143
Clindamycin hydrochloride, 133, 143
Clomid, 79, 84
Cold stress, preventing, 138, 146
Colostrum, 86–87, 102
Complete blood count (CBC), 77, 111,
    116, 157, 316, 335
Complete breech position, 284–285, 298
Complete hydatidiform mole, 174,
    177–178
Condoms. See Female condom; and Male
    condom

Conjugate/conjugata vera, 91, 105
Continuous positive airway pressure
    (CPAP), 287, 291, 293, 294,
    307, 328
Coombs test, 218, 223
Corticosteroid. *See* Betamethasone
CPR training, 310, 312
Crepitus, 19, 37
Cryopreservation, 80, 98
Cryotherapy/laser therapy
    for retinopathy of prematurity (ROP),
    308, 312
Cryptorchidism, 22, 39, 291, 301

Danger signs and causes, 51, 65–66,
    84–85, 101
Decidua basalis, 81, 99
Decidua capsularis, 81, 99
Decidua vera, 81, 99
Deep tendon reflexes (DTR), 175, 178,
    193, 201
Deep vein thrombosis (DVT), 57, 71
Deltasone. *See* Prednisone
Depo-provera®, 51, 53, 66–67
    administration, 53
Dextrose, 27, 43
Diabeta. *See* Glyburide
Diabetes. *See also* Gestational
    diabetes (GD)
    type I, 206, 213
    type II, 206, 213
Diaphragm, 52, 66–67
Diclofenac, 97
Diethylstilbestrol (DES), 180, 185
Discharge instructions for patient
    ABO incompatibility, 221
    cardiac disease, 257, 262
    hyperemesis gravidarum (HG), 114, 118
    newborn nursing care, 31
    postpartum care, 50–51
    preterm labor (PTL), 246, 252
    sickle cell anemia, 274, 276
Disseminated intravascular coagulation
    (DIC), 182–183, 187
Down syndrome, 85, 86, 101
Doxycycline, 122, 126
Drug usage, during pregnancy, 78, 79, 97
Dysmenorrhea, 74, 95

Ear placement, 18, 36
Eclampsia, 175, 191, 197, 200, 204
Ectoderm, 82, 100
Ectopic pregnancy
    drug dosage, 169, 172
    human Chorionic Gonadotropin (hCG)
        in, 169, 170
    IV infusion, 168, 171
    methotrexate for, 169, 171–172
    nausea and vomiting, 169
    nursing diagnosis, 168, 171
    risk factors for, 167, 171
    salpingostomy for, 168, 171
Efavirenz, 278
Electronic medical records (EMR), 14
Endoderm, 82, 100
Endometrial biopsy test, 75
Endotracheal (ET) tube size, 232, 238,
    330, 332
Engorgement. *See* Breast-feeding
Enzyme-linked immunosorbent assay
    (ELISA), 277, 279, 281, 282
Epidural anesthesia, 134
    position for, 135, 144
    side effects of, 135, 144
Epispadias, 22, 39
Erb's palsy. *See* Brachial plexus injury
Erythema toxicum, 16, 34
Erythromycin ointment, 18
Expected date of delivery (EDD), 84, 100,
    152, 161
Extracorporeal membrane oxygenation
    (ECMO), 330, 333

Feeding methods. *See* Bottle-feeding;
    and Breast-feeding
Female condom, 51, 66–67
Female surgical sterilization, 52,
    66–67
Femoral artery and vein, 23
Fencing reflex. *See* Tonic neck reflex
Fertility awareness, 51, 66–67
Fetal alcohol effects (FAE), 345, 351
Fetal alcohol syndrome (FAS)
    facial features of, 345, 351
    occurrence of, 346, 351
Fetal circulation, 82, 99–100
Fetal demise, 84–85, 101

Fetal development, 81
  teratogens effects on, 78
Fetal heart tones (FHT), 85, 101, 107
Fetal-maternal hemorrhage, 182, 186
Fetal meconium, 134, 143
Fetal movements (FMs), 105, 208, 214
First trimester bleeding and previa
  administering blood/blood products,
      steps for, 157, 165
  cause of, 149, 159
  Cesarean birth, preparation for,
      154–155, 163
  fetal monitor strip for, 154, 163
  getting out of bed, 149, 159
  infant in distress at birth, 157, 165
  IV infusion, 150, 154, 159, 163
  last menstrual period (LMP) and
      expected date of delivery (EDD),
      152, 161
  low-transverse uterine incision,
      155, 164
  marginal previa, 153, 162
  normal blood loss for delivery, 157, 165
  nursing diagnosis, 149, 159
  placenta previa
    diagnosis with, 152–153, 161
    risk factors for, 154, 162
  spontaneous abortion, risk factor for,
      150–151, 160
  ultrasound assessment of, 152, 161
Focal seizures, 336
Folic acid, 83, 100, 266, 269
Follicular stimulating hormone (FSH),
      75, 96
  blood level test, 75
Fontanels, on infants, 17, 35
Footling breech position, 284–285, 298
Frank breech position, 284–285, 298
Fraternal twins, 288, 299

Gamete intrafallopian transfer (GIFT),
      80, 98
Garamycin. See Gentamicin
Gardasil, 122–123
Genetic abnormalities, 149, 159
Genetic and inborn errors of metabolism
      screening, 28
Genital herpes, 123, 127

Gentamicin, 324, 326
GERD (Gastroesophageal reflux), 110, 115
Germ layer developments, 82, 83, 100
Gestational diabetes (GD), 205–216
  diet history, 210, 215–216
  fetal heart accelerations, 208, 215
  fetal movements, 208, 214
  glucose intolerance in pregnancy,
      206, 214
  glucose tolerance test (GTT), 205,
      207, 213
  glycosylated hemoglobin (HbA1C),
      207, 214
  grams of carbohydrates, 209, 215
  IV infusion, 176
  lecithin-sphingomyelin ratio, 210, 216
  maternal and fetal risks, 207, 214
  medication, 207–208
  patient education, 209, 215
  phosphatidylglycerol (PG), 211, 216
  placental hormones in pregnancy,
      206, 213
Gestational diabetes mellitus (GDM),
      206, 213
Gestational hypertension
  cerebral signs with, 192, 201
  clinical signs of, 189, 199
  deep tendon reflexes (DTR), 193, 201
  diagnosis of, 190, 191, 200
  drug dosage, 194, 202
  eclampsia, 191, 200
  fetal heart rate, 195, 203
  and HELLP syndrome, 195–196, 203
  IV infusion, 194
  liver function tests, 192, 201
  mild preeclampsia, 191, 200
  nursing interventions for, 194, 202
  priority during seizure, 194, 195, 203
  risk factors for, 192, 200
  severe preeclampsia, 191, 200
  sims position, 192, 201
  toxemia, 191, 200
Gestational trophoblastic disease (GTD)
  drug dosage, 176, 178
  etiology, 174, 177–178
  headache and spilling protein urine,
      complains of, 175, 178
  hormonal abnormality with molar
      pregnancy, 174, 177

patient education, 176, 178
risk factors for, 175, 178
symptoms of, 173, 177
Glucose intolerance, in pregnancy, 206, 214
Glucose sample, steps for obtaining, 25, 42
Glutamine, 114, 118
Glyburide, 207–208
Glycerophospholipids, 216
Glycosylated hemoglobin (HbA1C),
    207–214
Gonorrhea, 120–121, 125, 126
Group B streptococcus (GBS), 131,
    132, 142

Habits and study skills, 1, 2–4
Habitual aborter, 151, 160
Harlequin sign, 16, 34
Head circumference, for age, 17, 35,
    338, 342
Heart murmur, infant, 20–21, 38
Hegar's sign, 81, 99
HELLP syndrome, gestational
    hypertension and, 195–196, 203
Hematopoiesis structure, 82, 99
Hemorrhage, 264, 268
Heparin, 58, 71
Hepatitis B vaccine, administering,
    323, 326
Herpes, 120, 123, 125, 127
HIV. *See* Human immunodeficiency
    virus (HIV)
Human chorionic gonadotropin (hCG),
    109, 115, 174, 177
  in ectopic pregnancy, 169
Human immunodeficiency virus (HIV)
  antiretroviral therapy during
      pregnancy, 278, 281
  attacking T4 cells, 277, 281
  CD4, normal levels of, 280, 282
  drug dosage, 278
  enzyme-linked immunosorbent assay
      (ELISA), 277, 281
  fetal and newborn risks, 279, 282
  goal of delivery for HIV-positive
      patient, 280, 282
  heterosexual females, 278, 281
  patient education, 278
  screening, 279, 282

transmitting by breast milk, 278, 282
treatment for infants born, to HIV-
    positive mother, 280, 282
Western Blot/immunofluorescence
    assay, 279, 282
Human papillomavirus (HPV)
    immunization, 122–123, 127
Hurt, Insulted, Threatened with harm,
    and Screamed at them (HITS)
    screening tool, 77
Hydatidiform mole. *See* Gestational
    trophoblastic disease (GTD)
Hydrazaline, 194
Hydrocephalus, 339, 343
Hydrops fetalis, 220, 225
Hyperaeration, 328, 331
Hyperbilirubinemia, 17, 35
Hypercoagulable state, 59, 72
Hyperemesis gravidarum (HG), 84–85,
    101, 109–121
  addressing issues, upon admission,
      110–111, 116
  discharge teaching, 114, 118
  drug dosage, 112, 113–114, 117–118
  gravid and para, 110, 115
  high-risk perinatal unit for treatment,
      admitted to, 110–111, 116
  human chorionic gonadotropin (hCG),
      109, 115
  IV infusion, 111, 116
  rectal suppository administration, steps
      in intervention of, 112, 117
  risk factors for, 110, 115
  SBAR communication tool, 113, 117
  Tomiko's fall risks, 112, 117
  total parental nutrition (TPN),
      114, 118
  vomiting and dehydration, 111, 116
Hypertonicity symptom, 26, 43
Hypertrophy, 88, 103
Hypoglycemia, 19, 26, 37, 43, 157, 165
Hypomenorrhea, 74, 95
Hypospadias, 22, 39
Hypotension, 48, 63, 232, 238, 247, 252
Hypothermia
  in neonate, 335, 341
  in newborn, 13, 33
Hypotonicity symptom, 26, 43
Hysterosalpingography, 77

Ibuprofen, 49, 64, 74, 97
Identifiers, to matching mothers and
    infants, 24, 41
IgA, 25, 41–42
IgG, 25, 41–42
IgM, 25, 41–42
Impaired glucose tolerance, 206, 213
Implanon, 51–52, 66–67
In vitro fertilization (IVF), 80, 98
Inborn errors of metabolism
    amino acid deficiency, 356, 359
    arterial blood gas (ABG), 355, 359
    maple syrup urine disease (MSUD),
        356, 359, 360
    parents education, 357, 360
    urine test, 356, 359
Incompetent cervix
    abruption and, 181, 186
    disseminated intravascular coagulation
        (DIC) and, 182–183
    fetal heart rate, 181, 186
    gravid and para, 179, 185
    internal cervical, spotting, 179, 185
    IV infusion, 181
    Kleihauer-Betke test, 182, 184,
        186, 187
    nursing interventions, 180, 186
    platelets, normal count of,
        183, 187
    risk factors for, 180, 185
    Shirodkar procedure, 180
Inderal. See Propranolol
Indocin. See Indomethacin
Indomethacin, 97, 295, 304
Induced abortion, 151, 160
Inevitable abortion, 151, 160
Infants. See Newborns
Infection, possible causes of, 84–85, 101
Infertility/preconception/conception
    amnion structure, 82, 99
    artificial reproductive therapies and
        description, 80, 98
    cervical mucosa ferns, 75, 96
    Chadwick's sign, 81, 99
    childbirth preparation classes, 91, 106
    chorion structure, 82, 99
    complaints affecting integumentary
        system changes, 86–87, 102

conjugate/conjugata vera, 91, 105
diagnostic tests, 76, 96
    endometrial biopsy, 75
    FSH blood level, 75
    progesterone blood level, 75
    ultrasound, 75
Down syndrome, 85, 86, 101
drug dosage, 92, 106–107
endometrial lining layers and
    functions, 81, 99
fetal circulation, 82, 100
fetal heart rate (FHR), 90, 104–105
Fetal Heart Tones (FHT), 85, 86,
    101, 102
follicular stimulating hormone
    (FSH), 75
    blood level, 75
germ layer developments, 82, 83, 100
Hegar's sign, 81, 99
hematopoiesis structure, 82, 99
Hurt, Insulted, Threatened with harm,
    and Screamed at them (HITS)
    screening tool, 77
implantation, 81, 98
intimate partner violence (IPV) risk,
    77, 97
IV infusion, 92, 93, 107
last menstrual period (LMP) and
    expected date of delivery (EDD),
    84, 100
Leopold maneuvers, 89, 104
leutinizing hormone (LH), 75
men's lower sperm count, risk factors
    for, 76, 96–97
menstrual cycle, 73, 74, 75, 95, 96
    patient teaching about, 75, 96
mittelschmerz symptom, 75, 96
neural tube developments, 83, 100
nonsteroidal anti-inflammatory drugs
    (NSAID), 77, 78, 97
nonstress test (NST), 89–90, 104–105
nursing diagnosis, 91, 106
patient education, 75, 76, 96
pregnancy
    carpal tunnel syndrome in, 88, 104
    danger signs of, 84–85, 101
    drug usage during, 78, 79, 97
    FDA, categories for drugs, 79, 97

monilia/vaginal yeast infections, 87, 103
physiological anemia of, 89, 104
quickening in, 87, 103
recommended weight gain, 88, 103
systolic murmurs during, 88, 103
premature rupture of membranes, 93, 107
preterm labor and, 84, 93, 101, 107
priority diagnosis for couple, 81, 98
progesterone injections, side effects of, 80, 98
teratogens effects, on fetal development, 78
true labor, 92, 106
uterine fundus, 83, 100
Wharton's jelly structure, 82, 99
white blood cells (WBCs) increases during labor, 89, 104
Intact hard palate, Epstein pearls, and intact soft palate, 18, 36
Intimate partner violence (IPV) risk, 77, 97, 150, 160
Intrauterine pressure catheter (IUPC), 133, 134, 143
Iron deficiency anemia, 274, 276
IVPB (IV Piggyback), 133, 143, 272, 276

Jaundice, 219, 220, 224

Kernicterus, 220, 225
Kidneys, 100
Kleihauer-Betke test, 182, 184, 186, 187

Labor and delivery
   allergies, 130–131, 142
   angiocatheter size, 133, 143
   Apgar score, 138, 147
   assessments in priority order, 130, 141
   birth plan, 129, 141
   checking woman's fundus postdelivery, 140, 147
   drug dosage, 133, 136, 139, 143, 145, 147
   epidural/spinal anesthesia, 134

   position for, 135, 144
   side effects of, 135, 144
   fetal meconium, 134, 143
   fetal monitor strip, 132, 136–137, 145
   gravid and para, 130, 142
   group B streptococcus (GBS), 131, 132, 142
   intrauterine pressure catheter (IUPC), 133, 134, 143
   IV infusion, 133, 143
   last stage of labor (stage 3), 139, 147
   nuchal cord, 138, 146
   nursing diagnosis in, 129, 141
   nursing interventions, 130, 135, 137, 142, 144, 145–146
   patient safety, step for, 138, 146
   placental separation, four signs of, 139, 147
   precautions using in delivery room, 137, 146
   risk factors for infant weight loss, 140, 148
   Ritgen's maneuver, 138, 146
   stage and phase of, 134, 139, 144, 147
   uterine contractions (UCs), 129, 132, 136, 142–143, 144
Lanugo, 87, 103
Laser therapy/cryotherapy
   for retinopathy of prematurity (ROP), 308, 312
Last menstrual period (LMP) and expected date of delivery (EDD), 84, 100, 152, 161
Lateral ventricle, spotting, 337, 341
Leading up to test day, 1, 9–11
   checklist, 11
Lecithin-sphingomyelin ratio, 210, 216
Leopold maneuvers, 89, 104
Lethargy symptom, 26, 43
Leukorrhea, 86–87, 102
Leutinizing hormone (LH), 75, 96
Lifesavers, anchors and, 1, 7–9
Linea nigra, 86–87, 102
Liver function tests, 192, 201
Low forceps delivery, 257, 262
Low-lying placenta previa, 152–153, 161
Low-transverse uterine incision, 155, 164
Lunelle injectable, 52, 66–67

Magnesium sulfate (MgSO$_4$), 175, 176, 178, 194, 195, 202, 242, 243, 245–246, 249, 252

Male condom, 51–52, 66–67

Male genital condition, abnormalities of, 22, 39

Male sterilization, 52, 66–67

Maple syrup urine disease (MSUD), 356, 359, 360

Marginal placenta previa, 152–153, 161

Marginal previa, 153, 162

Maternal hypertension, 327, 331

Meconium, 134, 143

Meconium aspiration syndrome (MAS)
  antibiotics, starting, 329, 332
  chest X-ray, findings on, 328, 331
  endotracheal (ET) tube size, 330, 332
  extracorporeal membrane oxygenation (ECMO), 330, 333
  nursing intervention, 328, 331
  persistent pulmonary hypertension (PPHN), diagnosis of, 329, 332
  precipitous delivery, 327, 331
  respiratory acidosis, 329, 332
  risk factors for, 327, 331

Medroxyprogesterone acetate. *See* Depo-provera®

Menometrorrhagia, 74, 95

Menorrhagia, 74, 95

Men's lower sperm count, risk factors for, 76, 96–97

Menstrual cycle, 73, 74, 75, 95, 96

Mesoderm, 82, 100

Metabolic acidosis, 355, 359

Metabolism, inborn errors of. *See* Inborn errors of metabolism

Methotrexate, 169, 171–172

Mild anxiety, 219, 224

Mild preeclampsia, 191, 200

Milia, 15–16, 34

Mirena IUD, 52, 53, 66–67

Miscarriage. *See* Spontaneous abortion

Missed abortion, 151, 160

Mittelschmerz symptom, 75, 96

Mnemonics, 7–9

Mongolian spot, 15–16, 34

Montgomery tubercles, 86–87, 102

Moro reflex, 23–24, 40–41

Morphine, 330, 333

Mother-infant interaction in NICU, 288, 299

Multifocal clonic seizures, 336

Muscle twitching symptom, 26–27, 43

Myoclonic seizures, 336

Naproxen, 78, 97

Nasal flaring and grunting
  in newborns, 20, 38, 287, 299

Nausea and vomiting, 169
  in pregnancy, 110, 111, 116

NCLEX-RN®
  anchors and lifesavers, 1, 7–9
  guide for students, by students, 1–11
  introduction, importance of, 1–2
  leading up to test day, 1, 9–11
  preparation for, 1, 4–7
    Authorization to Test (ATT), 4
    planning for examination, 5–7
    register for the test, 4–5
    tip to reducing test-taking anxiety, 5
  study skills and habits, 1, 2–4

Neck assessment, for newborns, 19, 37

Neonatal abstinence syndrome (NAS), 347
  caretaker education, 349, 353
  clinical signs, 347, 352
  drug dosage, 348, 352
  fetal alcohol syndrome (FAS). *See* Fetal alcohol syndrome (FAS)
  nursing diagnosis, 348, 352
  nursing intervention, 348–349, 352–353
  ruddy/plethoric appearance, 346, 351

Neonatal intensive care unit (NICU), 93, 157, 233, 285, 288, 295, 299, 304, 309, 312

Neonatal polycythemia, 214

Neonatal respiratory distress syndrome, 214

Neonatal sepsis, 132, 142

Neural tube defects (NTD), 266, 269

Neural tube developments, 83, 100

Neurological exams, for infants, 23–24, 40–41

Neutral thermal environment (NTE), 19, 37

Nevus flammeus, 16, 34

Nevus vasculosus, 16, 34

Newborn assessment, in electronic medical records (EMR), 14

Newborn rash. *See* Erythema toxicum
Newborn respiratory distress, 287, 299
Newborns
  AGA (appropriate for gestational age), 14, 33
  anterior fontanel shape of, 17, 35
  bilirubin test, 28, 29, 44
  birth trauma, incidence of, 19, 37
  blood specimen, correct spot to obtaining, 26, 42
  body heat loss methods, 24, 41
  breast-feeding, 25, 31, 41, 45
  clavicle, palpation of, 19
  drug dosage, 27, 43
  ear placement, 18, 36
  fontanels on, 17, 35
  fourth intercostals space in midclavicular line, spotting, 20, 38
  glucose sample, steps for obtaining, 25, 42
  head shape for, 17, 35
  hypoglycemia symptoms, 26, 43
  hypothermia in, 13, 33
  identifiers, to matching mothers and infants, 24, 41
  infant weigh (lost 10% of birth weight), 28, 43
  intravenous (IV) glucose infusion, 27, 43
  IV infusion, 27, 43
  low/high limit of glucose, calculating, 26, 43
  male genital condition, abnormalities of, 22, 39
  nasal flaring and grunting in, 20, 38
  neck assessment for, 19, 37
  neurological exams for, 23–24, 40–41
  neutral thermal environment (NTE) for, 19, 37
  normal lab values for, 15
  nursing interventions placement, with heart murmur, 20–21, 38
  observations in, 22, 39
  oral assessment for, 18, 36
  patient education, 23, 30, 40, 44
  polycythemia in, 15, 33, 34
  posterior fontanel shape of, 17, 35
  postpartum maternal and newborn discharge, 31
  prone position, placing in, 31, 45
  pseudomenstruation in, 21, 39
  radiant warmers, 14, 33
  respiratory rate (RR) for, 19, 21, 37, 39
  safety, 30, 44
  screening tests, 28
  skin variations on, 15–16, 34
  suggestions for parents with infants crying, 30, 45
  talc powder for, 30, 44
  Turner syndrome, 19, 37
  umbilical cords, 21, 39
  vital signs, 16, 34
  vitamin K administration to, 23, 40
  weight conversion, 13–14, 33
Nidation, 81, 98
Nifedipine, 246, 252
Nipples, sore, 59, 71
Nonsteroidal anti-inflammatory drugs (NSAID), 77, 78, 97
Nonstress tests (NSTs), 89–90, 104–105, 208
Normal labor curve for nullipara, 283, 297–298
Nuchal cord, 138, 146
NuvaRing®, 51–52, 66–67

Observations, in newborns, 22, 39
Occiput posterior, 284, 298
Odansetran, 113, 114, 117–118
Oligohydramnios, 229, 236
Oligomenorrhea, 74, 95
Oligoovulation, 75, 96
Ophthalmia neonatorum, 18
Ophthalmoscope, 243, 250
Oracit, 155, 163
Oral assessment, for newborns, 18, 36
Oral contraceptives, 52, 53, 66–67
Ortho Erva patch, 52, 53, 66–67
Oxytocin, 136, 139, 145, 147

Pale, 315, 319
Palmer erythema, 86–87, 102
Palmer grasp reflex, 23–24, 40–41
ParaGard IUD, 51–52, 66–67
Paregoric (camphorated opium tincture), 348, 352

Partial birth abortion, 151, 160
Partial hydatidiform mole, 174, 177–178
Partial placenta previa, 152–153, 161
Patent ductus arteriosus (PDA), 255–256, 261, 295
Paternal behavior, 50, 65
PCA (patient-controlled analgesia), 54, 68
Pedal edema, 254, 260
Pediculosis pubis, 120–121, 125
Perineal discomfort, decreasing, 49, 64
Peripartum cardiomyopathy, 257, 262
Periventricular-intraventicular hemorrhage
  C-reactive protein, 335, 341
  causative factors of, 337, 342
  drug dosage, 338, 342
  environmental interventions, 339, 342
  grades, 338, 342
  hypothermia, in neonate, 335, 341
  lateral ventricle, spotting, 337, 341
  nursing intervention, 338, 342
  parents education, 339, 343
  seizures in infants, 336
Persistent pulmonary hypertension (PPHN), 329, 332
Phenergan, 112, 117
Phenobarbital, 338, 342
Phenylalanine, 28
Phosphatidylglycerol (PG), 211, 216
Physical examination, of newborn, 16, 34
Physiological anemia, of pregnancy, 89, 104
Pitocin. *See* Oxytocin
Placenta, 315, 319
Placenta previa, diagnosis with, 152–153, 161
Placental hormones in pregnancy, 206, 213
Placental separation, four signs of, 139, 147
Planter grasp reflex, 23–24, 40–41
Platelets, normal count of, 183, 187
Point of maximum impact (PMI), 20
Polycythemia, 15, 33, 34
  anemia and, 315–320. *See also* Twin-to-twin transfusion syndrome (TTTS)
Polydactyly, 22, 39
Polymenorrhea, 74, 95

Port wine stain. *See* Nevus flammeus
Postcoital emergency contraceptive (EC), 51–52, 66–67
Posterior fontanel shape, 17, 35
Postpartum care
  B-U-B-B-L-E-H-E format, 47
  birth control (BC) method, 51–53, 66–67
  bowel movement, 56, 70
  breast- and bottle-feeding, 49, 64–65
  breast engorgement, therapeutic intervention for, 59, 71
  Cesarean birth patient, 54, 56, 68, 70
  danger signs, 51, 65–66
  decrease in pulse in patients, 54, 69
  deep vein thrombosis (DVT), interventions for, 57, 71
  discharge instructions, 50–51
  drug dosage, 49, 53, 54, 64, 67–68
  fluids intake, 55, 69
  hypercoagulable state, 59, 72
  hypotension, 48, 63
  IV infusion, 55, 69
  nursing diagnosis, 57, 70–71
    for patient self-reporting loss of confidence and tearfulness, 61, 72
  paternal behavior, 50, 65
  patient education, 49, 51, 55, 64, 66, 69
  PCA (patient-controlled analgesia), 54, 68
  perineal discomfort, decreasing, 49, 64
  postpartum depression
    risk factors for, 60, 72
    self-report, 61, 72
  R-E-E-D-A assessment, 47, 56
  Rh_o(D) Immune Globulin, 55, 56, 70
  right/left mediolateral episiotomy, 48, 63
  SBAR communication tool, 57
  sore nipples, nursing interventions for, 59, 71
  taking-hold phase, 50, 65
  urinary retention, 48, 64
Postpartum depression
  risk factors for, 60, 72
  self-report, 61, 72
Postpartum maternal and newborn discharge, 31
Precipitous delivery, 327, 331

Prednisone, 263, 267
Preeclampsia, 191, 200
Pregnancy. *See also* Ectopic pregnancy
  antiretroviral therapy during
     pregnancy, 278, 281
  blood volume increases during,
     253, 259
  carpal tunnel syndrome in, 88, 104
  danger signs of, 84–85, 101
  drug usage during, 78, 79, 97
  FDA, categories for drugs, 79, 97
  glucose intolerance in, 206, 207, 214
  heart problems and, 253–262
  hemodynamic changes during,
     253, 259
  hormonal abnormality with molar
     pregnancy, 174, 177
  maternal complications, during
     pregnancy, 264, 268
  monilia/vaginal yeast infections, 87, 103
  nausea and vomiting in, 110, 111, 116
  physiological anemia of, 89, 104
  placental hormones in, 206, 213
  pregnancy effects, on respiratory
     system, 264, 267
  quickening in, 87, 103
  recommended weight gain, 88, 103
  on respiratory system, 264, 267
  systolic murmurs during, 88, 103
  worsening during pregnancy, 264, 267
Pregnancy-induced hypertension, 84–85,
    101, 264, 268
Premature rupture of membranes,
    93, 107
Prenatal classes, 91, 106
Preterm infant care
  apnea, 292, 294, 302
  blood gases, 293–294, 303
  bottle-feeding, duration of, 296, 304
  breech presentation, 284–285, 298
  cryptorchidism, 291, 301
  drug dosage, 295, 304
  dry diaper, 294, 303
  fraternal twins, 288, 299
  infant umbilical cords, cleaning,
    289, 300
  infants' weight on growth chart,
    286, 298
  IV infusion, 295, 304

  lower back/sacral pain, complains of,
    284, 298
  maintaining environment, 292, 302
  NG tube, measuring, 293, 302
  normal labor curve for nullipara, 283,
    297–298
  nursing diagnosis, 288, 299
  nursing intervention, 288, 299
  occiput posterior position, 284, 298
  oxygen therapy goal for, 288, 300
  physical assessment findings, 290,
    300, 301
  pulse oximetry, 286, 299
  referrals for, 296, 305
  respiratory distress, 287, 299
  supraclavicular retractions, assessing,
    289, 300
  vital signs, 289–290, 300
Preterm labor (PTL), 84–85, 93, 101, 107
  betamethasone administration,
    243, 250
  discharge instructions for, 246, 252
  drug dosage, 242, 246, 249, 252
  IV infusion, 242, 249
  lab reports, 245, 251–252
  magnesium sulfate (MgSO$_4$), 242, 243,
    245–246, 249, 252
  nifedipine side effects, 247, 252
  nursing diagnosis, 245, 251
  nursing interventions, 245, 251
  risk factors for, 241, 249
  sterile catheterization procedure, steps
    requiring for, 244, 251
Preterm premature rupture of
    membranes (PPROM), 84–85, 101,
    227, 235
Preterm rupture of membranes (PROM),
    227, 235
  risk factors for, 228, 235
Previa, 84–85, 101
Previous spontaneous abortion, 150, 160
Procardia. *See* Nifedipine
Progesterone blood level test, 75
Progesterone injections, side effects of,
    80, 98
Prolonged rupture of membranes,
    227, 235
Promethazine, 112
Propranolol, 256

Protection from abuse (PFA), 129, 131, 142
Proventil. *See* Albuterol
Pseudomenstruation, in infants, 21, 39
Pulmonary vascular vasoconstriction, 329, 332
Pulse oximetry, 20, 38, 286, 299
Pupil, dilation of, 308, 311
Purified protein derivative (PPD) test, 265
Pyrexia, 317, 320

Quickening, in pregnancy, 87, 103

R-E-E-D-A assessment, 47, 56
Radiant warmers, 14, 33
Rash, newborn. *See* Erythema toxicum
Rectal suppository administration, steps in intervention of, 112, 117
Rectus femoris, 23
Red blood cell (RBC), normal life span of, 275
Reflex hammer, 243, 250
Reproductive therapies, 80, 98
Respiratory acidosis, 329, 332
Respiratory distress, 13, 33
Respiratory rate (RR) for infants, 19, 21, 37, 39
Retinopathy of prematurity (ROP)
  and bronchopulmonary dysplasia (BPD), 309, 312
  CPR training, 310, 312
  cryotherapy/laser therapy treatment, 308, 312
  eye pupils, dilating, 308, 311
  nursing diagnosis, for patient's family, 310, 313
  parents education, 308, 310, 311, 312
  risk factor, 307, 311
    for developing, 308, 311
  screening for, 308, 311
Rh negative, 217, 223
Rheumatic heart disease, 256, 261
Rh$_o$(D) Immune Globulin (RhoGAM), 55, 56, 70, 217, 218, 223
Right occipital posterior (ROP), 86, 102

Right/left mediolateral episiotomy, 48, 63
Ritgen's maneuver, 138, 146
Rooting reflex, 23–24, 40–41
Rupture of the membranes (ROM), 227–239
  advantages of breast milk to preterm infants, 233, 239
  betamethasone administration, 230, 231, 237
  elevation in FHR, 227, 235
  fetal heart rate, 230–232, 237–238
  hypotension and, 232, 238
  IV infusion, 229, 236
  nursing interventions, 230, 237
  parents education, 233, 239
  positive ROM, 228–229, 236
  risk factors for PROM, 228, 235
  by transvaginal ultrasound, 229, 236
RUQ pain, 196, 203

Salpingostomy, for ectopic pregnancy, 168, 171
SBAR communication tool, 57, 113, 117
Scabies, 120–121, 125
Screening tests, newborn, 28
Seizures, in infants, 336
Semi-Fowler's position, 135, 144
Severe preeclampsia, 191, 200
Sexually transmitted disease (STD)
  bacterial STD, 119, 125
  decrease spreading of, 121, 126
  diagnosis, 120, 125
  drug dosage, 122, 126
  genital herpes infection, 123, 127
  gonorrhea, 120–121, 125, 126
  human papillomavirus (HPV) immunization, 122–123, 127
  patient education regarding, 121, 123, 126, 127
  symptoms, 120–121, 125
Shaking baby syndrome (SBS), 30
Shirodkar procedure, 180
Sickle cell anemia
  complaining of pain in right knee, 272, 275
  discharge instructions for patient, 274, 276

drug dosage, 272, 276
fetal heart rate, 273, 276
HbA replacing with HbS, 271, 275
inherited disease, 271, 275
iron deficiency anemia and, 274, 276
IV infusion, 272, 276
life span of, 272, 275
red blood cell (RBC), normal life span
    of, 272, 275
SIDS (sudden infant death), 317, 320
Simian crease, 22, 39
Sims position, for gestational
    hypertension, 192, 201
Skin breakdown on infants, 348, 352
Skin variations, on newborns, 15–16, 34
Sodium citrate. *See* Oracit
Sore nipples, 59, 71
Sperm, problem with, 76, 96–97
Sponge, 52, 66–67
Spontaneous abortion, 109, 151, 160
    cause of first trimester, 149, 159
    risk factor for, 150, 160
Stadol. *See* Butorphanol
Stepping reflex, 23–24, 40–41
Sterile vaginal exam (SVE), 92, 130, 141
Stork bite, 15, 34
Strawberry hemangioma. *See* Nevus
    vasculosus
Stress, defined, 2–3
Striae gravidarum, 86–87, 102
Study skills and habits, 1, 2–4
Subtle, 336
Sucking reflex, 23–24, 40–41
Sudden infant death syndrome (SIDS),
    prevention against, 31, 45
Sufentanil, 135
Supraventricular Tachycardia, 256, 261
Surfactant, 87, 103
Syndactyly, 22, 39
Syphilis, 120–121, 125
Systolic murmurs during pregnancy, 88, 103

T4 cells, 277, 281
Taking-hold phase, 50, 65
Talc powder, 30, 44
Teratogens effects, on fetal
    development, 78

Terbutaline, 92, 106, 231
Tetralogy of Fallot, 255, 260
Tomiko's fall risks, 112, 117
Tonic neck reflex, 23–24, 40–41
Tonic seizures, 336
Total parental nutrition (TPN), 113,
    114, 118
Total placenta previa, 152–153, 161
Toxemia, 191, 200
Transient tachypnea of the
    newborn (TTN)
    breast-feeding, for first time,
        323, 326
    hepatitis B vaccine, administering,
        323, 326
    nursing interventions, 321, 325
    parents education, 322, 326
    risk factors for, 322, 325
    screen tests, 323, 326
    universal newborn hearing screen
        (UNHS) and, 324, 326
Trisomy, 85
True labor, 92, 106
Tubal embryo transfer (TET), 80, 98
Tuberculosis (TB), 265, 268
Turner syndrome, 19, 37
Twin-to-twin transfusion syndrome
    (TTTS), 315–320
    risk factors, 316, 319
    SIDS (sudden infant death) and,
        317, 320
    steps to blood administration, 316–317,
        319–320
Type I diabetes, 206, 213
Type II diabetes, 206, 213

Ultrasound, 75
    of first trimester bleeding and previa,
        152, 161
    transvaginal ultrasound, 229, 236
Umbilical cords, 21, 39, 82, 99
Umbilicus, 83, 100
Universal newborn hearing screen
    (UNHS), 28, 324, 326
Urinary retention, 48, 64
Urinary tract infections (UTIs), 84–85,
    101, 214, 252

Uterine contractions (UCs), 129, 132, 136, 142–143, 144, 283
Uterine fundus, 83, 100

Vaginal yeast infections, 214
Valacyclovir, 123
Valtrex. *See* Valacyclovir
Vastus lateralus, 23
Ventricle septal defect (VSD), 255–256, 261
Vernix, 87, 103
Vernix caseosa, 15–16, 34
Vital signs, newborn, 16, 34
Vitamin C, 266, 269

Vitamin K administration, to newborns, 23, 40
Voluntary commitment statement (VCS), 30

Weight conversion, newborn, 13–14, 33
Western Blot/immunofluorescence assay, 279, 282
Wharton's jelly structure, 82, 99
White blood cells (WBCs), 89, 104

Zofran, 113, 114, 117–118
Zygote intrafallopian transfer (ZIFT), 80, 98